W9-BRG-801

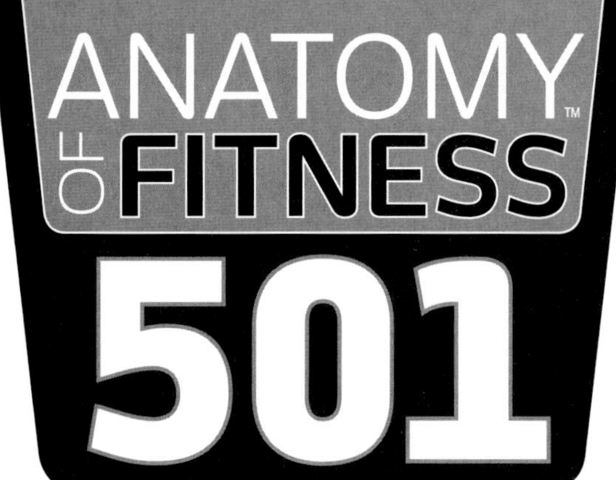

Strength Exercises

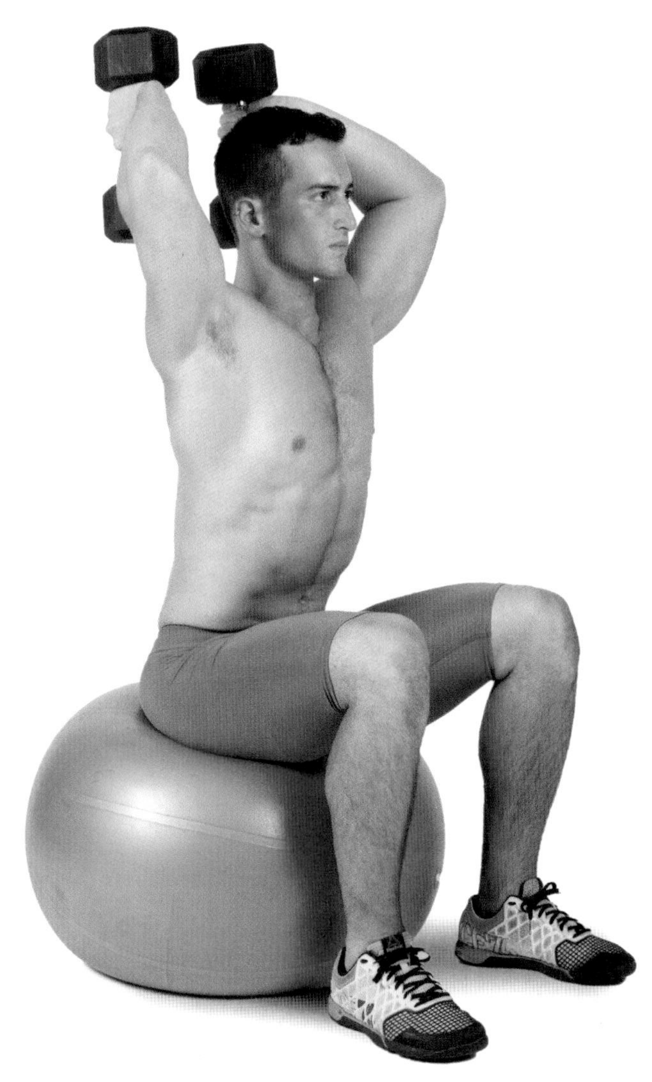

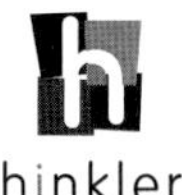

Published by Hinkler Books Pty Ltd 2018
45–55 Fairchild Street
Heatherton Victoria 3202 Australia
www.hinkler.com

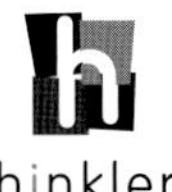

Created by Moseley Road Inc.
Cover Designer: Sam Grimmer
Prepress: Splitting Image
Production Director: Adam Moore
Designer: Nicola Plumb
Photographer: Naila Ruechel
Author: Natasha Diamond-Walker

ISBN: 978 1 4889 3412 4

Printed and bound in Canada

ANATOMY OF FITNESS™

501

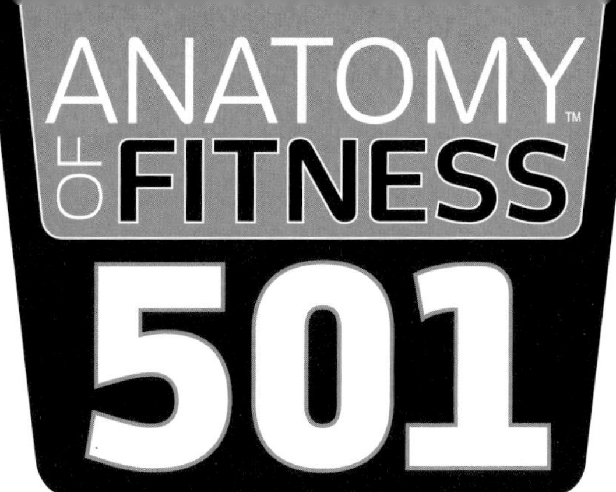

Strength Exercises

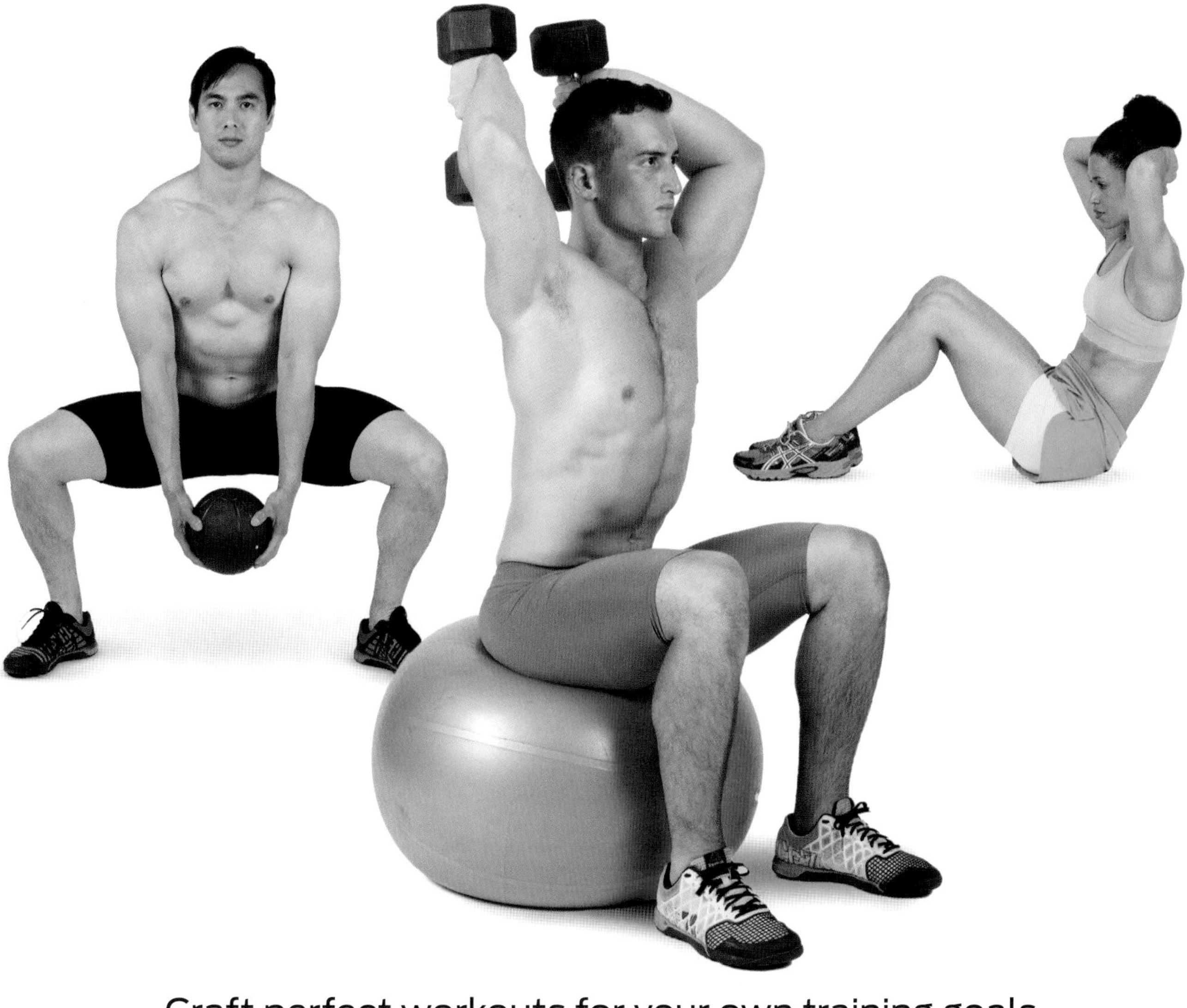

Craft perfect workouts for your own training goals and discover the amazing hidden structure of your body

Contents

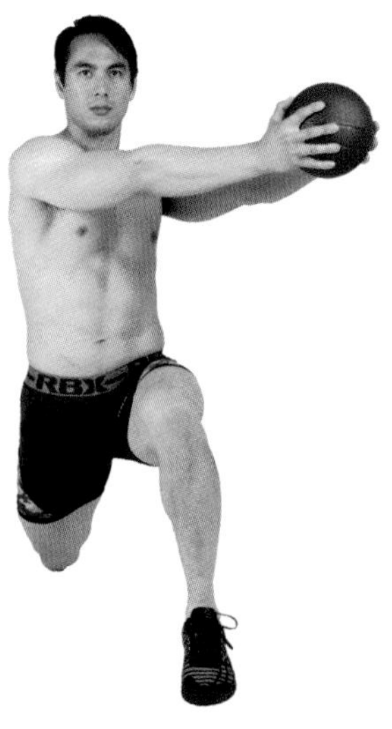

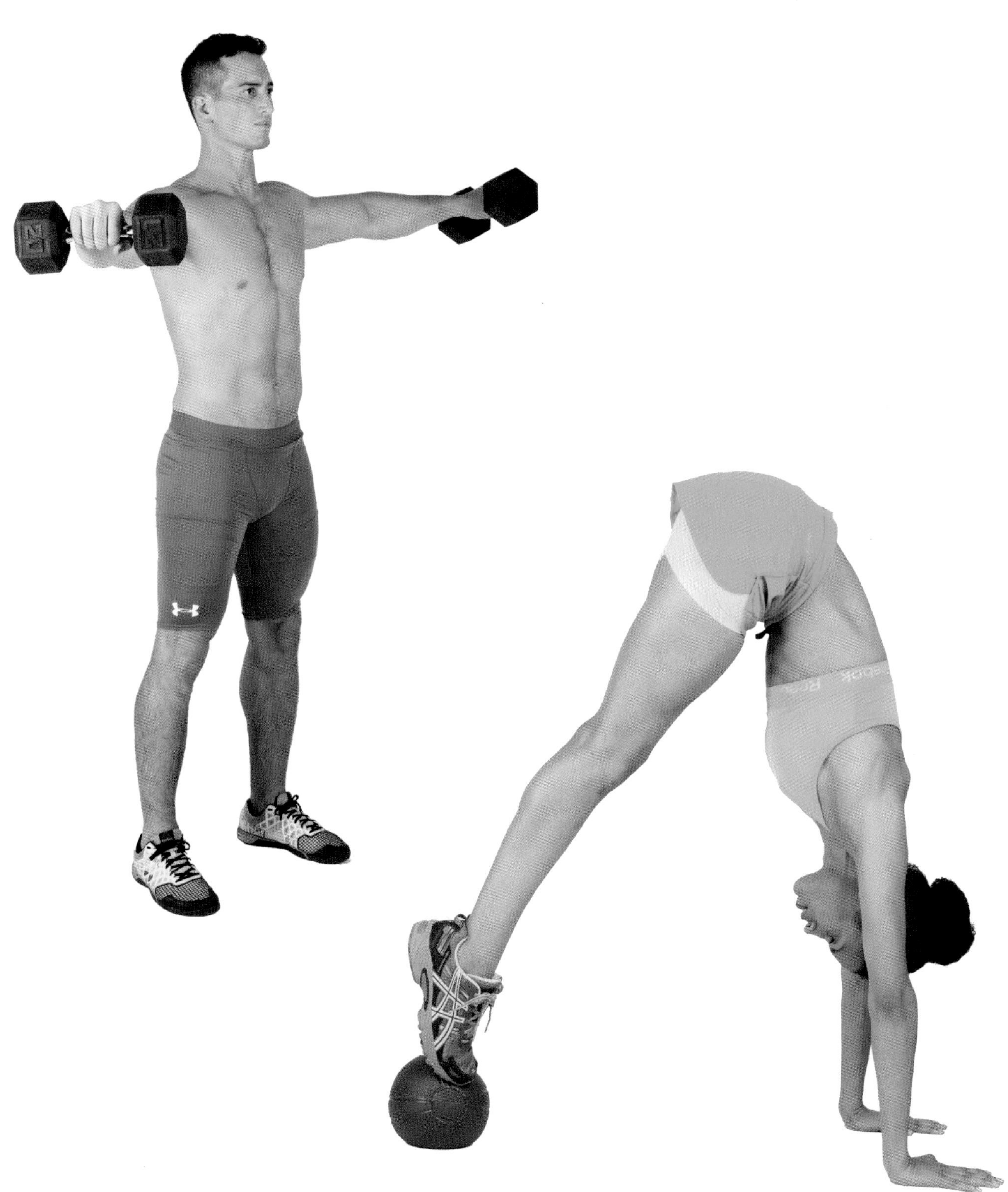

Introduction

Why exercise?

There is so much talk nowadays, more than ever, about working out. Everyone seems to be getting their Hollywood bodies hand-crafted by doctors, joining shiny fads such as Monster Cycle, or signing up for those acrobatic pole-dance cardio classes. But, truly, what does it really mean to work out? To exercise, to take interest in your health and wellness? Well, the meaning of what it is to work out is definitely personal and individual to each of us. Whether you are someone who enjoys an intense, sweaty, one-hour heavy-lifting session or prefer a high-intensity short-burst mix-up, take care to spend time crafting your need-specific workout routine. And feel free to mix it up a little bit as you go, trying different moves and tempos along the way.

At the core

When it comes to fitness and working out we often hear a lot about the core. But what does "core" mean? It sounds mysterious and a little bit hard to place, if you think about it. For starters, we can assume that the core is located in the center somewhere; after all, the core of an apple is at its center. So, we have an idea of where it is, but a little information about what it is, exactly, would be nice. In fitness, it is commonly understood that the core encompasses all of the abdominal muscle groups, the middle and lower back muscles, and, in most cases, the pelvis as well. Core-based workouts are plentiful and often focus on routines based around working the abdominals. Our cores are important because, in order to support optimal function throughout the rest of the body, our cores must be healthy and strong.

The great spine

In order to live a healthy life, we need a healthy spinal column to support our bones, muscles, and organs. Made up of 33 individual bones interjoined with our nervous system, our spines and our spinal health dictate very much of our day-to-day lives. The spine traverses more than 50 percent of our body's length and connects to over 120 muscles and has more than 100 joints. So, when you move through your workout, and daily activities, remember to thank your spine for all its support!

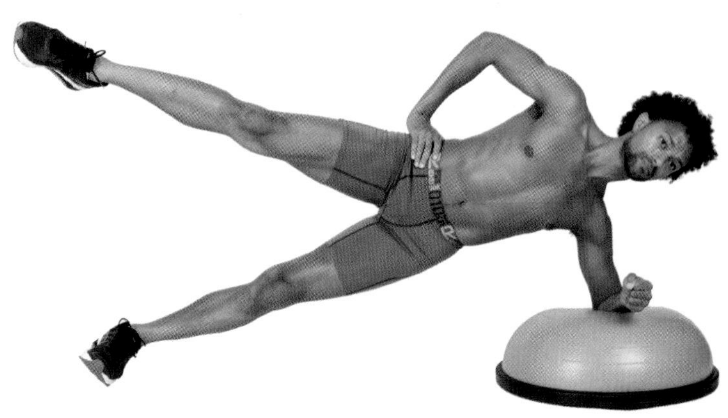

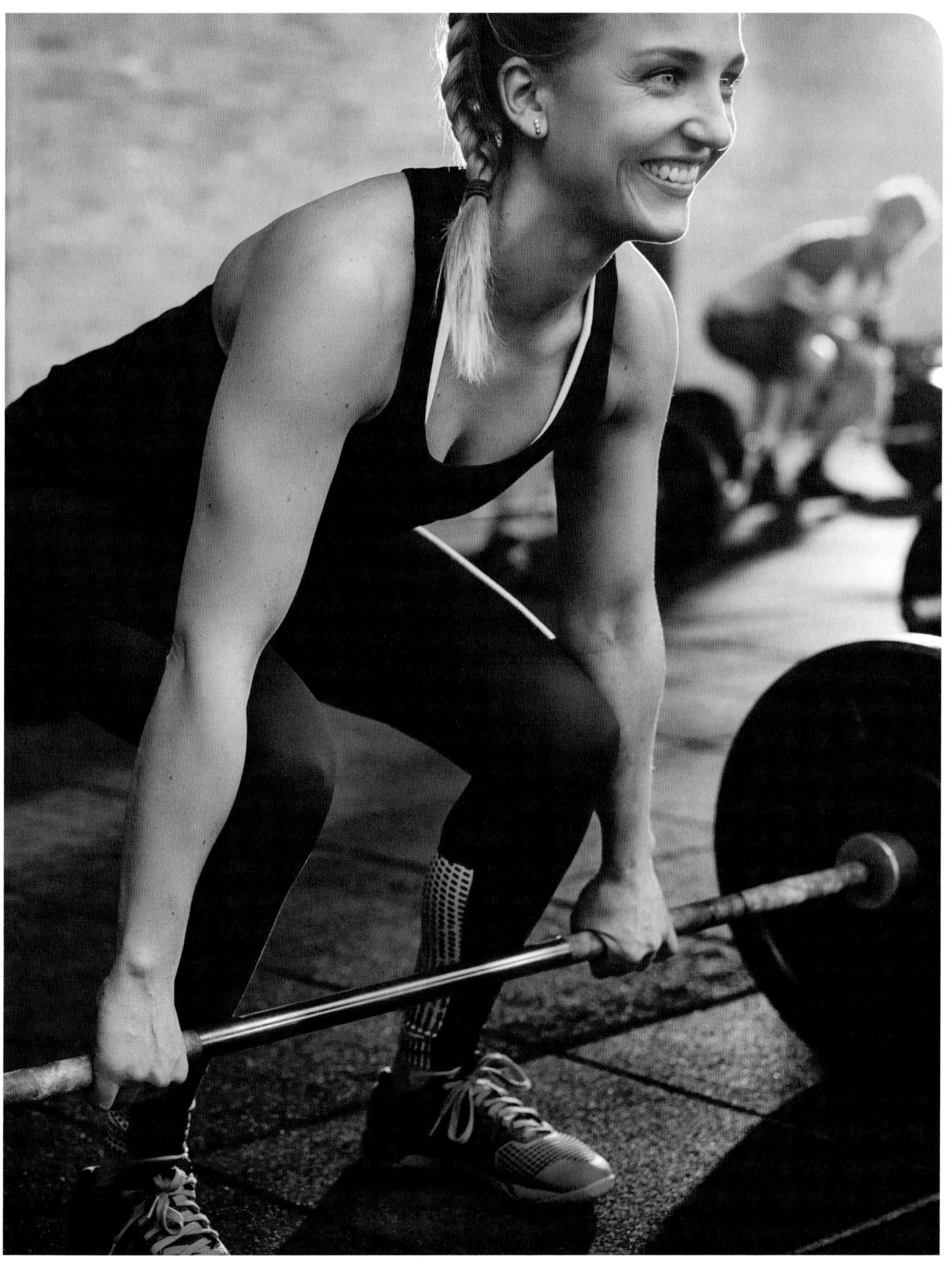

Back to back

Moving on from the spine, and all of its fun facts, we should discuss the back. When we say "back," we are using a blanket term for the total area that makes up the distance from the shoulders down to the tailbone or sacrum. The muscles of the middle back and the lower back are all supported by the spine, at the deepest level, and then by the muscles that make up the core on a more superficial level. Our backs are responsible for carrying a lot of weight and, thus, require a sufficient amount of attention, development, and care. When you are formatting your workouts, take time to include exercises that strengthen your back so that it may be healthy, pain-free, and reliable.

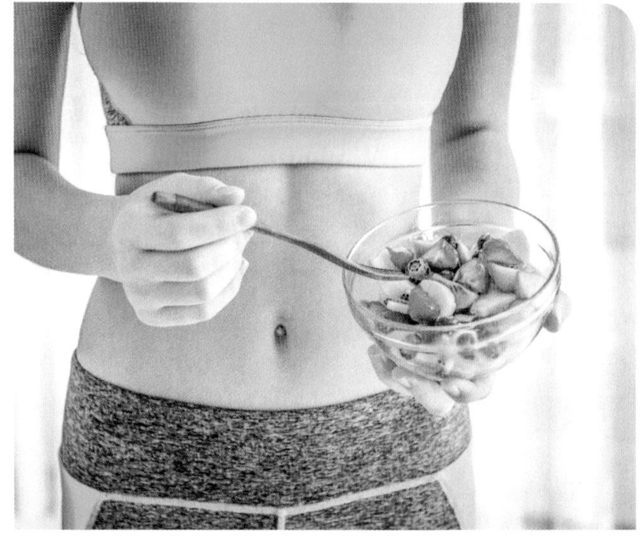

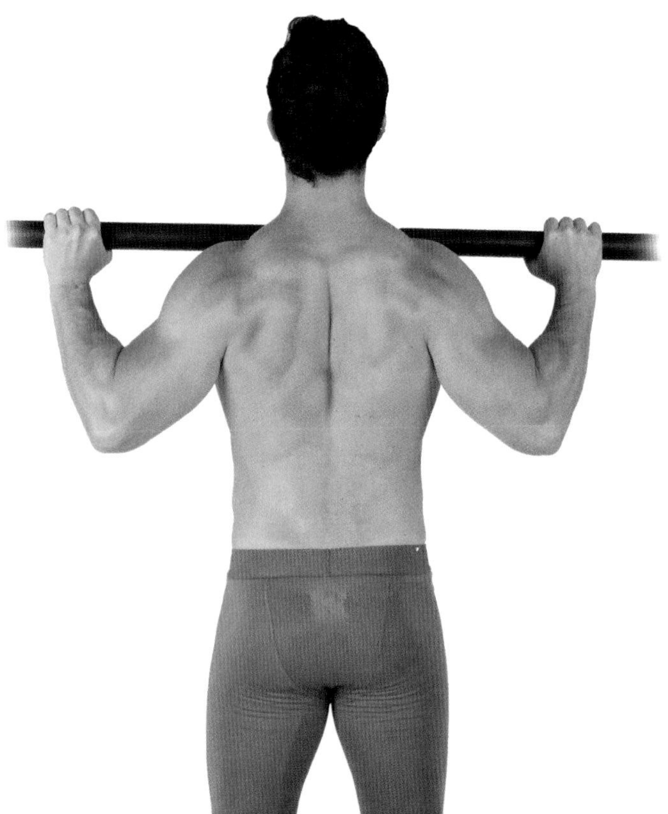

Food as fuel

What to eat, what to eat, what to eat? So much talk about diet! And not to mention losing weight, gaining weight, organic, holistic, vegan, vegetarian, gluten-free this, sugar-free that, and Paleo (what does Paleo even mean, really?). But, honestly, all fun aside–your diet, and what you choose to put into your body, is important. If you intend to have a successful life of working out, feeling good, and living up to your best potential, you should take care to develop a sustainable diet that works best for you and your individual needs. Information abounds via the internet about all things diet-related–it is a great resource for researching and catering to a lifestyle that suits you fully.

Moving with your breath

Whether the focus of your workouts is to put on muscle mass, to lose weight, to tone, to feel better, or to gain flexibility, all require you to have an optimal flow of breath. Breathing is so important when it come to working out. There are so many ways to breathe and discovering the right pairing of breath with each exercise is a personal journey. However, you should keep in mind that breathing regulates the oxygen flow throughout the body. This includes oxygen in the lungs and also to and from the muscles. For optimal workout results, you must remember to breathe deeply and frequently, usually exhaling at the beginning of a movement and inhaling as you move.

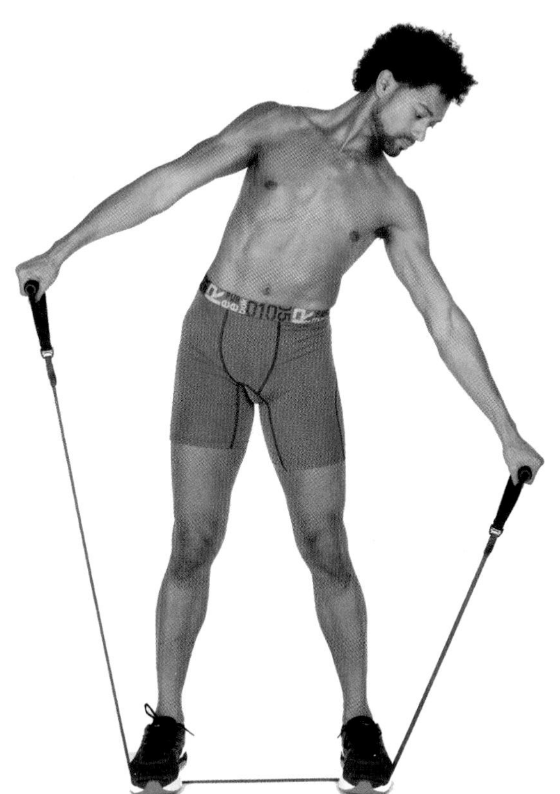

Props on top of props

The vast, abundant world of props! You might be thinking that you do not need to include props in any of your workouts, and you are right, you don't! But, if you do, your exercise results could far exceed what you even dreamed possible. Incorporating props into your workout regime can be fun, challenging, and highly aerobic. The great thing about using props is that they add all sorts of dimensions into your moves. However, planking with your forearm centered on a balance ball, while holding a dumbbell in the other hand, out to the side, will invite the muscles to work in a whole new way! Some of the props you will find utilized in this book are: resistance bands, cables, balance balls, kettlebells, dumbbells, Medicine balls, Swiss balls, and step platforms.

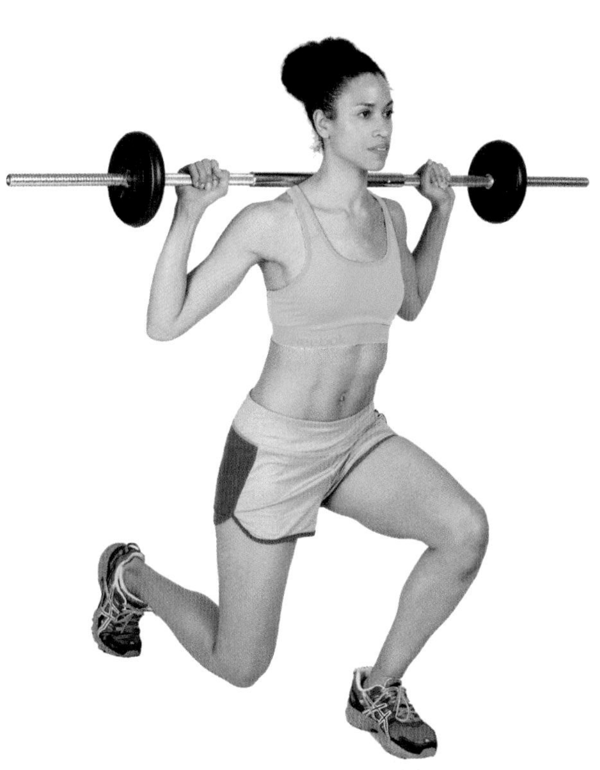

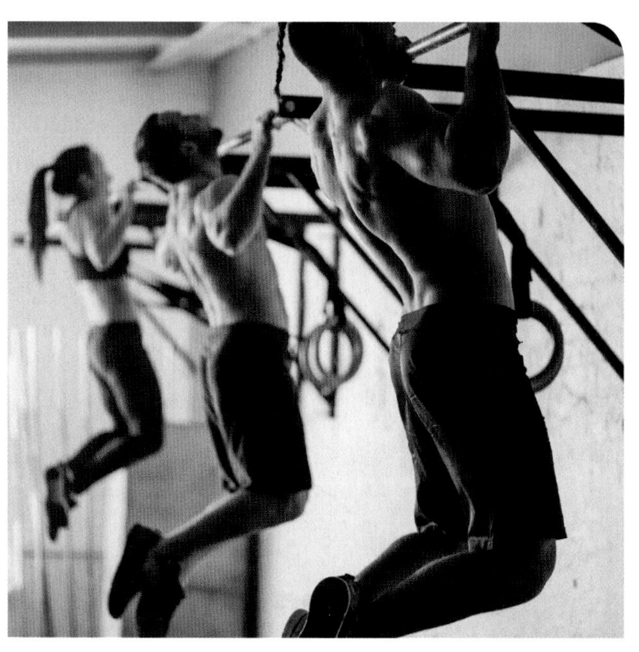

Plyometric play

You will see the word "plyometric" sprinkled throughout this book, as you move through the exercises. A "plyometric" exercise is defined as a quick, powerful movement that starts with a muscle- lengthening (eccentric) movement that is immediately followed by a muscle-shortening (concentric) movement. Or, more simply, you can think of it as jump training. Plyometric exercises require you to move quickly into your range in a short amount of time, but with the maximum amount of speed and power. Incorporating plyometric exercises one to three times a week can increase your tone and strength, as well as allow you to move more quickly and powerfully.

Stay home or hit the gym?

Whether you choose to work out at home or to work out at the gym, either way you are choosing the path of bettering your health. Both are good options that provide different benefits, depending on the type of gym or home-workout system you have in place. Some people find it useful to get up and go out to a public space, like a gym. The idea that there are other people in a joint setting, doing the same things as themselves or moving in the direction of wellness, is inspiring. Other people, however, prefer to exercise in the privacy of their own home, or are just unable to attend the gym because of monetary or time restrictions. It is your personal choice. However, with the availability of books like this one, online workout routines, and the ability to pick up just about any sort of exercise prop at the store, working out at home has become just as simple as hitting the gym.

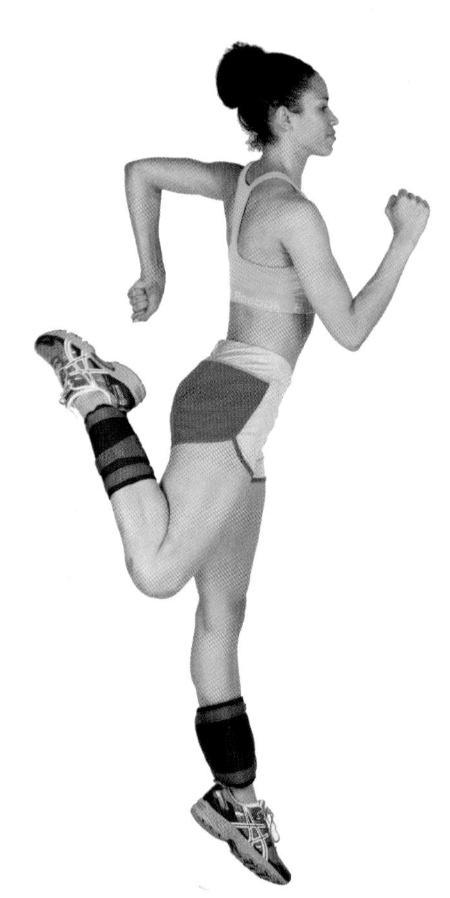

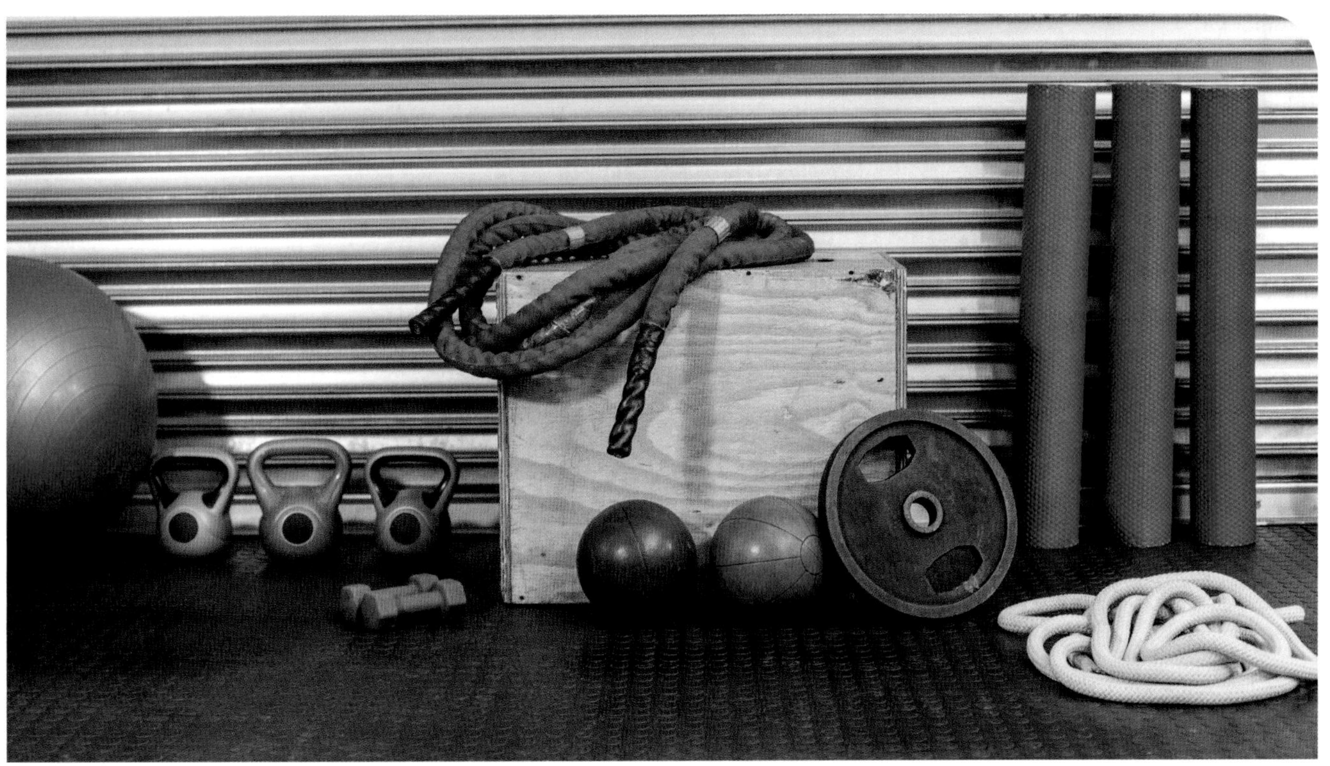

Getting organized

So, here you are, you have the book in hand, you have thought about your diet and you have thought about what parts of your physique you would like to chisel out and strengthen. What next? The next thing that needs to be sorted out is what kind of routine you are going to set up. Some things to keep in mind are: what your work schedule is like, how much time you would like to spend exercising, what times of day you have the most energy, whether you would like a personal trainer, and if you think working out at home or the gym is a good choice for you. Planning your work and working your plan are two major aspects of the path to health and wellness. Making a plan for your workout routines is also vitally important—most trainers advise exercising every other day if you prefer a total body workout, but you could also alternate lower and upper body routines, or strength with cardio. One of the main reasons people give up on their gym membership, or exercise in general, is boredom; this book allows you to add variety to your workout by offering multiple versions of each exercise. Instead of doing the same push-ups every other day, you can choose from the 43 different push-ups described in this book! Have fun planning each week's routine. There are infinite variations you can devise—your workout need never be boring again.

Full-Body Anatomy

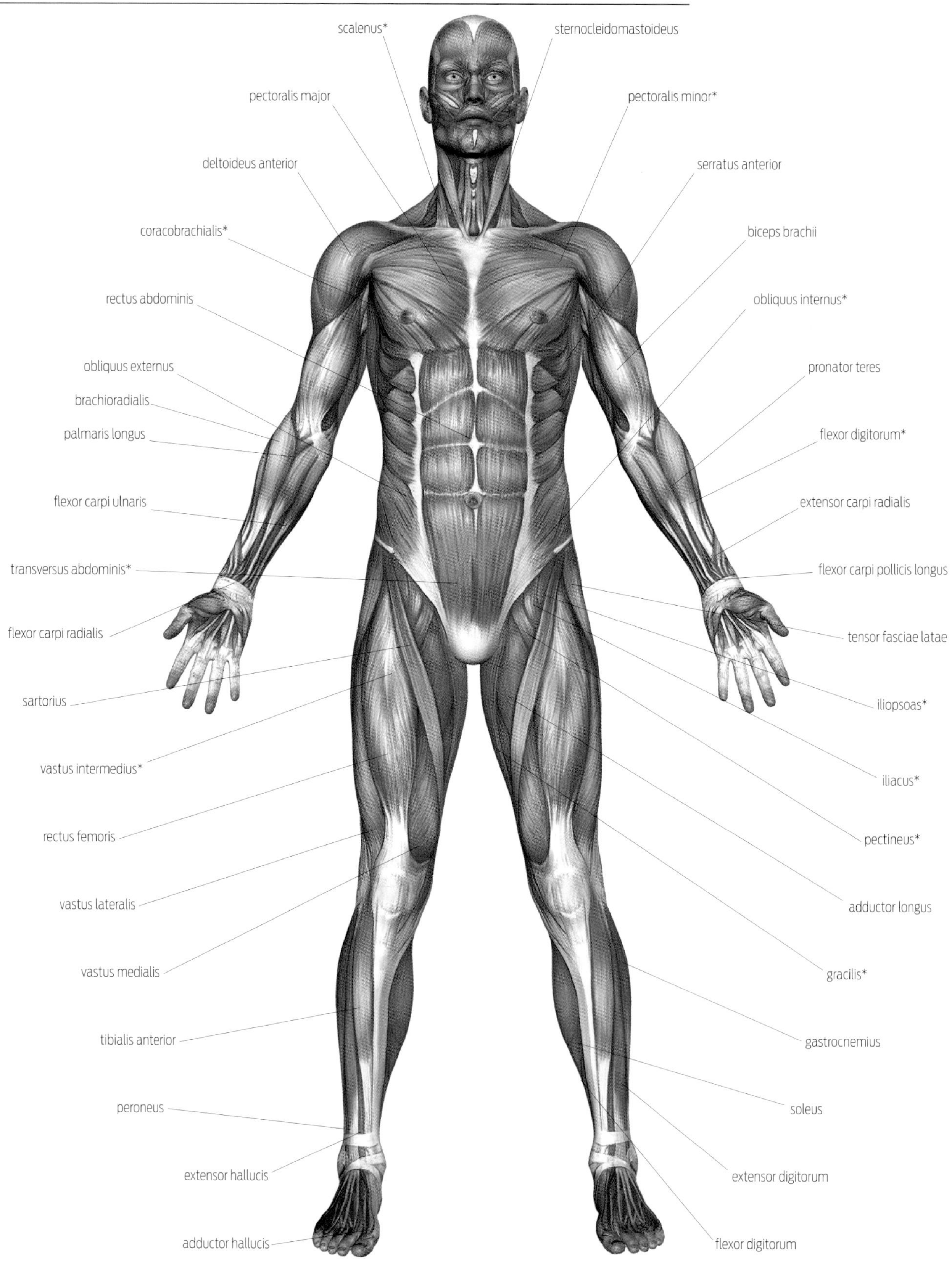

Annotation Key
* indicates deep muscles

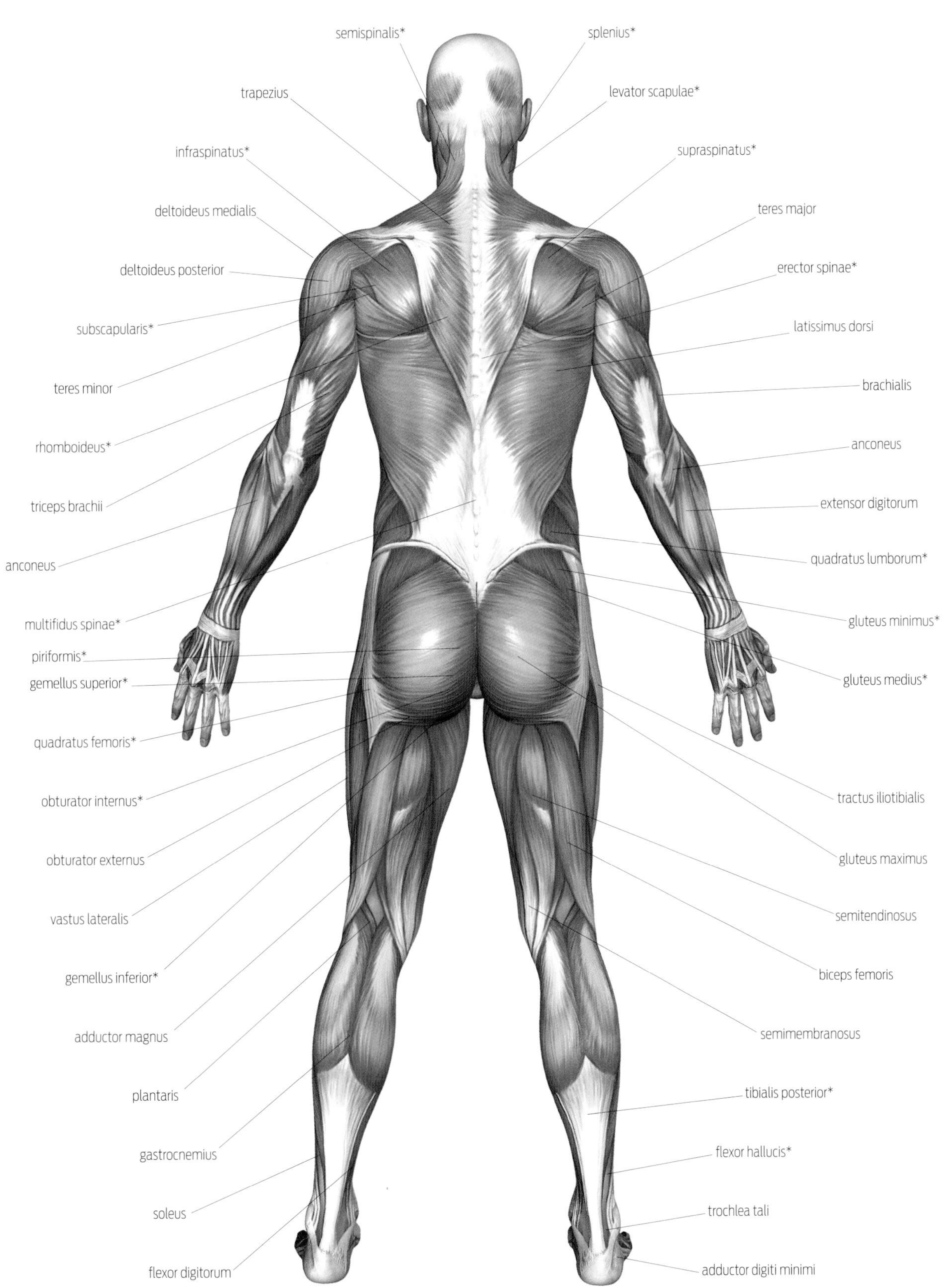

CHAPTER ONE

Upper Body

Our bodies can be divided, generally, into two parts: The upper body and the lower body. Molded along the top and middle of the spine is the upper body. It contains the head, neck, shoulders, chest, muscle groups in your back, and the front of the body abdominal groups. Additionally, we have all of our organs housed here! Needless to say, a balanced and strong upper body is very important to our general health and contributes greatly to how we feel day to day. A dynamic workout routine that includes attention to each part of your upper body will be sure to keep you functioning at your best, both inside and out!

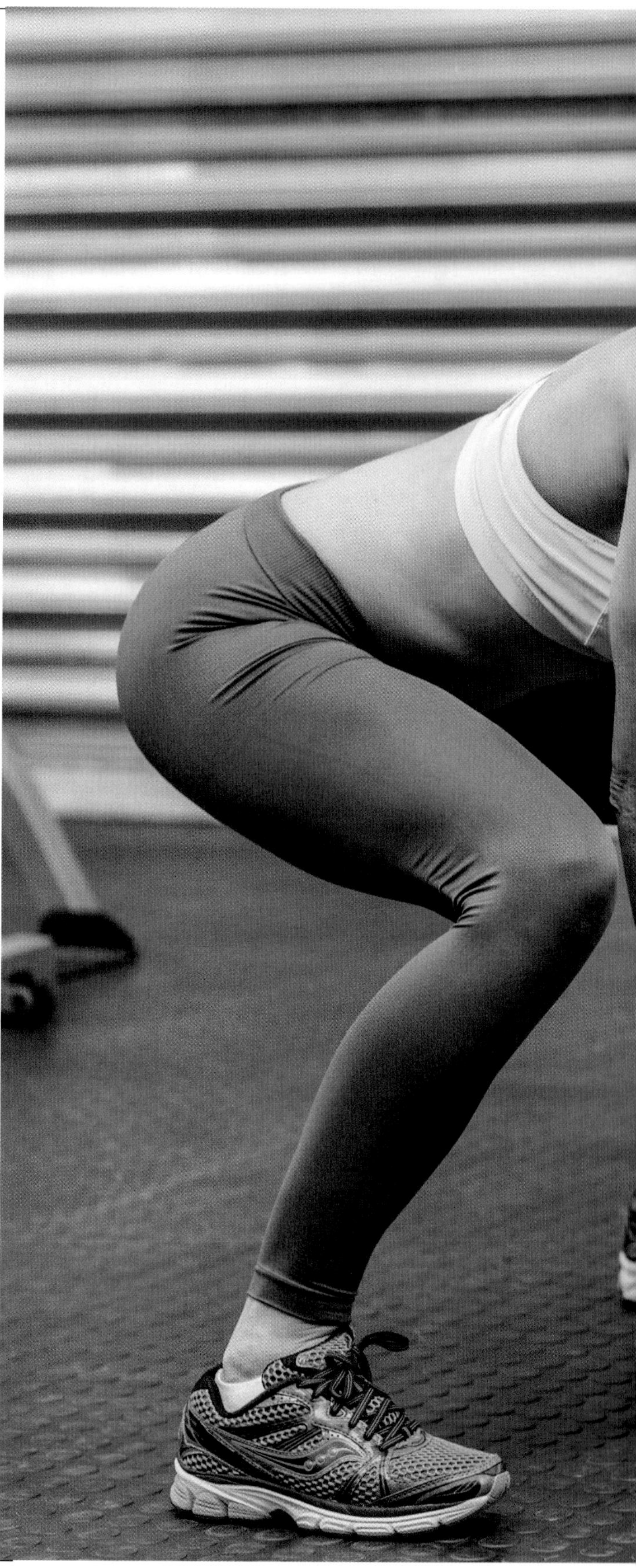

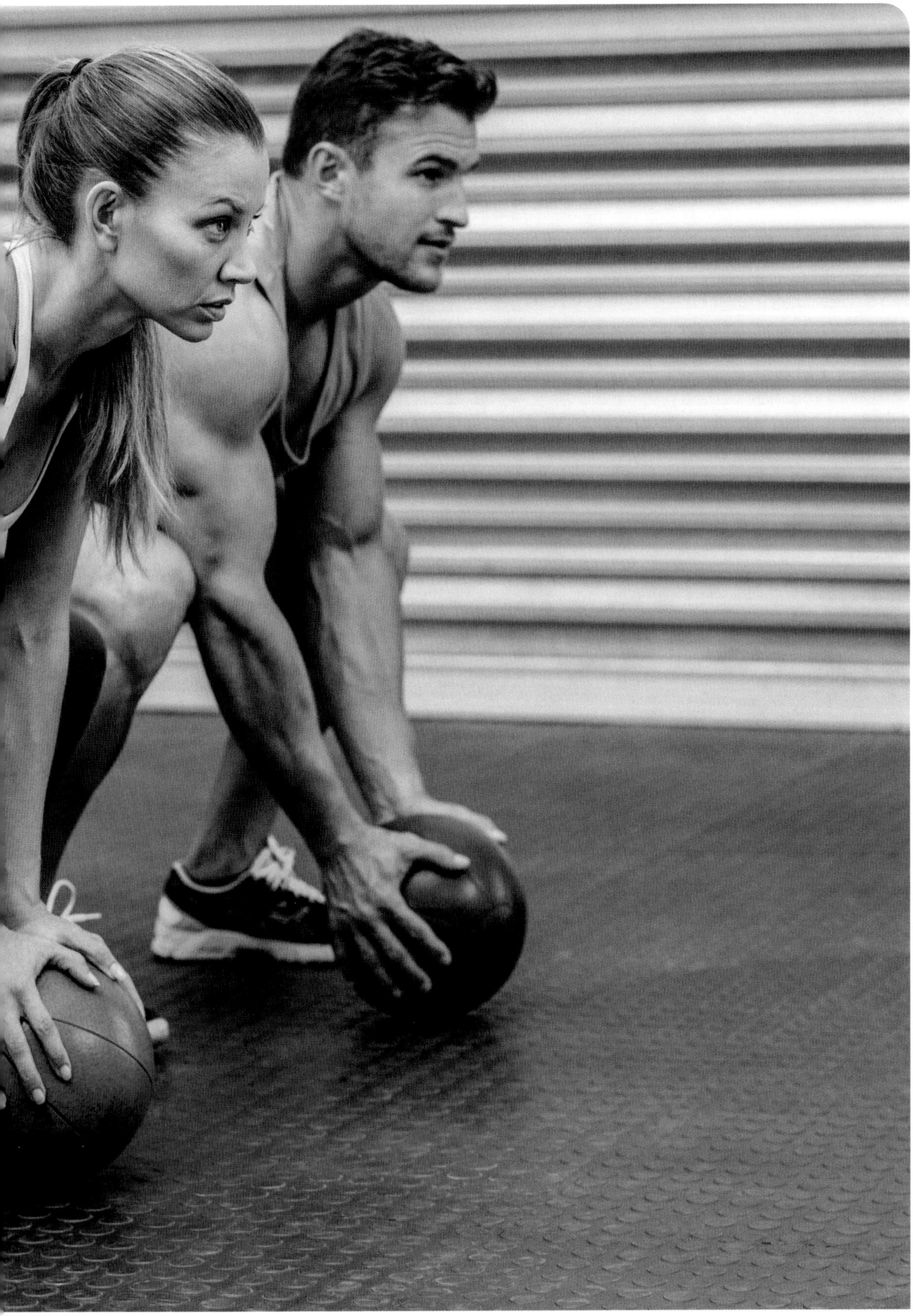

Upper Body

001

Pull-Up

Working all of the main muscles in the upper-body region, including the chest, back, shoulders, and both arms is the tried and true Pull-Up. This move is particularly challenging because in performing it, you must be able to lift the entire weight of the lower body up off the ground by strongly gripping a bar overhead and pulling with the back and arms. Indeed, you are levitating with the base of your power in the torso!

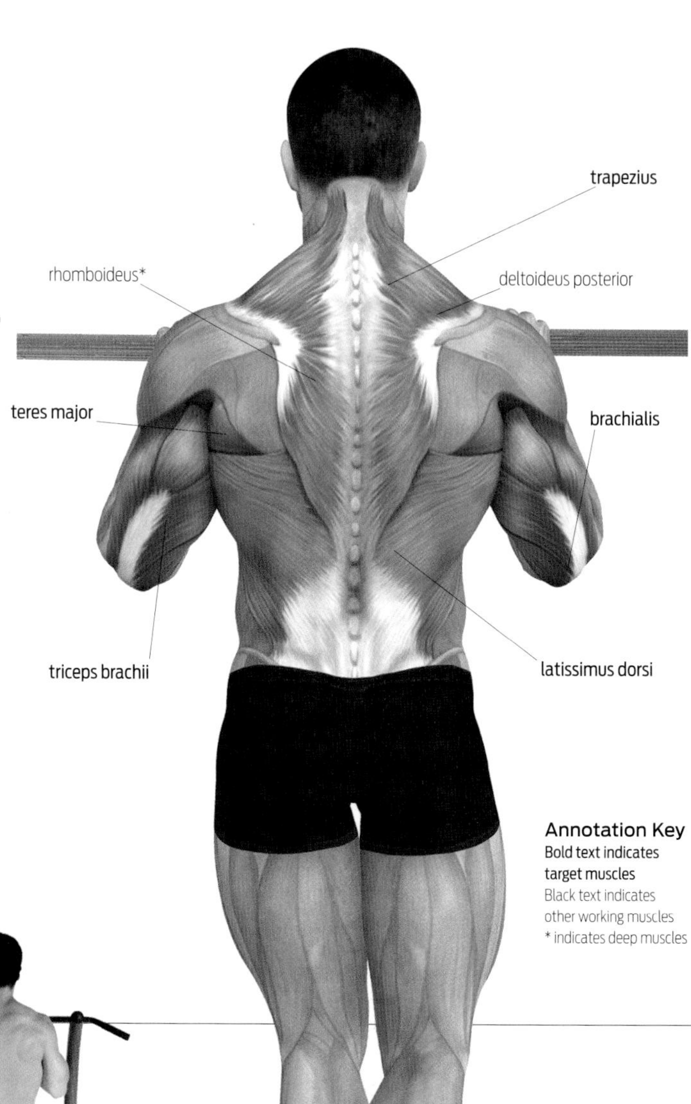

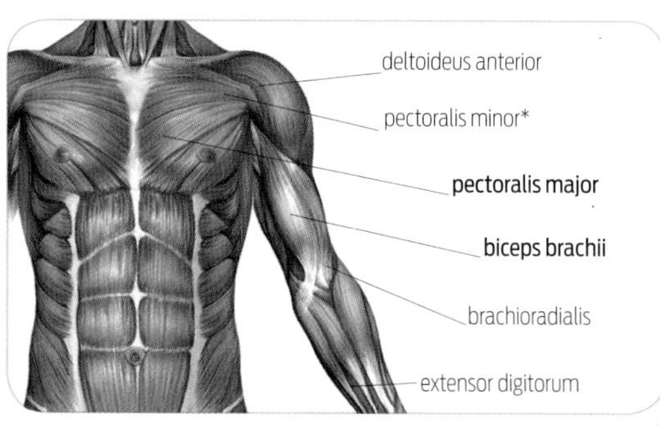

Annotation Key
Bold text indicates target muscles
Black text indicates other working muscles
* indicates deep muscles

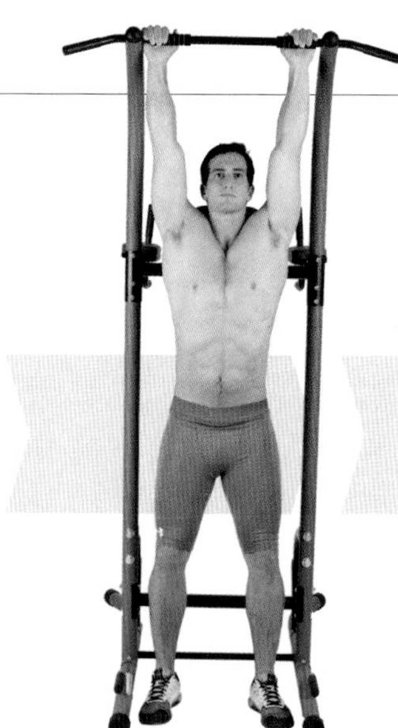

- Stand tall with your arms extended up holding the pull-up bar directly above. Engage your back and abs and pull your body up.

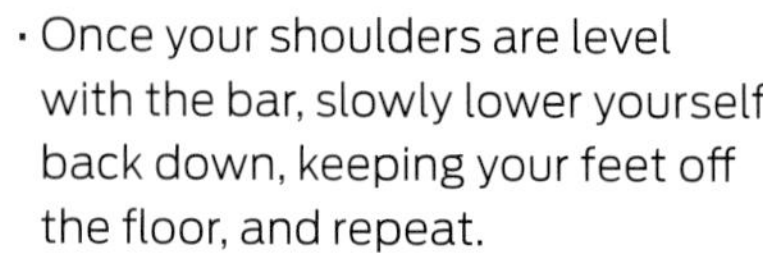

- Once your shoulders are level with the bar, slowly lower yourself back down, keeping your feet off the floor, and repeat.

Correct form

Focus on your back moving primarily. Your arms should only serve as levers to lift your weight up and down.

Avoid

Don't move your grip around too much once you have established your position. You want the hands, wrists, and forearms to be in a straight line.

002 Weighted Pull-Up

Adding weight to your Pull-Up increases the amount of work for the arms and chest. In this exercise, try using a weighted ball. Place it between the thighs, squeezing in on the ball, thus engaging the upper legs and abs.

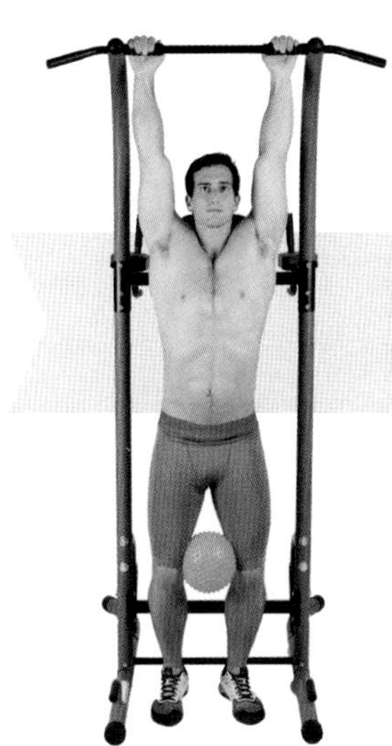

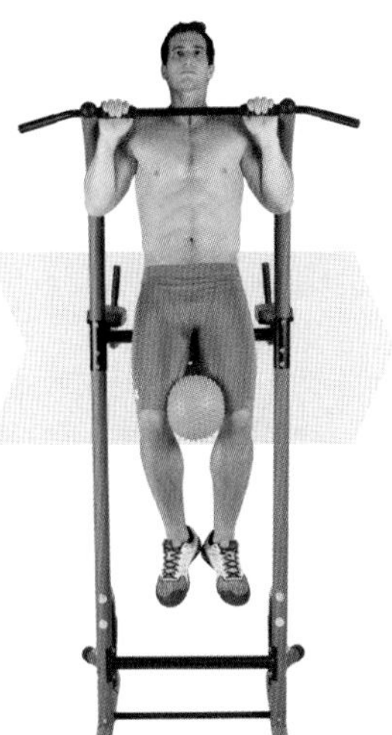

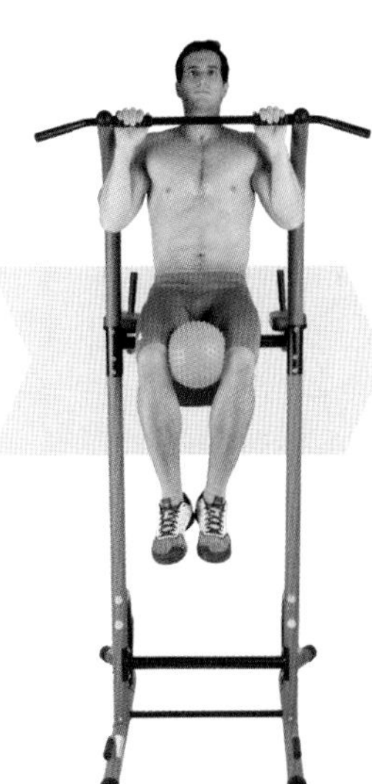

- With a long spine and a ball held between your legs, reach up for your bar.
- Holding the bar firmly, pull your body up, squeezing in tightly on the weighted ball.
- Once at the top of your Pull-Up, challenge your lower abs by bending your knees to a 90-degree angle, keeping the ball in between your thighs.

003 Chin-Up

For your Chin-Up, reverse the grip of your Pull-Up. Using an underhand grip, hold the bar tightly and pull the body up. Keep the feet crossed at the ankles while suspended and the shoulders aligned with the hands.

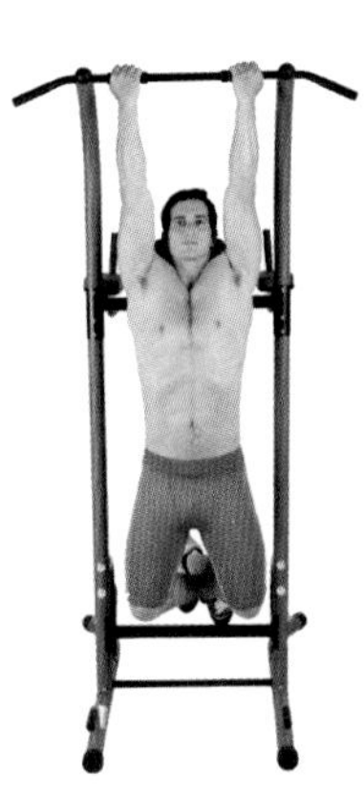

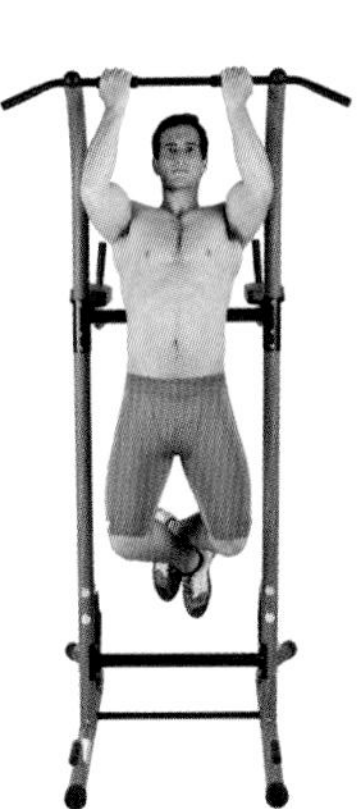

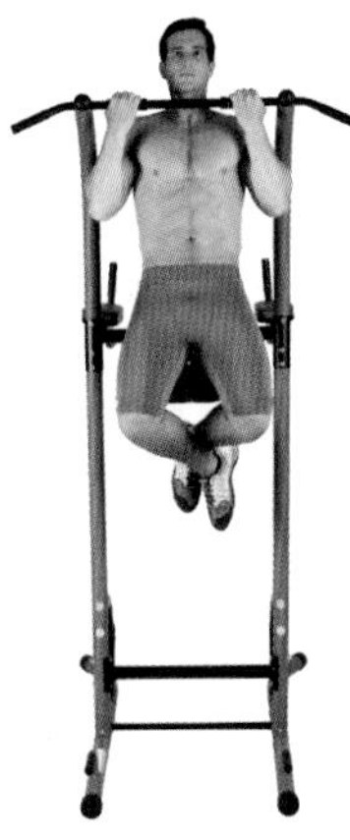

004 Weighted Chin-Up

Place a weighted ball between your legs at the lower thigh. Hang long from the bar while squeezing in on the ball with your inner legs. Bend at the knee, lifting your feet behind you. Engage your back and abs strongly and move into your Chin-Up.

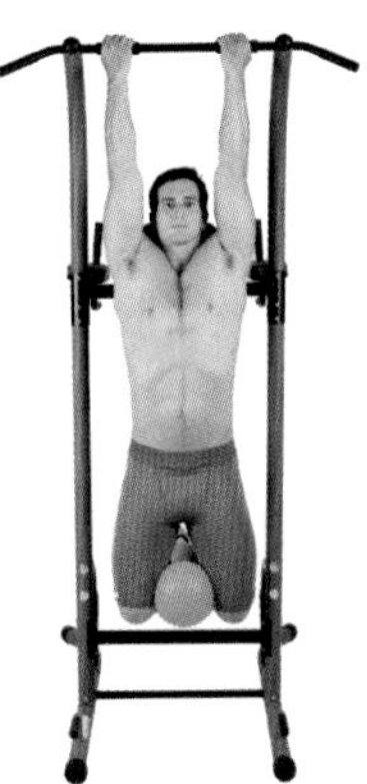

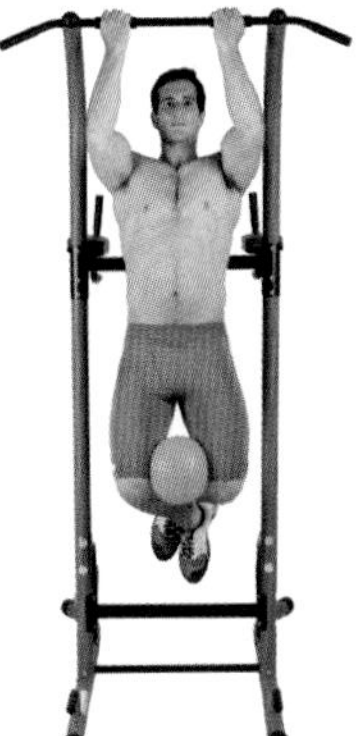

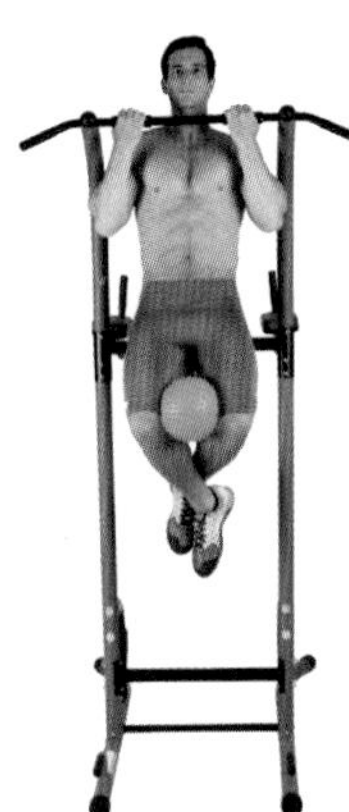

005 Wide-Grip Pull-Up

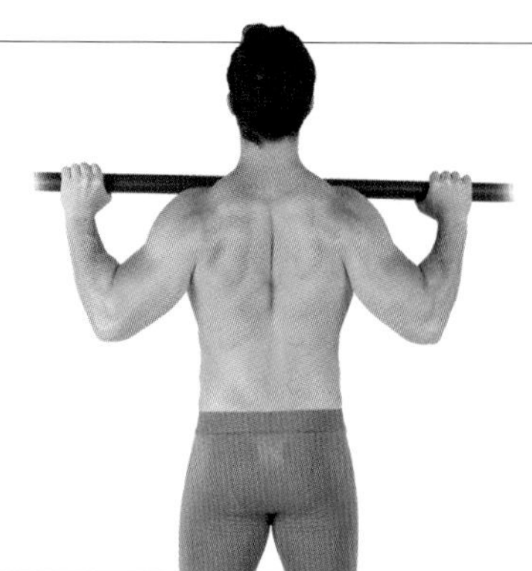

Doing a Pull-Up while holding the bar in a wider grip works your latissimus dorsi more than the rhomboids, as you would in a closer grip Pull-Up. Start by standing tall and open your arms to a wide V-shape at either end of the bar. Perform your Pull-Up there.

006 Assisted Pull-Up

Position your arms on the bar as for a Pull-Up (#001). Perform your Pull-Up while someone assists you. Have them stand directly to the side of your body while keeping their hands under your lower legs for support until you have completed the desired amount of repetitions.

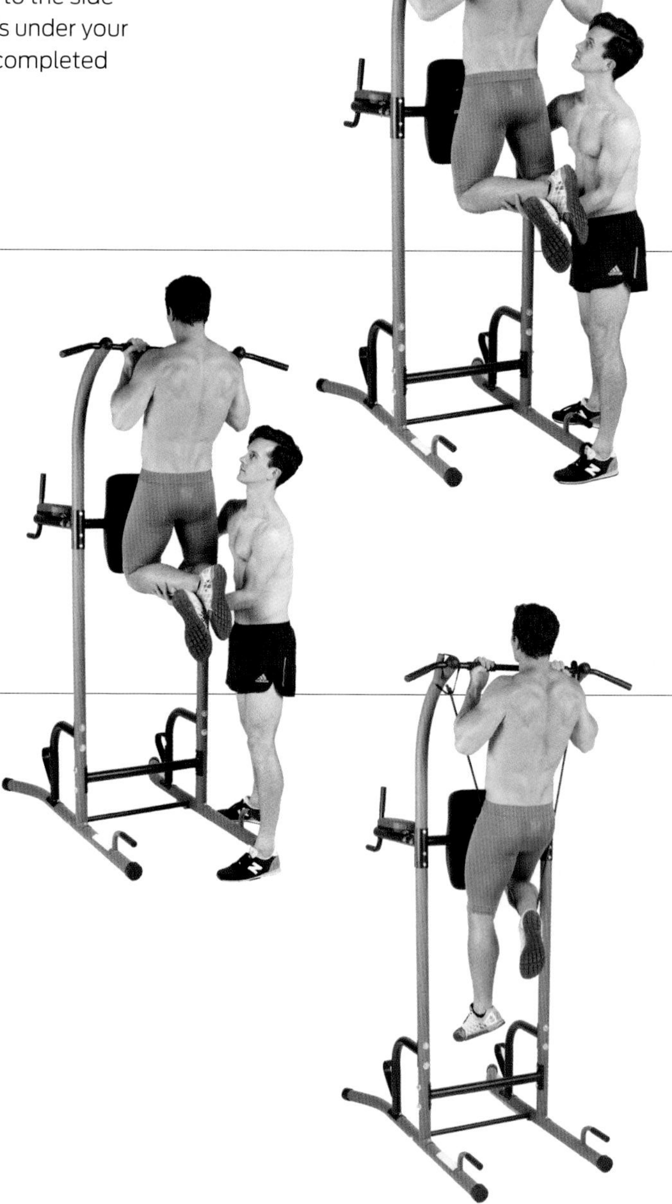

007 Assisted Chin-Up

With a reverse grip, go for your Chin-Up with someone supporting the weight of your lower legs with their hands under your shins until you have completed the desired amount of repetitions.

008 Assisted Chin-Up with Bands

Secure a band by looping the handles on either end of your pull-up bar. Stand tall in front of your bar and place your right knee down onto the suspended band. Perform your Chin-Up with the help of the band's support.

009 Assisted Pull-Up with Bands

Perform as you would your Assisted Chin-Up with Bands (#008). For your Pull-Up, note that your hands should be on the outside of your band handles, for a wider grip.

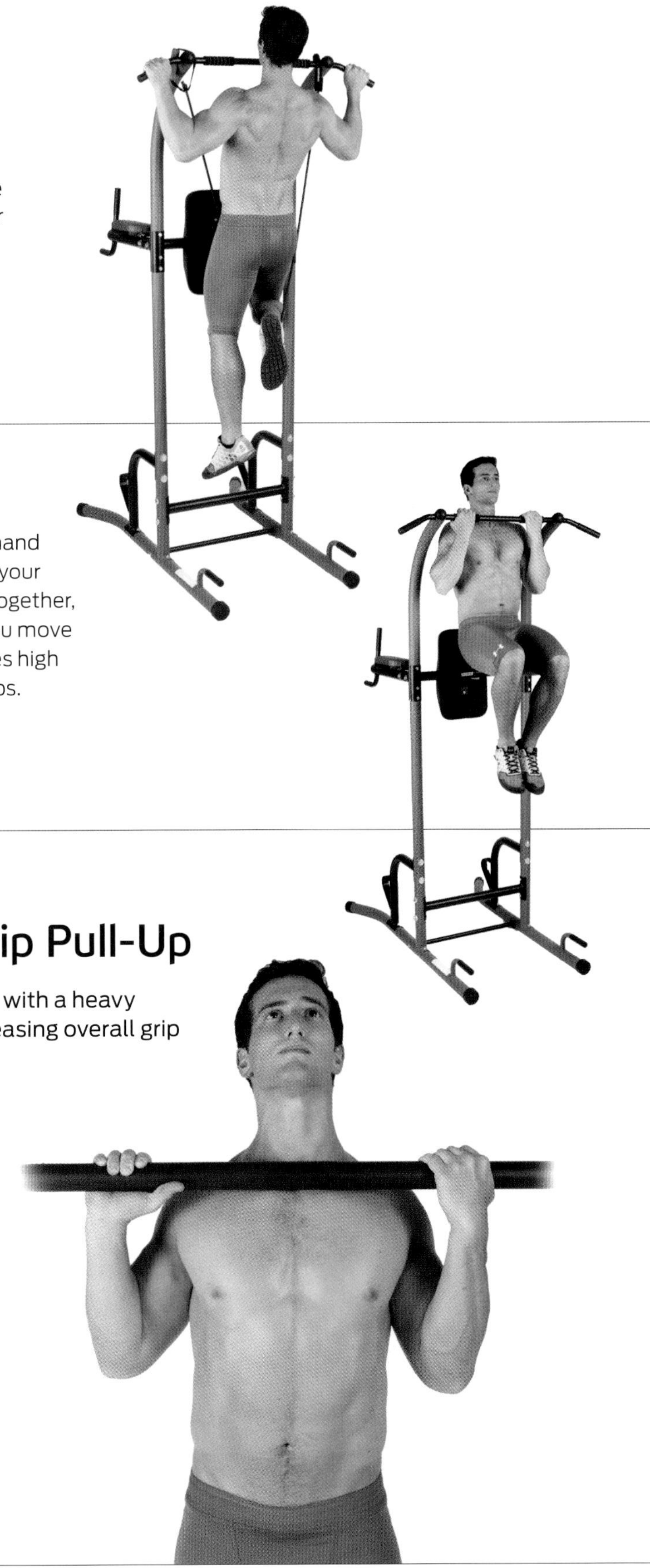

010 Chin-Up with Hanging Leg Raise

Stand at your bar with an underhand grip. Hold the bar and hang with your arms straight. Bring your knees together, squeezing the inner thighs. As you move into your Chin-Up, bring the knees high into the chest, challenging the abs.

011 Alternating-Grip Pull-Up

This is the preferred grip to use in conjunction with a heavy body belt and/or weighted ankle straps—increasing overall grip strength in the hands.

- Put one hand over the top of the bar and the other hand underneath it.
- With arms shoulder-width apart, in opposing grips, go for your Pull-Up.
- Track your elbows down and into the body while moving in and out of your Pull-Up.

012 Mountain-Climber Grip Pull-Up

Standing tall to one side of the bar, reach up and place one hand in front of the other. With a strong grip, pull your body up so that your shoulder comes to touch the bar. Try the Pull-Up alternating your body to either side of the bar for a challenge.

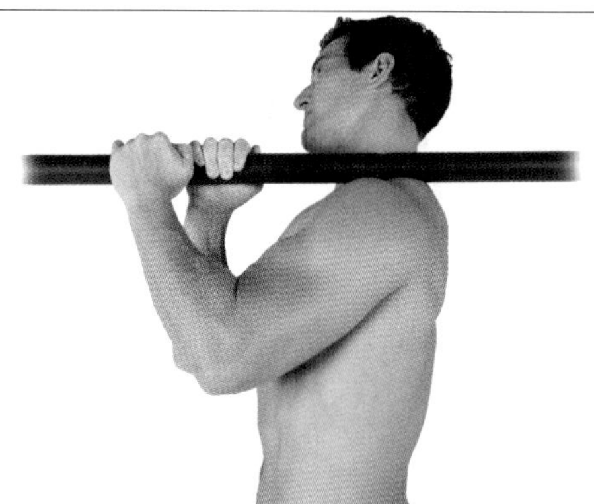

013 Neutral-Grip Pull-Up

Locate the set of parallel handles on your pull-up bar and place your hands firmly around them. Go for your Pull-Up here. Be sure to track your arm movements evenly: straight, then into right angles, then fully bent at the elbow with your head above the bar.

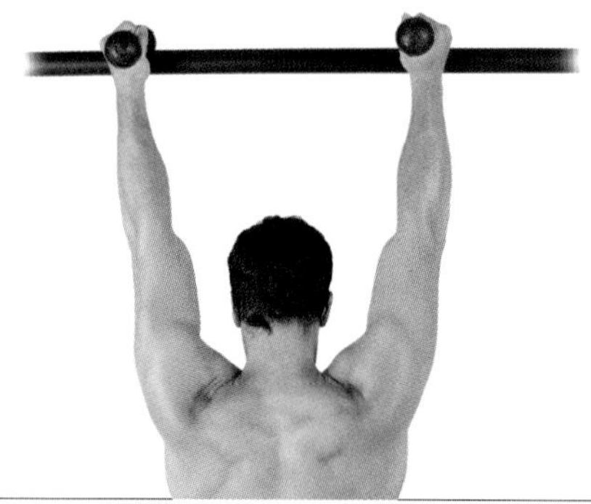

014 Close-Grip Pull-Up

Place your hands close together, gripping the bar on the underside. Sqeeze your abs in and lengthen your back. Your arms and upper body will have an increase of activation with this closer grip.

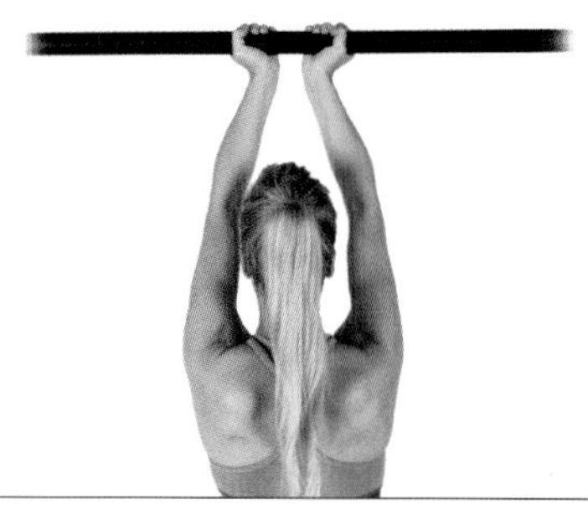

015 Body Row

Sit under a low bar with your arms straight up at an angle from your body, holding the bar. Walk your feet out so that your body comes to hang in a straight line. Pushing your heels firmly into the floor, engage your abs and pull your body up to meet the bar.

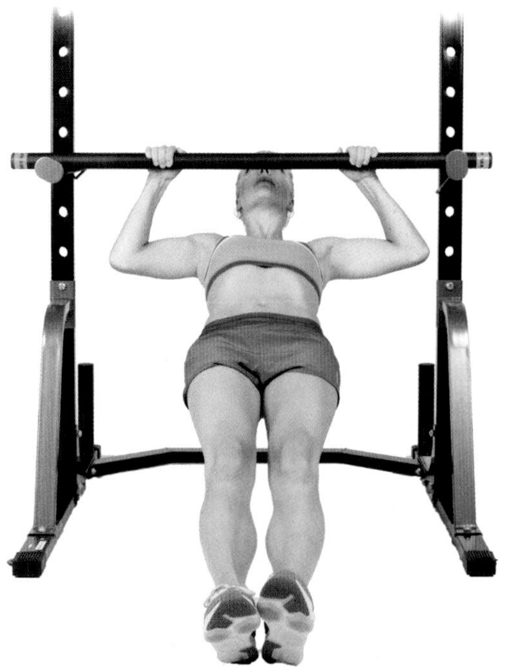

016 Vertical Rope with Alternating Grip

Incorporating the vertical rope into your pull-up routine will add a dynamic challenge of being off balance. Holding the rope tightly, it becomes a vector and you are able to swing your hips back, while keeping your feet in contact with a secure base, challenging your arms to climb up and down.

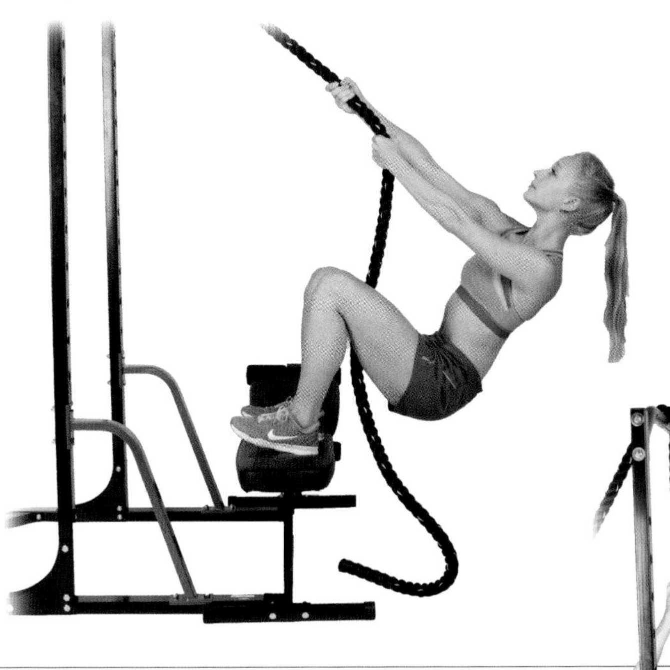

- Stand with your feet on a bench and the rope hanging through your legs. Place one hand above the other, up on the rope, in an alternating grip.
- Bend your knees and walk your hands quite a way down the rope. Lean back from the bench, straightening your arms.
- Working against your lower-body weight, climb up and down the rope with your arms, keeping your legs bent the whole time.

017 Lateral Rope Pull

With your feet firmly planted on top of a bench, hold high up on the vertical rope with one hand above the other. Bend the knees and slowly sway your body out to one side until you are sideways, suspended in the air. Walk up and down the rope, keeping your feet weighted into the bench. This is a lot of core and arm work.

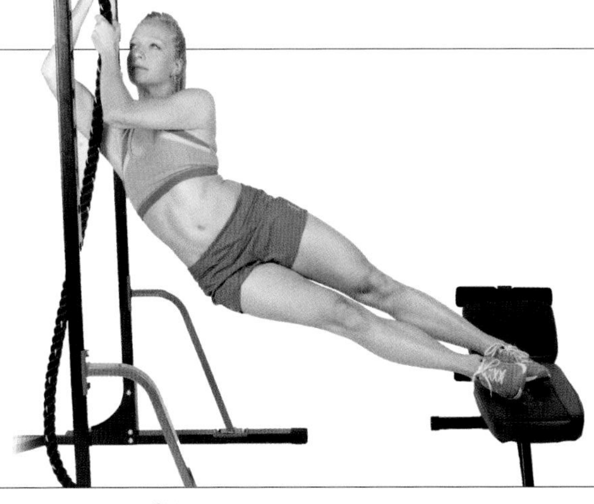

018 Rope Chin

Stand tall behind a vertical hanging rope. With an alternating grip, take the rope into your hands. Walk your top arm up high so it is straight and the lower one is bent. Pull up your body with the top arm so that it bends, bringing your chin to that hand.

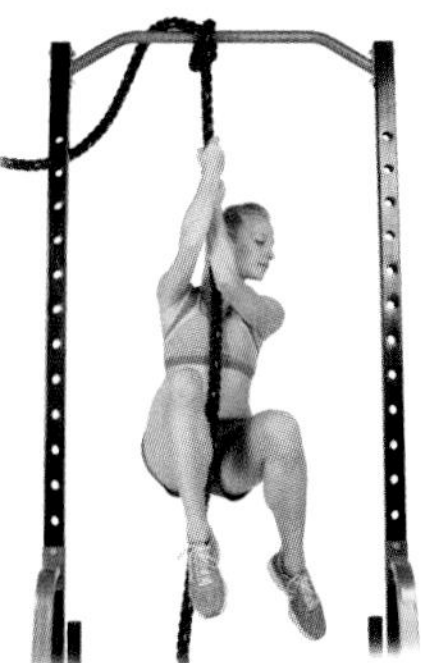

019

Push-Up

The simple and beautiful, standard Push-Up is one of the very best movements to master. Whether you are looking to have chiseled sleek arms or tight, strong abs, doing Push-Ups will give you both, and so much more. From an upright planked position, the Push-Up requires you to lower slowly into and away from gravity, all while isolating the bend of your elbows.

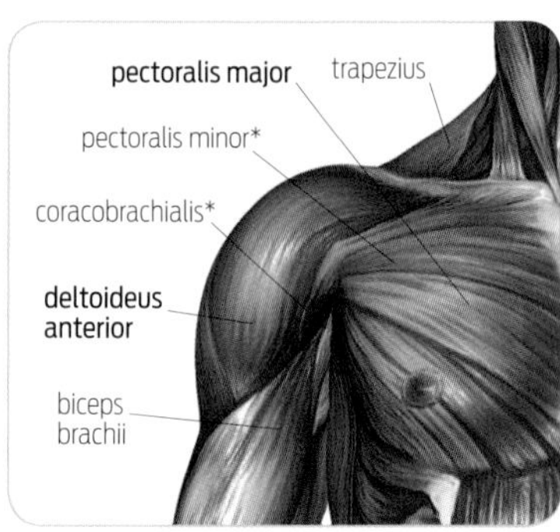

Annotation Key
Bold text indicates target muscles
Black text indicates other working muscles
* indicates deep muscles

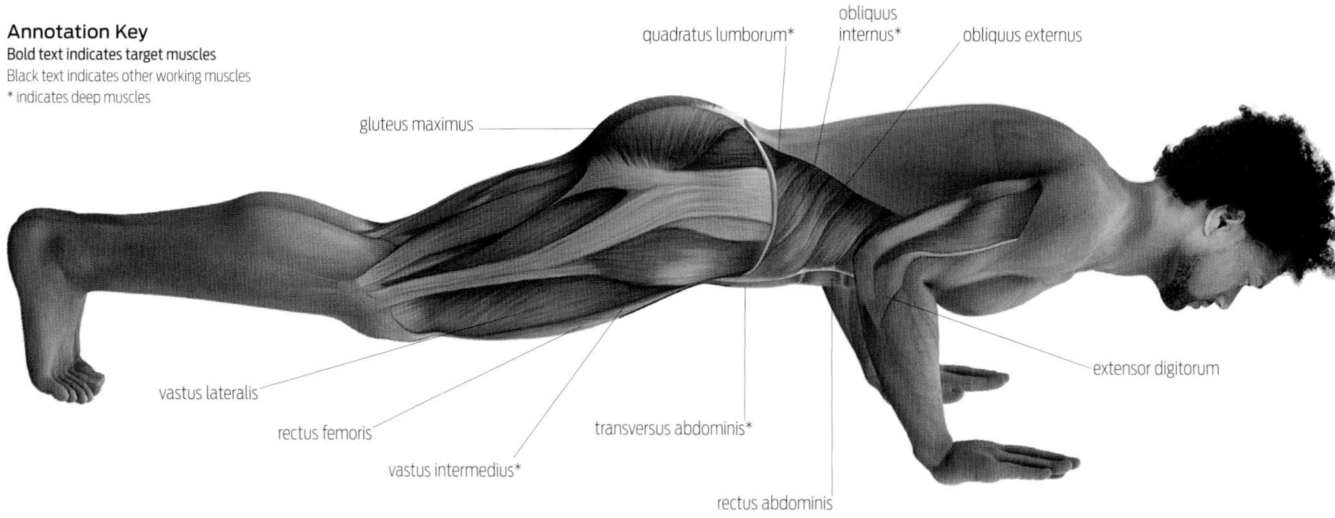

- Start with your body long and parallel to the floor, balanced on your hands and the balls of your feet.
- Keep the sensation of floating by pulling up the abs tightly into the back body. Slowly, isolate the elbows, bending at the joint, and bringing your chest to meet the ground below you.

Correct form

Be sure to keep the body in one straight line the entire time you perform your Push-Up! This challenging stance requires you to work your abdominals a lot while, simultaneously, engaging your arms isometrically.

Avoid

Avoid arching your pelvis back behind you or tucking it forward. Maintain a neutral pelvis. Pay special attention to your lower-back region and your tailbone.

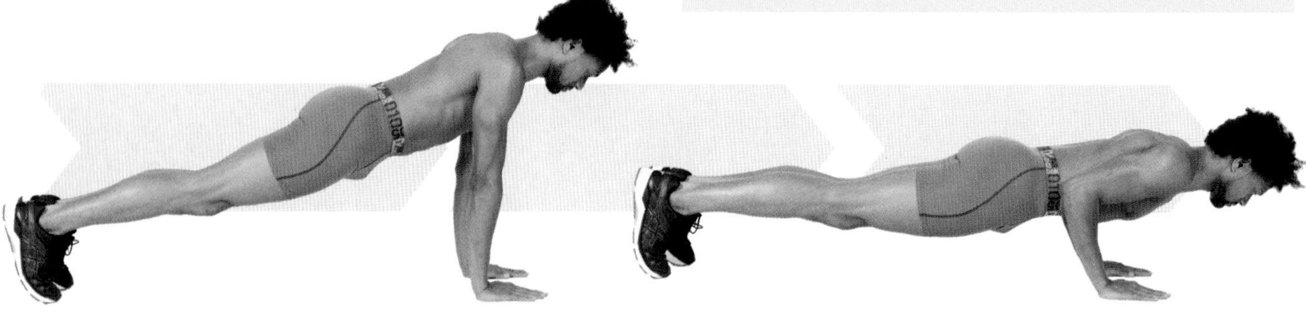

020 Swiss Ball Push-Up

Come to your hands and knees and place one foot, then the other, on top of a Swiss ball. With your body in one straight line, your arms at a 90-degree angle, and your hands shoulder-width apart, bend your elbows and lower your chest to the floor.

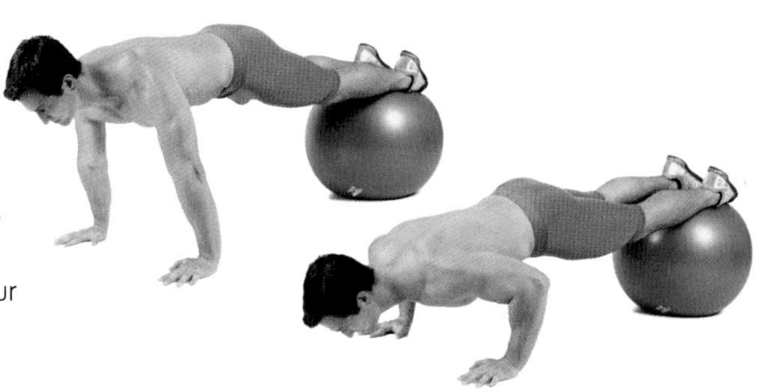

021 Single-Arm Medicine Ball Push-Up

Start in your straight-armed Push-Up position. Place a firm Medicine ball under your right hand. Slowly, without moving the ball, and keeping your weight even on both hands and feet, perform your Push-Up. Switch the ball to the left and repeat.

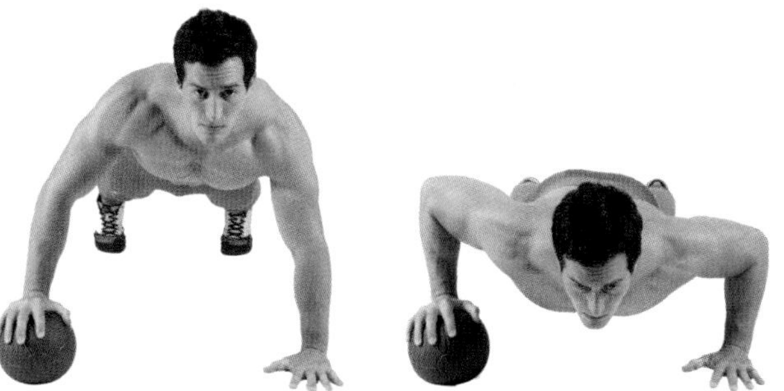

022 Hand-Weight Push-Up

Holding your hand weights with the flat side down, flush with the floor, come into your Push-Up stance with a long spine and very straight arms. Bend your elbows slowly into a Push-Up. Squeeze the abs up and into the body the whole time!

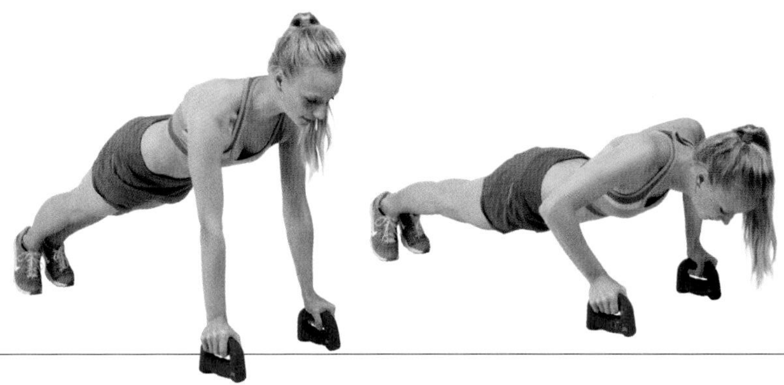

023 Plyo Kettlebell Push-Up

This variation of a Push-Up maximizes force with its quick intervals between moves.

- Start in your Push-Up form with the right hand over the top of the kettlebell.
- Bend the arms into a Push-Up, quickly straighten the arms, and switch the kettlebell into the left hand. Repeat.

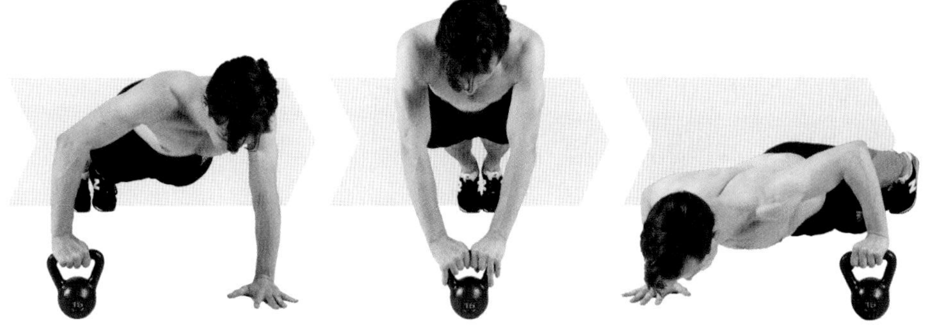

024 Swiss Ball Incline Dumbbell Push-Up

By incorporating both the Swiss ball and dumbbells into your Push-Up, you will maximize muscle intelligence and agility. The Swiss ball adds the challenge of instability, challenging all the muscles in the body to engage and pull up, while the dumbbells give you an element of alternate hand grip.

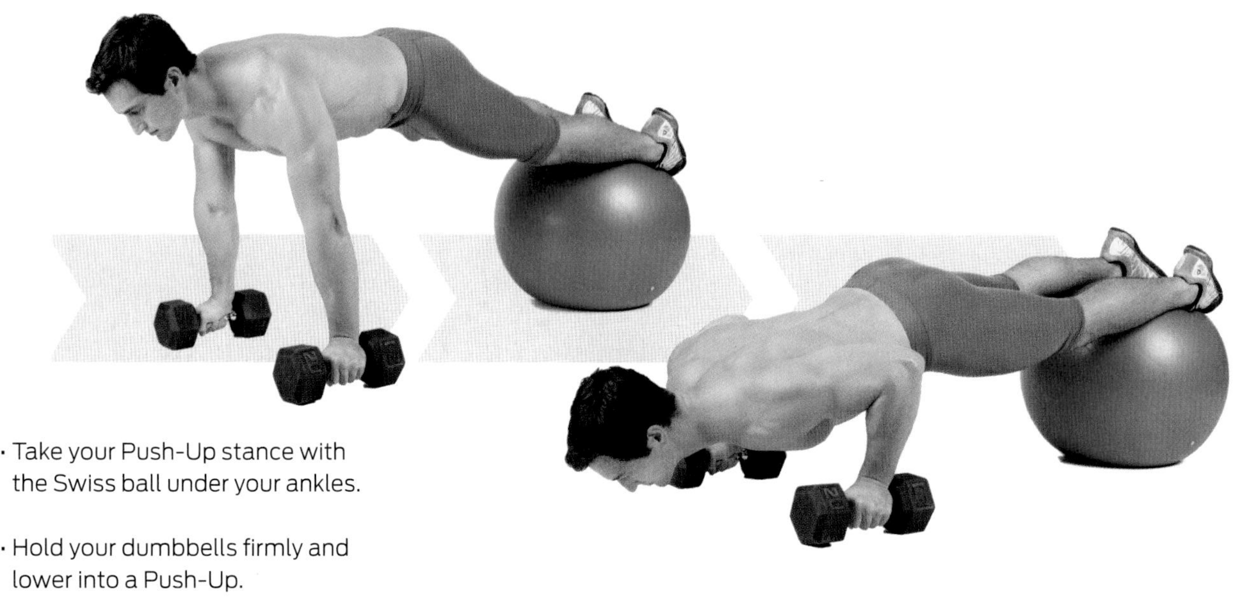

- Take your Push-Up stance with the Swiss ball under your ankles.
- Hold your dumbbells firmly and lower into a Push-Up.

025 Diamond Push-Up

With your palms down on the floor, make a diamond shape by extending your two thumbs together and your index fingers together. Slowly press the elbows open into your Push-Up. The closeness of your hands works the pecs and triceps.

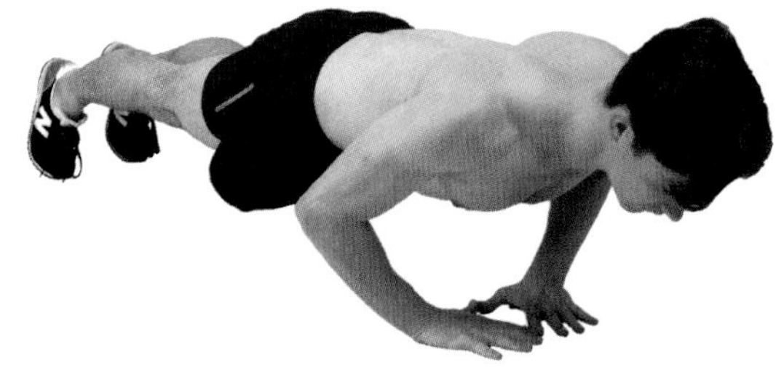

026 Plate Push-Up

Place a weighted plate between your shoulder blades, at the top of your back. With your arms open to shoulder-width, feel as if you are pushing up into the plate with your back while, simultaneously, lowering the body down.

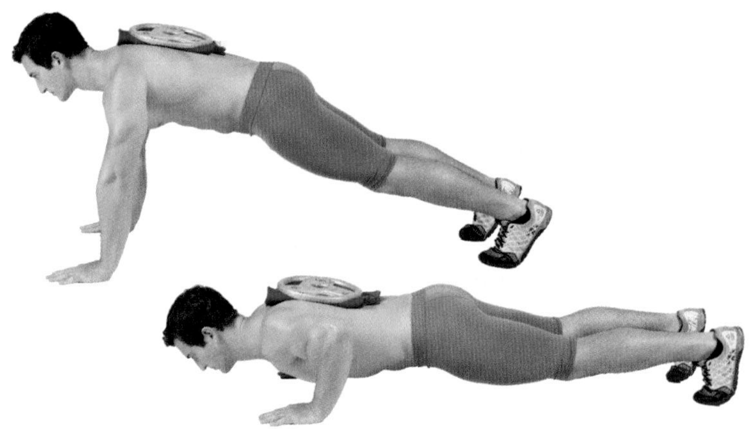

027 Close-Grip Swiss Ball Push-Up

Come to your hands and knees and place one foot, then the other, on top of a Swiss ball. With your body in one straight line, your arms at a 90-degree angle, and hands close together, bend your elbows and lower your chest to the floor.

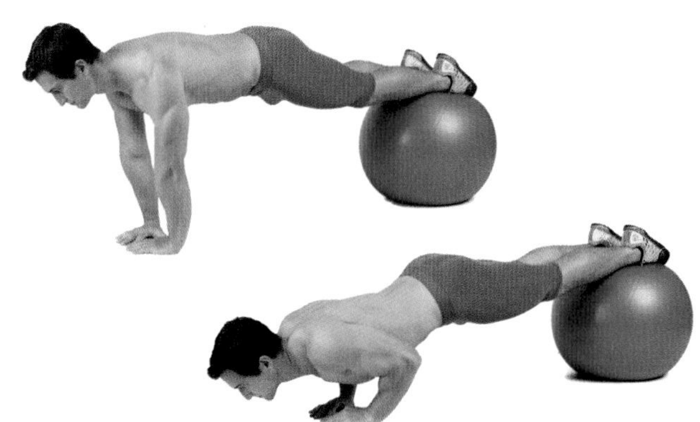

028 Medicine Ball Push-Up

Stand with your abs engaged, holding a Medicine ball in both hands. Bend forward, balancing your weight onto the ball with straight arms. Walk your feet back and perch in a wide stance on your tiptoes. Perform a Push-Up in this position, keeping your balance by pulling the abs in deeply and working the arms slowly from bent to straight.

Total Balance

Medicine balls are a great prop to incorporate into your workout routines! Supporting your body's weight on the top of a small sphere challenges your core and leg muscles to engage on a much deeper level.

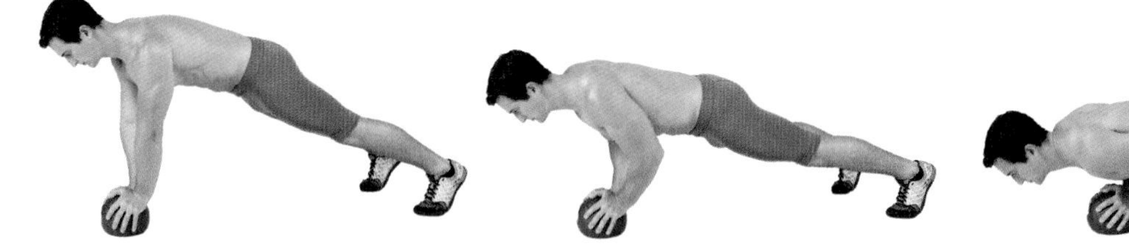

029 Foam-Roller Push-Up

Balance your body with your arms on a horizontal foam roller. Squeeze the upper arms into the sides of your body and slowly lower into your Push-Up. Be sure to keep the arms moving up and down along the sides of your body for optimal balance.

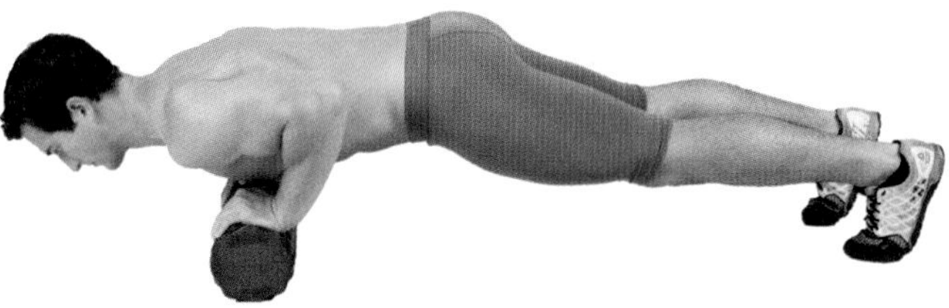

030 Balance Ball Push-Up

The balance ball creates an unstable base for your body in a Push-Up. Start with a balance ball flipped over onto the round side. Engage your abs strongly, squeeze the inner leg muscles together and, with your hands at each edge, balancing, perform a Push-Up.

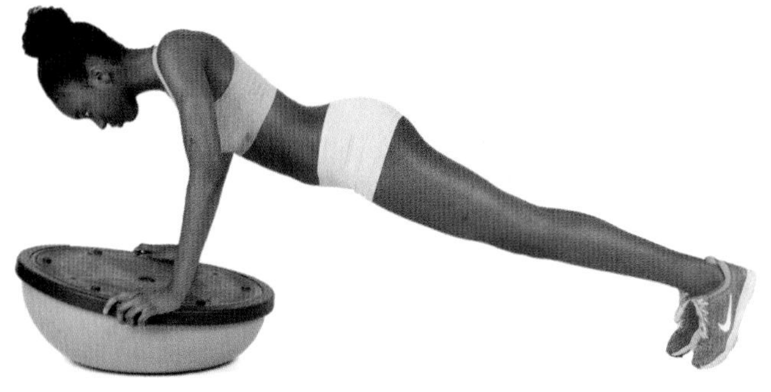

031 Balance Ball Diamond Push-Up

Put the flat side of the balance ball down onto the floor and come into your diamond hand position for your Push-Up. Keeping your focus on your abs and arms, lower into a Push-Up with the elbows opening to the sides.

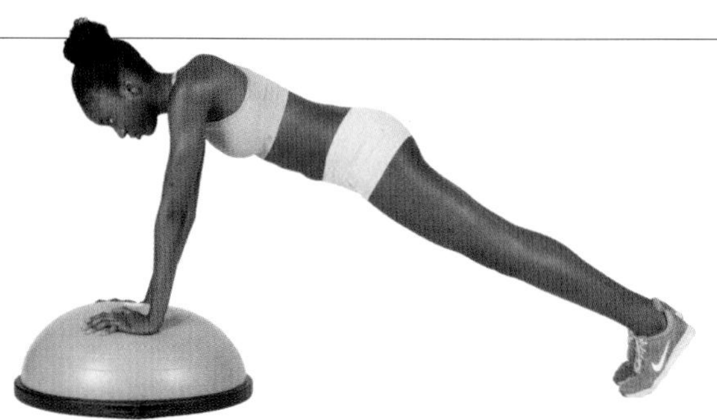

032 Medicine Ball Knee-Tuck Push-Up

Start in your straight armed Push-Up position. Place a firm Medicine ball under your left hand. Slowly, without moving the ball and keeping your weight even on both hands, perform your Push-Up, pulling the right knee across the torso to the left side. Switch the ball to the right hand and repeat.

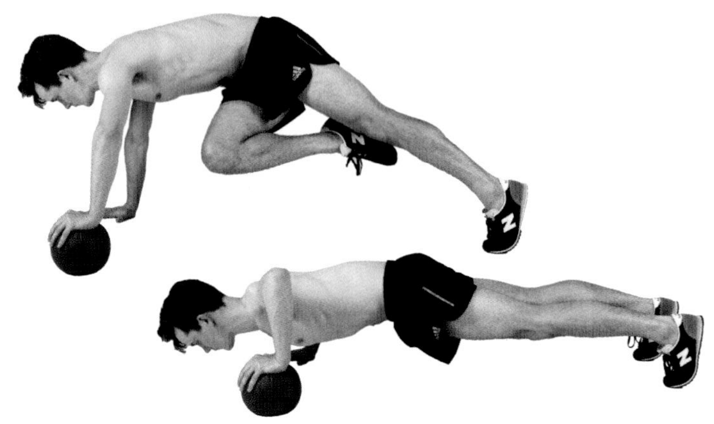

033 Suspended Push-Up

Come to your hands and knees and place one foot, then the other, into the suspension strap. With your body in one straight line, your arms at a 90-degree angle and hands shoulder-width apart, bend your elbows and lower your chest to the floor.

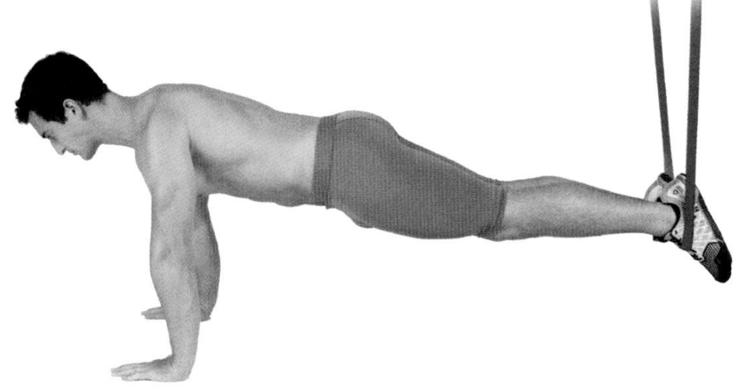

034 Suspended Atomic Push-Up

With your feet suspended off the ground in your strap, hold the arms very long and strong at a 90-degree angle to your body. Keep your upper body straight and engage the upper abs to pull your legs into your chest. Hold there for an added challenge.

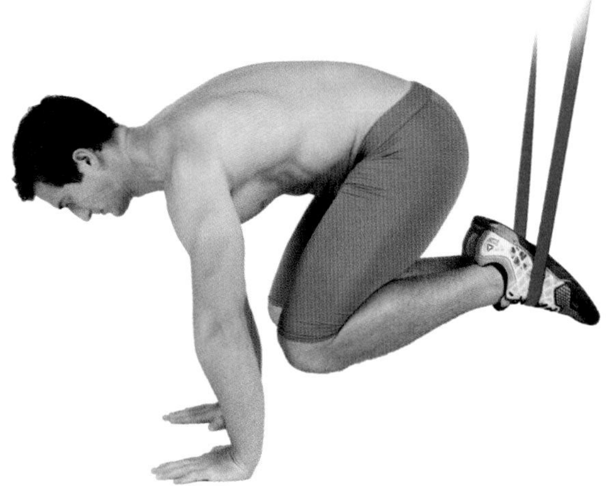

035 Mini-Medicine Ball Push-Up

Balanced atop your mini Medicine balls, one in each hand, come into your Push-Up stance with a long spine and very straight arms. Bend your elbows slowly into a Push-Up. Squeeze the abs up and into the body the whole time.

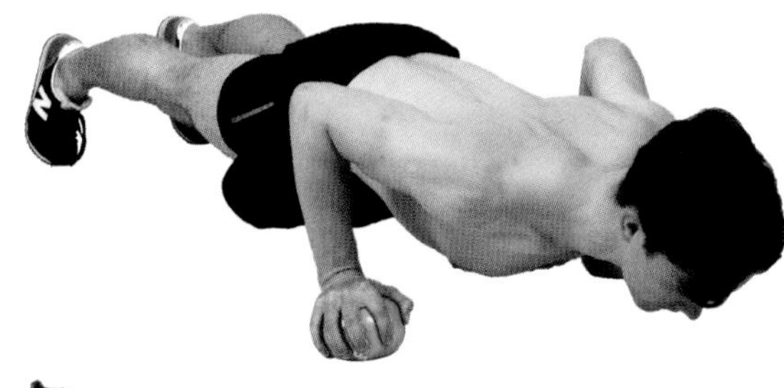

036 Knuckle Push-Up

Make two fists and rest them down on the floor, shoulder-width apart. Straighten your arms and come into a Push-Up position with your shoulders floating over your hands. Take a Push-Up here.

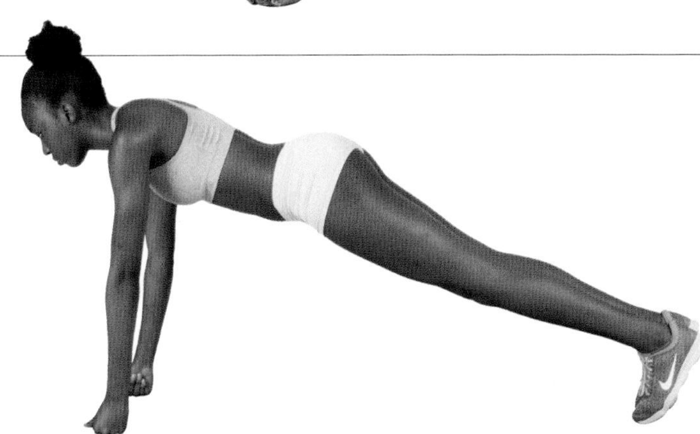

037 Kettlebell Push-Up

Kettlebells may look very stable, until you place them on the floor. Attempting to perform your Push-Ups on top of kettlebells requires you to super engage your core muscles and pecs while stabilizing your shoulders. This is a challenging exercise that will enhance your balance and overall alignment.

- Set your kettlebells down about shoulder-width apart and perch atop them with your hands securely balanced on the handles.
- Keeping your weight forward over the kettlebells slowly, lower into your Push-Up, just until your pecs are in line with the handles.

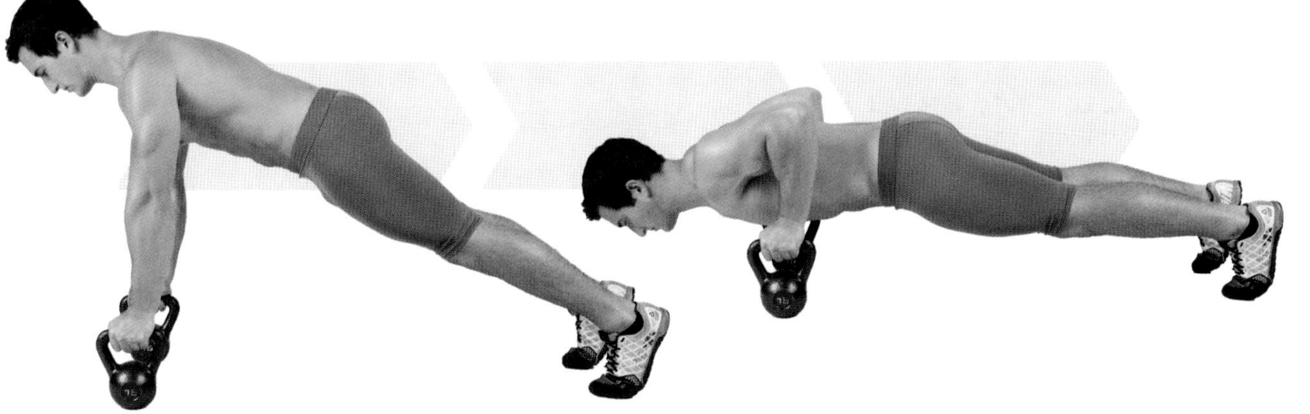

038 Rotational-Stand Push-Up

Start with your hands holding the rotational-stand handles straight in line with your body. As you start to lower into your Push-Up, turn the handles out so that they are flat to the sides, pause here in your Push-Up, then swivel the handles back straight to come up.

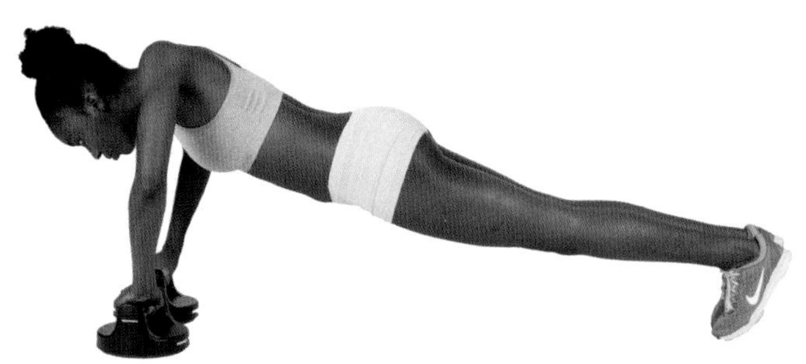

039 Pilates Magic Circle Push-Up

Place a magic circle directly under your belly button and come into your Push-Up stance. Using the resistance of your circle, lower down into your Push-Up, working against the circle. The circle will remind you to engage your abs.

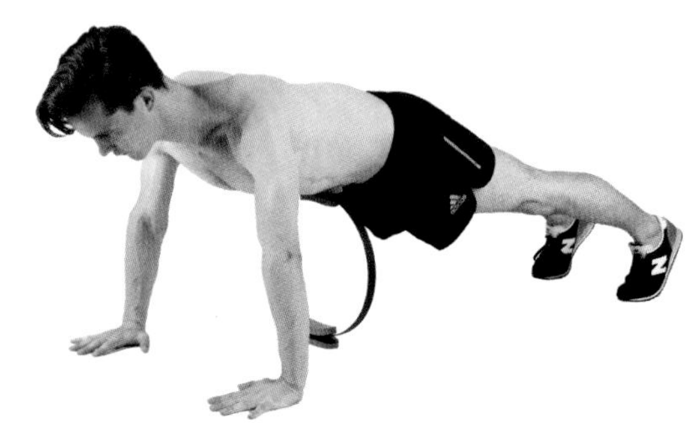

040 Alternating One-Arm Push-Up

This Push-Up with the arms wide and feet together challenges the stability of the shoulders and rotator cuffs. Performing this style of Push-Up will create deep stabilization in the shoulder girdles, rotator cuffs, and shoulder blades. Be sure to keep good alignment and move slowly.

- With your arms wider than shoulder-width apart, swing your palms open to the corners of the room. Squeeze your legs together, balanced on the balls of your feet.
- Slowly track your elbow out to the right side, engage the core, and lower into a Push-Up, bringing your chest far right.
- Lift the body back up to the middle, engage the core, and lower left. Repeat side to side.

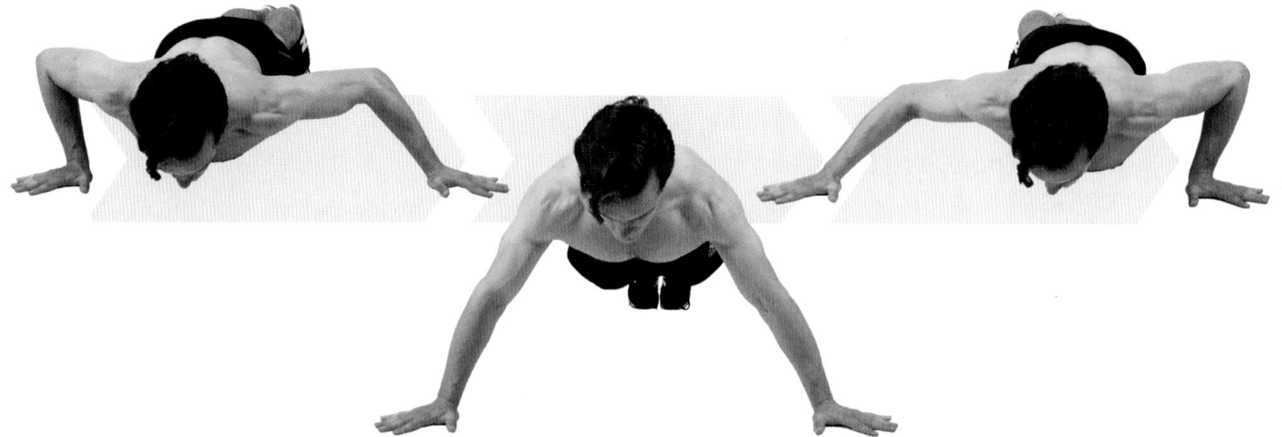

041 Weighted Santana Push-Up

This variation of Push-Up, continues to work on the stabilization of the shoulder joint, as well as maximizing the rotation of the chest, while holding in a twist with weights.

- Perform a Push-Up while balanced on top of dumbells.
- At the bottom of your Push-Up, hold.
- Spin open onto the right hand, lifting up the left dumbbell, and stacking the feet. Hold here for a beat, then push up again and switch sides.

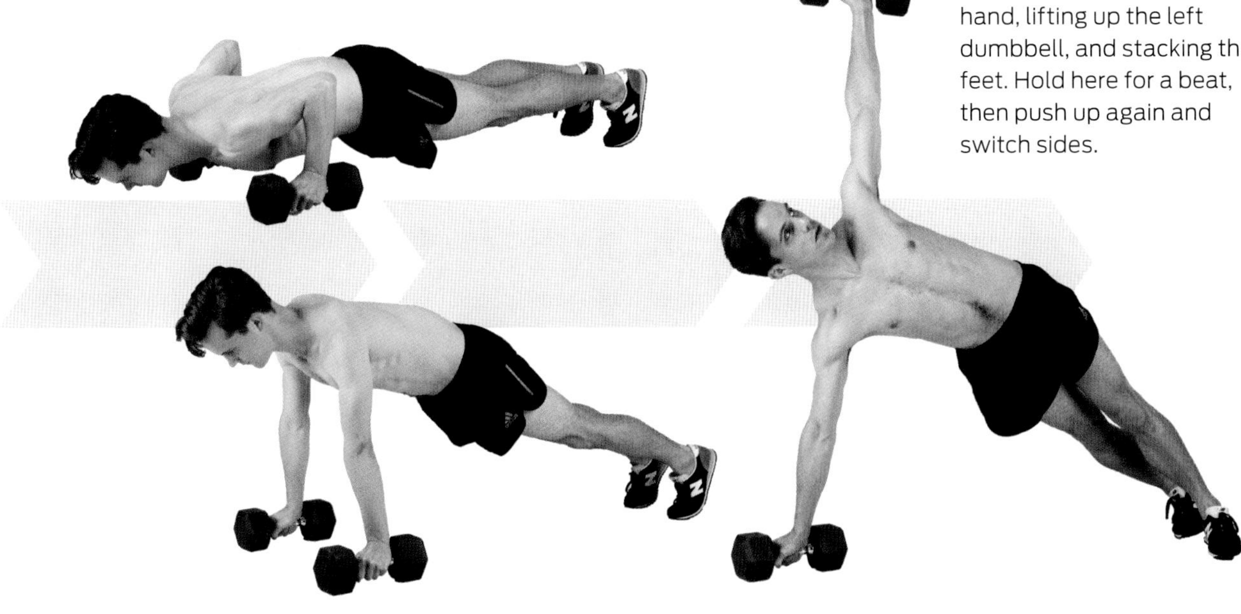

042 Push-Up with Lower-Body Rotation

Start off with stacked legs, one on top of the other. Place your hands down onto the floor in your Push-Up stance and perform a Push-Up, engaging both sides of your body. The lower-body rotation challenges your center of balance.

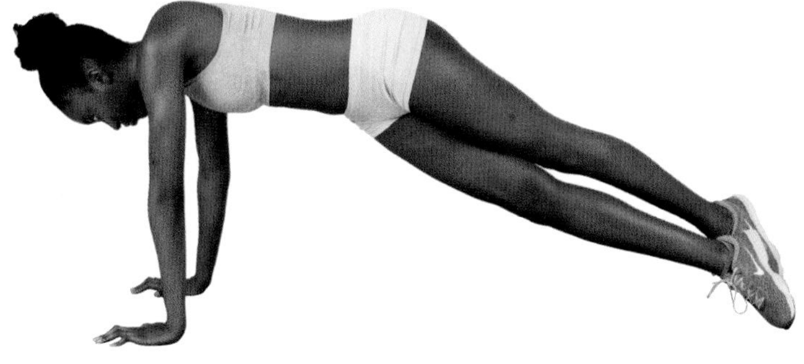

043 Single-Knee Push-Up

Begin on your hands and knees, with the weight evenly balanced on each point. Lift your left leg into a straight line with your torso. Lower into your Push-Up, allowing the weight of the body to shift forward, bringing your chest to the floor between your arms.

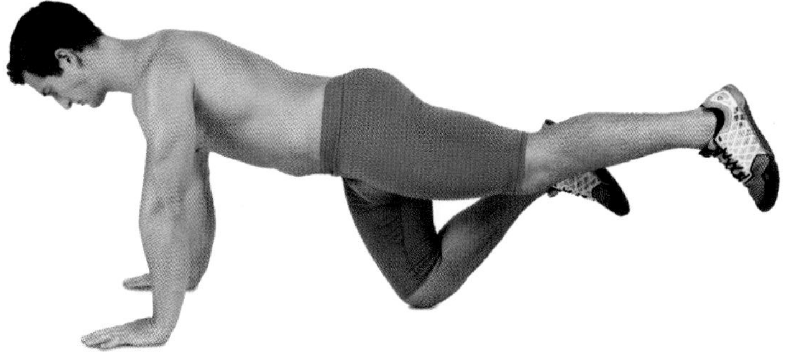

044 Single-Leg Push-Up

In Push-Up stance, squeeze the inner legs together while pulling the abs up and into the spine. Vertically, stack your left foot onto the back of the right heel. Lower into a Push-Up, return to the start position, and switch legs.

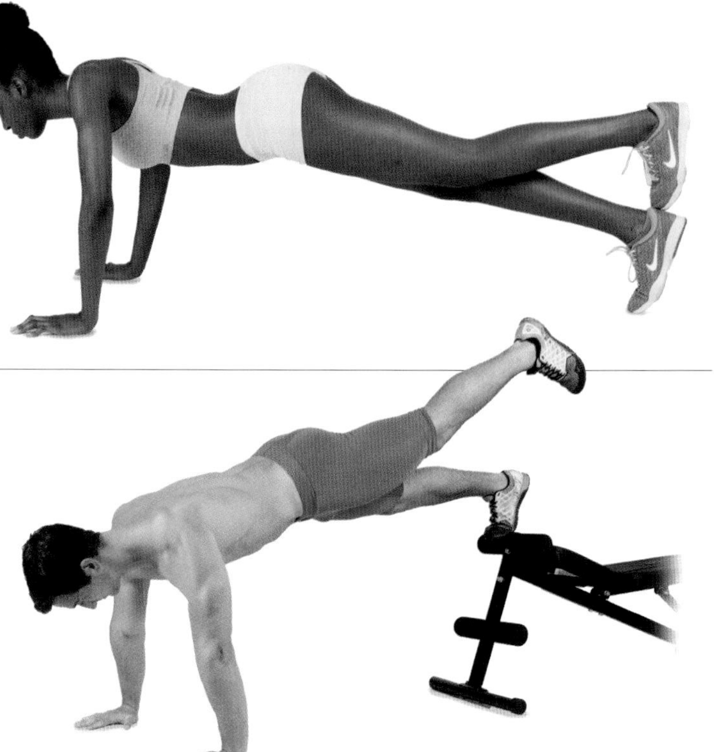

045 Single-Leg Decline Push-Up

Come to your hands and knees and place one foot on top of an elevated surface. With your body in one straight line, your arms at a 90-degree angle, and your hands shoulder-width apart, bend your elbows and lower your chest to the floor.

046 Single-Leg Roller Push-Up

In Push-Up stance, balanced on a roller, squeeze the inner legs together while pulling the abs up and into the spine. Raise your left foot off the floor and shift the weight into your arms. Lower into a Push-Up and switch legs.

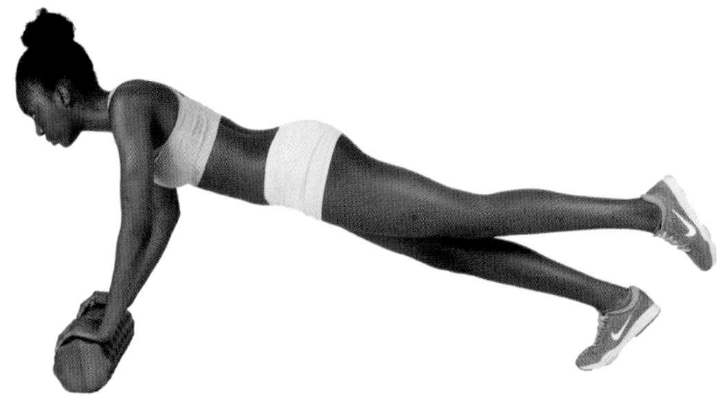

047 Push-Up on Swiss Ball and Blocks

Place a palm on each block so your hands are shoulder-width apart. Bring one foot, then the other, on top of a Swiss ball. With your body in one straight line, and your arms at a 90-degree angle to the body, bend your elbows and lower your chest until level with the blocks. Return to the start position, and repeat.

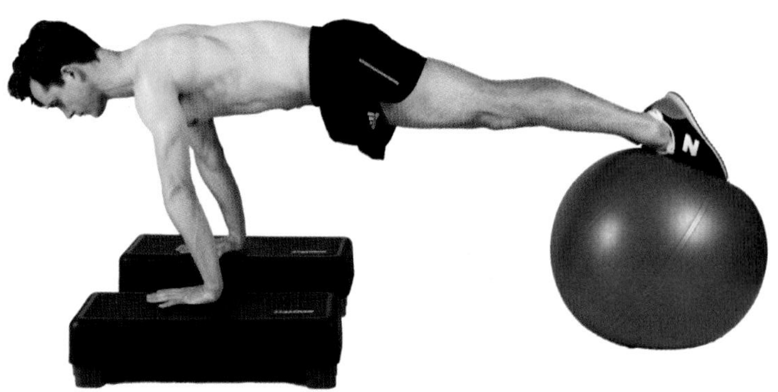

048 Single-Leg Push-Up on Swiss Ball and Blocks

With each hand on a block, bring your feet onto the Swiss ball. Keeping your body in one straight line, balance on your arms securely, and lift your left leg. Hold the leg steady and bend your elbows into a Push-Up.

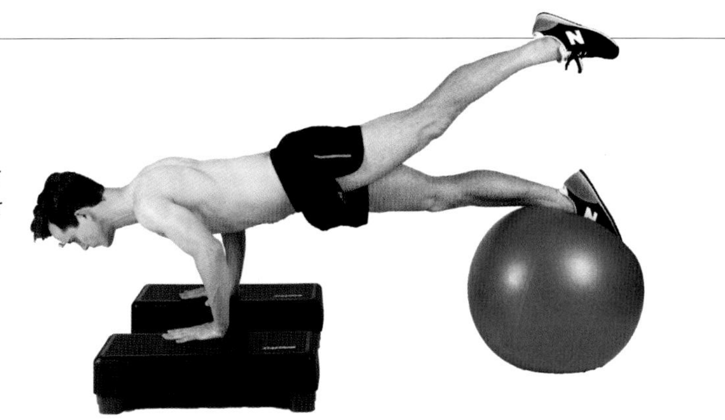

049 Box Push-Up

Start in your straight-armed Push-Up position. Place your right hand on top of the box. Slowly, keeping your weight even on both hands and feet, perform your Push-Up. Switch the box to the left side, and repeat.

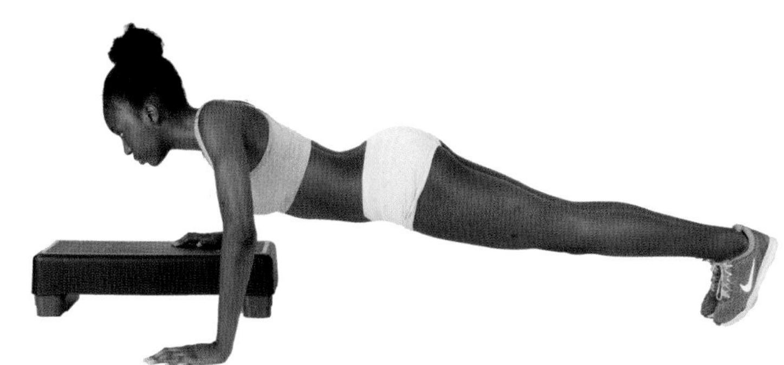

050 Crossover Box Push-Up

The Crossover Box Push-Up builds a high level of endurance, strengthens the pecs, and creates deep stabilization in the shoulder girdle. Not only are you performing a Push-Up, but you are also traveling back and forth across an unlevel surface! The peaks and valleys that you move through make this variation truly unique.

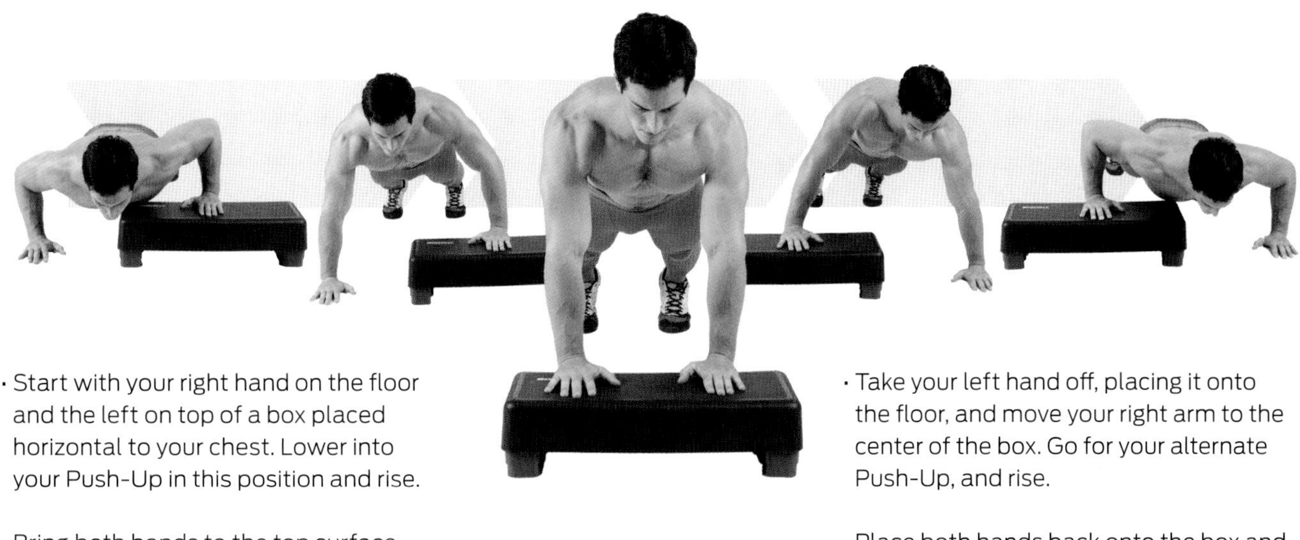

- Start with your right hand on the floor and the left on top of a box placed horizontal to your chest. Lower into your Push-Up in this position and rise.
- Bring both hands to the top surface of the box.
- Take your left hand off, placing it onto the floor, and move your right arm to the center of the box. Go for your alternate Push-Up, and rise.
- Place both hands back onto the box and continue alternating to each side.

051 Single-Arm Push-Up

Start in your straight-armed Push-Up position. Place your left hand behind your back. Slowly, while keeping the left shoulder in line with the right, perform your Push-Up. Switch arms, and repeat.

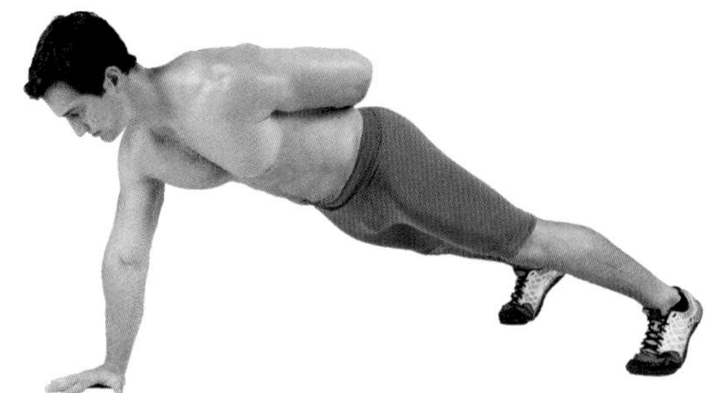

052 Single-Arm, Single-Leg Push-Up

With the weight evenly placed on both hands and the balls of your feet, in your Push-Up stance, raise the left arm off the floor, straight out in front of you. Then, raise the right leg straight out behind you. With balance, lower into your Push-Up.

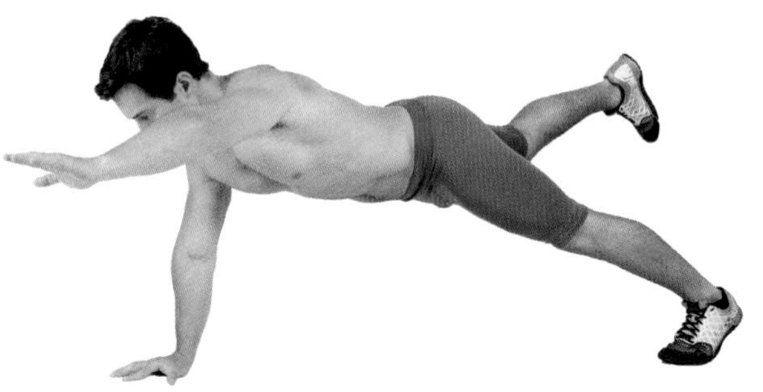

053 Dynamic Box Push-Up

This dynamic Push-Up gives you a good dose of plyometric and coordination work. Combining agility with quick, explosive, springing moves, you will develop incredible strength throughout the upper body and abdominals. Performing this exercise requires the ability to jump off the hands, from your lowest Push-Up level and land onto a box—all in one count!

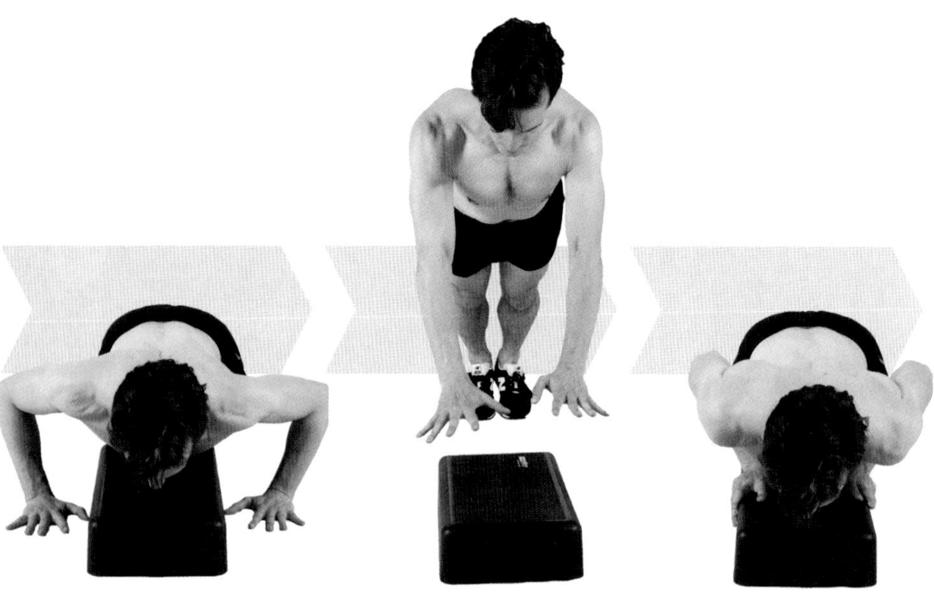

- Start in your Push-Up form with each hand on the outside of the box.
- Bend your arms into a Push-Up and quickly spring off the floor, bringing both hands together in the air and landing in a Push-Up on top of the box.
- Straighten up out of your Push-Up, still on top of the box.
- Then, lower into a Push-Up, and spring up off the box, opening the arms to land in your Push-Up, straddling the box, as you began.

054 Alternating Shuffle Push-Up

For maximum core and shoulder stabilization perform this challenging variation of the Push-Up (#019). By opening and closing your hands underneath the chest in a single repetition, you will work your upper-body coordination and engage your abdominals deeply, too.

- Start with your arms shoulder-width apart.
- Lower into your Push-Up and slide your right hand in along the floor to meet your left hand, all while staying low in your Push-Up.
- Straighten up with your hands together. Lower into a Push-Up again and slide the right hand out to open wide, staying low. Straighten up with wide arms and repeat from side to side.

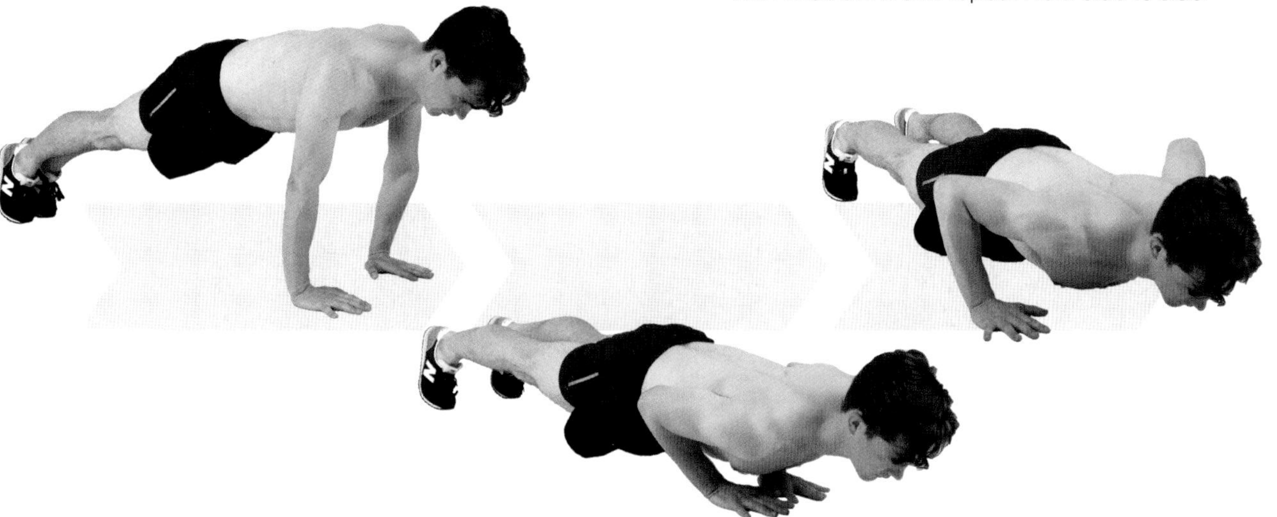

055 Alternating Medicine Ball Push-Up

Start in your straight-armed Push-Up position. Place a firm Medicine ball under your right hand. Slowly, without moving the ball and keeping your weight even on both hands and feet, perform your Push-Up. Switch the ball to the left hand, and repeat.

Benefits

Incorporating Medicine balls into your workouts is a great way to enhance your balance and work on coordination. Alternating the ball, with your hands, from side to side works the muscles in the body, but also works the brain's cross-axis circuits!

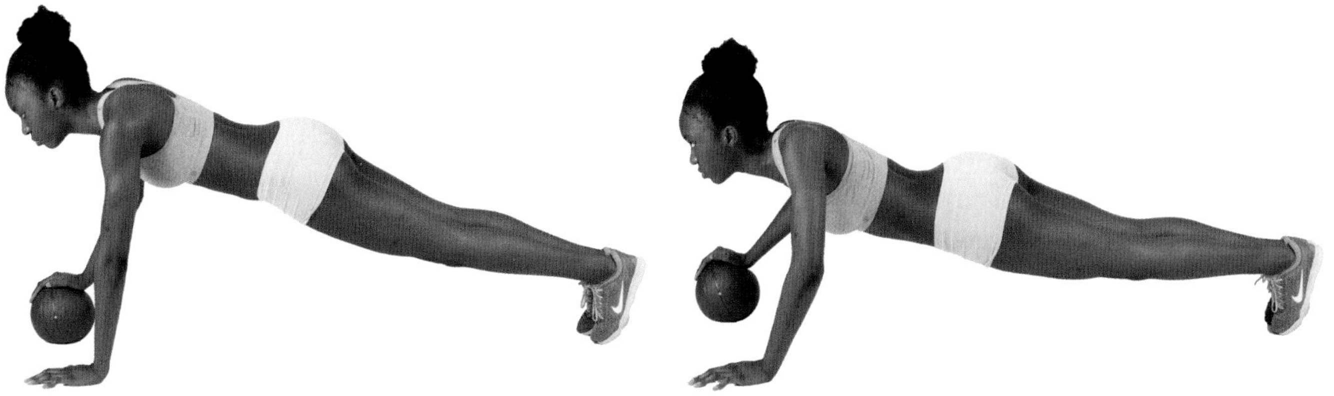

056

Clap Push-Up

Lower into your Push-Up and, in one explosive movement, push off the floor with both hands and clap them together quickly, in front of the chest. Open the hands and land again in your low Push-Up.

057

Knee Push-Up and Roll-Out

Hold onto a barbell with round weights at either end, and place both knees together on the floor. Lower out into your Push-Up while extending the torso long, keeping the arms straight, and rolling the barbell away from your body. Pull the barbell back toward your body to return to the starting position. Keep the core engaged at all times.

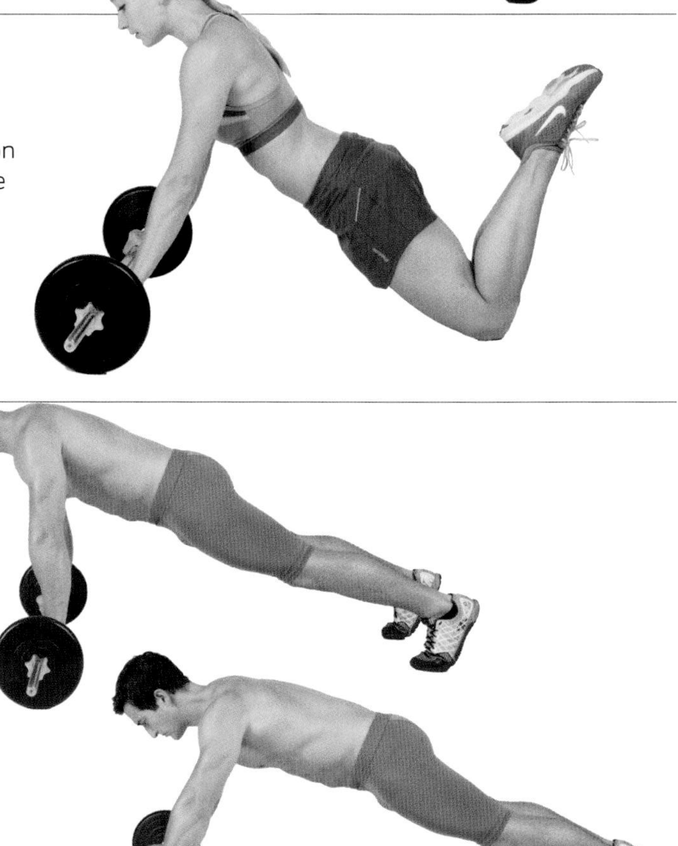

058

Push-Up and Roll-Out

Hold your barbell while in a balanced Push-Up stance. Lower out into your Push-Up while extending the torso long, keeping the arms straight, and rolling the barbell away from your body. Allow the chest to come as close to the floor as you can manage. Return to the start position. Keep the core engaged at all times.

Push-Up and Roll-Out Dumbbell Variation

Holding your dumbbells, come into your Push-Up stance with a long spine and very straight arms. Slowly bend your elbows into a Push-Up. Hold low in the Push-Up and take turns alternating rolling out: extending the dumbbell straight in front of you, and bringing it back in.

060 Push-Up and Walk-Over

The Push-Up and Walk-Over builds a high level of endurance, strengthens the pecs, and creates deep stabilization in the shoulder girdle. Not only are you performing a Push-Up, but you are also traveling back and forth across an unlevel surface.

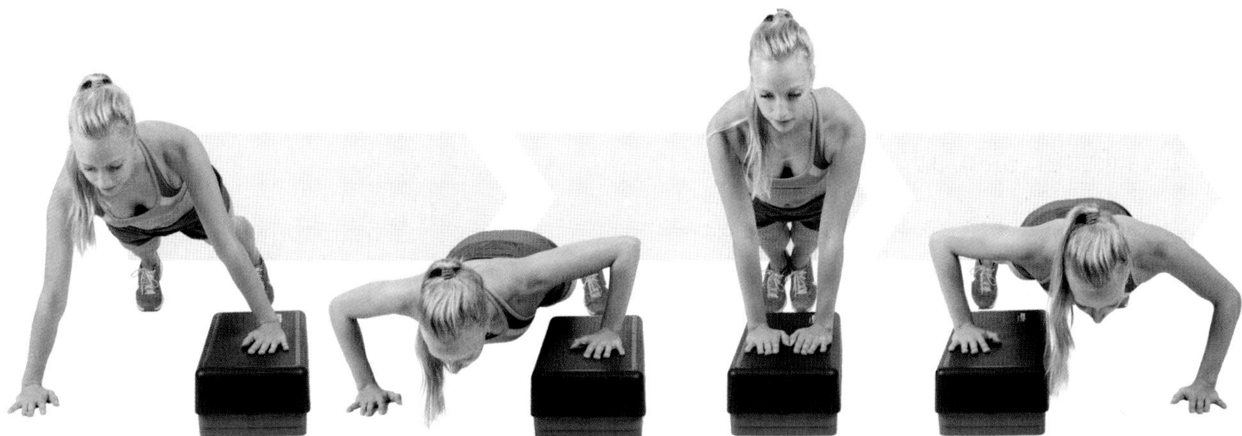

- Start with your right hand on the floor and the left on top of a box placed parallel to your chest. Lower into your Push-Up in this position, and rise.
- Bring both hands to the top surface of the box.
- Take your left hand off, placing it onto the floor, and keeping your right arm at the center of the box. Go for your alternating Push-Up, and rise.
- Place both hands back up onto the box and continue alternating to each side.

061 Gymnast Push-Up

This variation of the Push-Up maximizes level changes, combined with deep abdominal work. Start with the tops of the feet pointed into the floor. Bend your elbows deep into a Push-Up and hold. From there, place each forearm down onto the floor, and flex the ankles, coming onto the balls of the feet. Press back up and roll forward into the start position, and repeat.

Inspiration

Gymnasts are some of the hardest-working athletes. Their athleticism is borderline superhuman! Staying compact, tight, and in control requires a powerful core. Perform your "gymnast" Push-Up with this in mind!

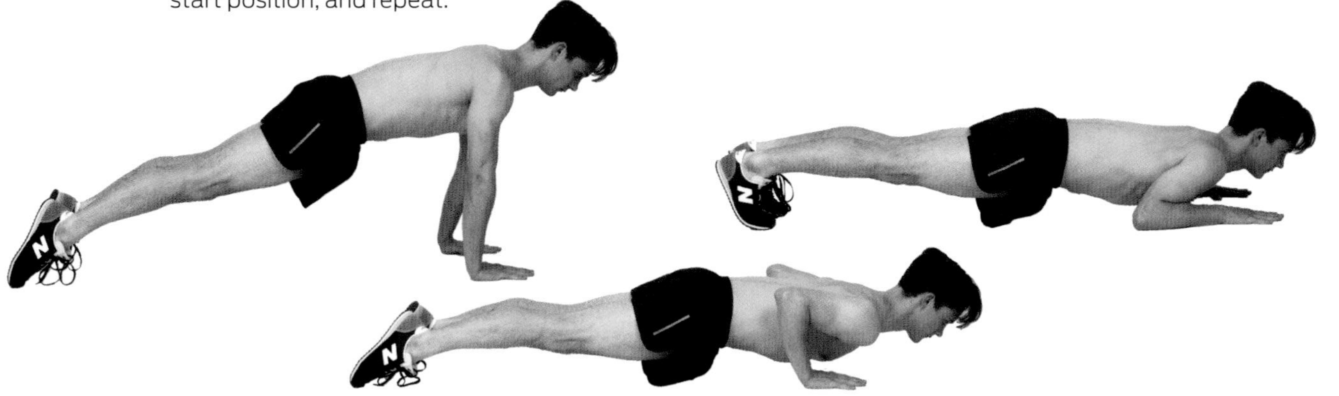

062

Lateral Raise

Executing the Lateral Raise in your best form will strengthen a few very important upper-body muscle groups, including the deltoids, trapezius, and pecs. Consequently, this movement also stabilizes the shoulders and scapula.

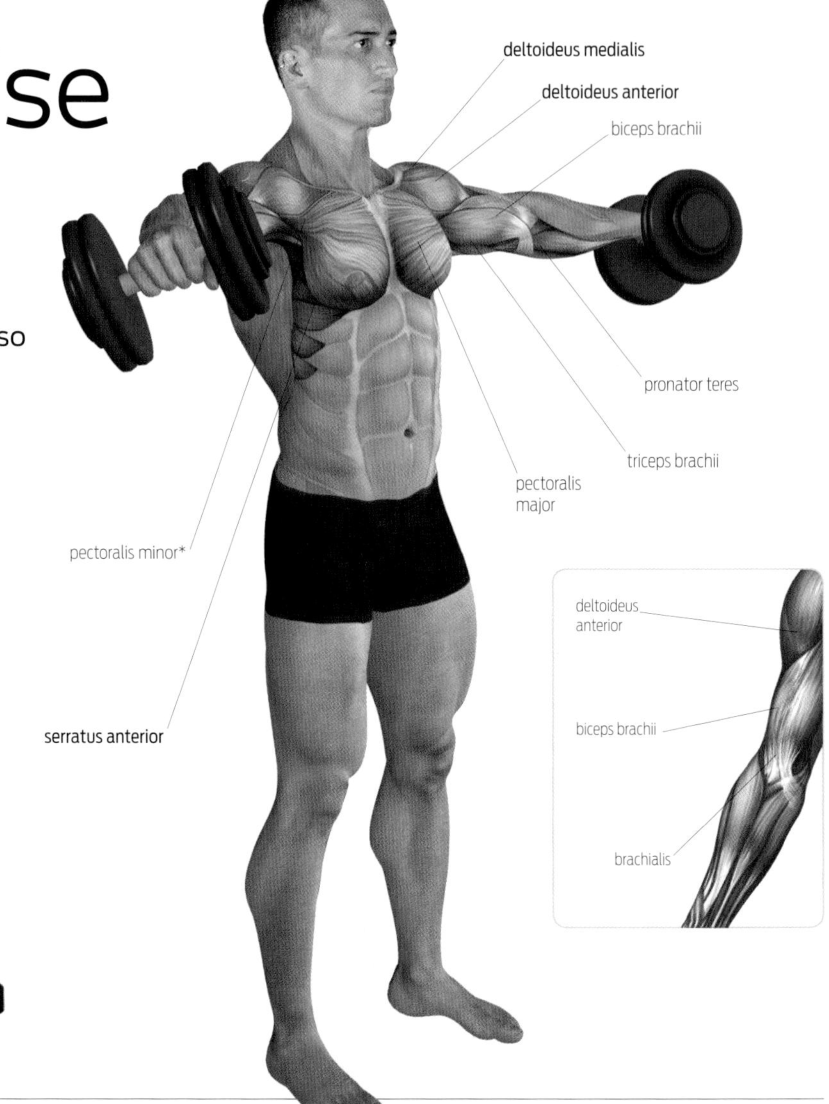

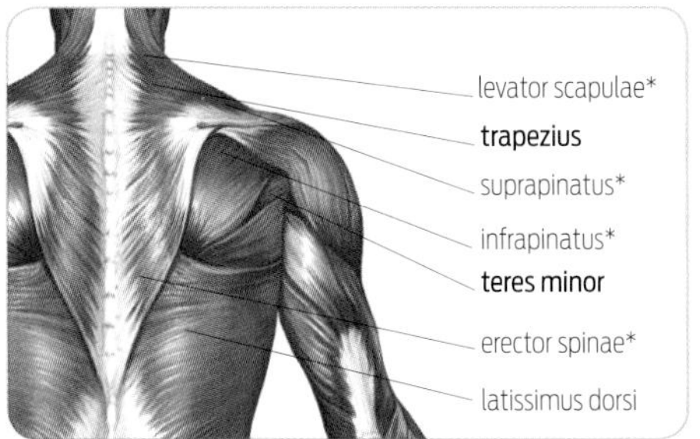

Annotation Key
Bold text indicates target muscles
Black text indicates other working muscles
* indicates deep muscles

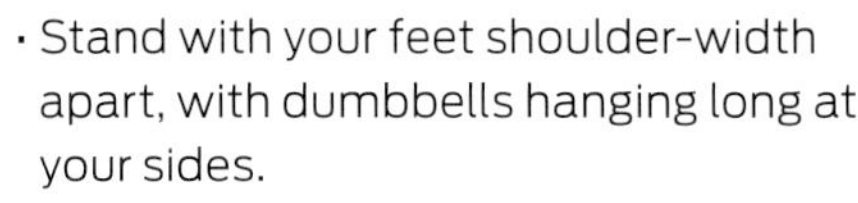

- Stand with your feet shoulder-width apart, with dumbbells hanging long at your sides.
- Keeping the core engaged, and the shoulders aligned with the hips, slowly raise your dumbbells out away from the body until they are parallel to the shoulders.
- Slowly lower the weights back down.

Correct form

Be sure to keep your elbows slightly bent throughout this exercise. The slight bend will allow the proper muscles to engage and work most efficiently. Exhale as you lift, inhale as you lower.

Avoid

Don't let your arms swing too far forward or backward. Track the movement of your arms directly in line with the sides of your hips.

063 Bent-Arm Lateral Raises

Adding a bend in the arms and knees while staying with the theme of the Lateral Raise gives an element of smaller, more focused muscle work. Additionally, maintaining a bent stance in the lower body, works the legs.

- From a tall, straight stance, bend the legs into a shallow squat position.
- Bend your elbows, bringing the dumbbells in front of your chest.
- Open the elbows out to each side, away from each other, until they are level with your shoulders.
- Lower the dumbbells back down, stand tall, and repeat.

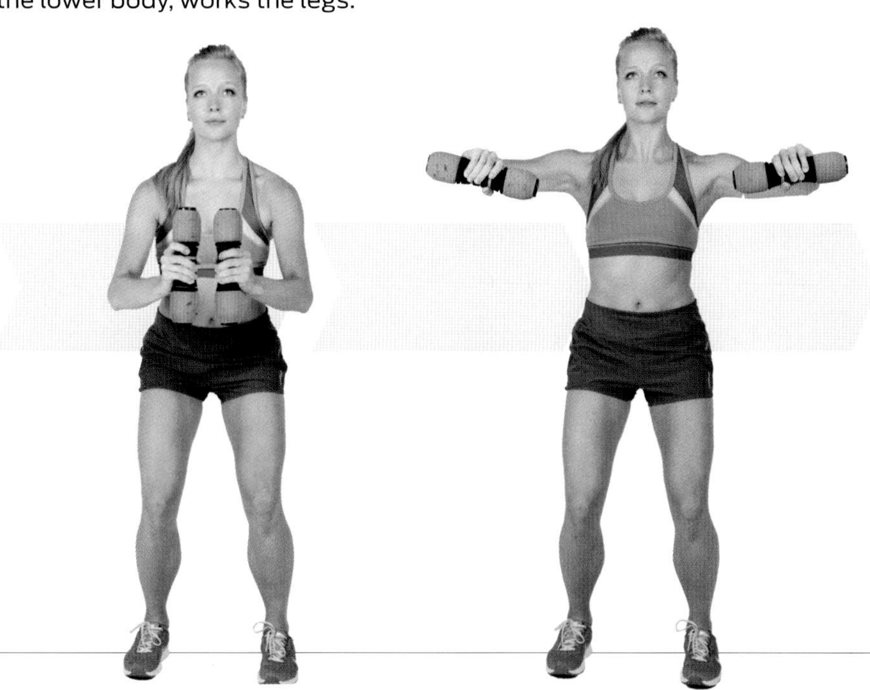

064 One-Arm Bent-Over Lateral Raises

Working each arm at a time, while keeping your balance on an incline bench, gives the core a major workout in this bent-over Lateral Raise variation.

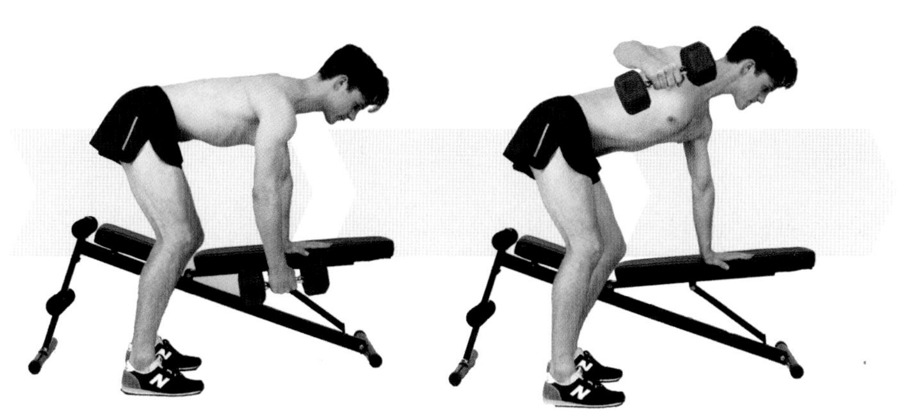

- With one hand on the incline bench, and a dumbbell in the other, bend the body over so it's just above a 90-degree angle.
- Using the bench to balance, open the dumbbell out to the side, parallel to your chest.
- Lower the dumbbell back alongside your bench, and repeat. Change sides after desired repetitions.

065 Front Raise with Plate

Stand with your feet shoulder-width apart. Grip a weighted plate with both hands, holding it in front of your hips. Let the shoulders be easy and keep the upper back long and straight. Slowly lift the plate up to shoulder height, then, lower.

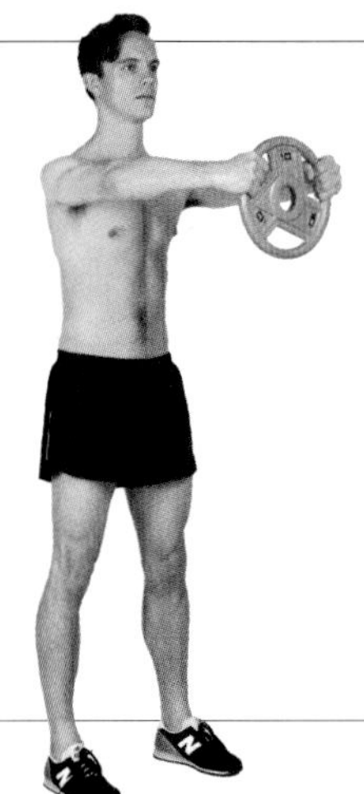

Take Care

Whenever you are working the upper-body muscles with hand weights or cables, remember to keep the larger muscle groups engaged, but not tense, while working the smaller muscles in that area. The neck and shoulder muscles are intricate and can be easily harmed if you use incorrect alignment or too much force.

066 One-Arm Dumbbell Raise

Hold onto the top of an incline bench or a chair with the left hand, and hold a dumbbell in the right hand. Bend the body over so it's just above a 90-degree angle. Using the bench to balance, open the dumbbell out and up, ending in line with your chest.

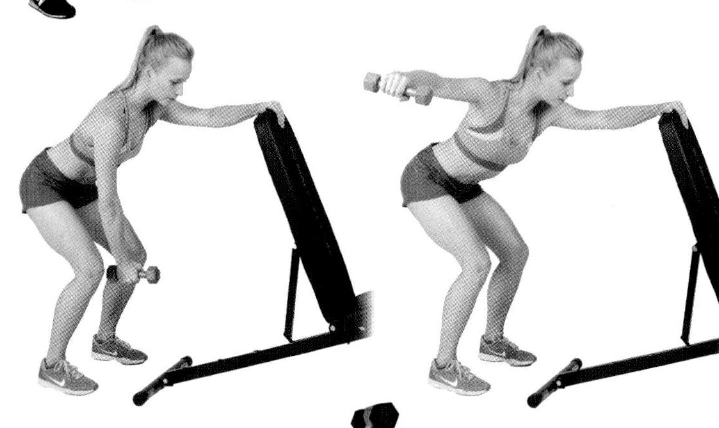

067 4-Count Overhead

Stand with your feet shoulder-width apart, holding a dumbbell with both hands at your right shoulder. Lift the weight overhead (count 1). Next, bring the dumbbell to your left shoulder (count 2), then back overhead (count 3). Return the dumbbell to your right shoulder (count 4). Repeat in this order each time.

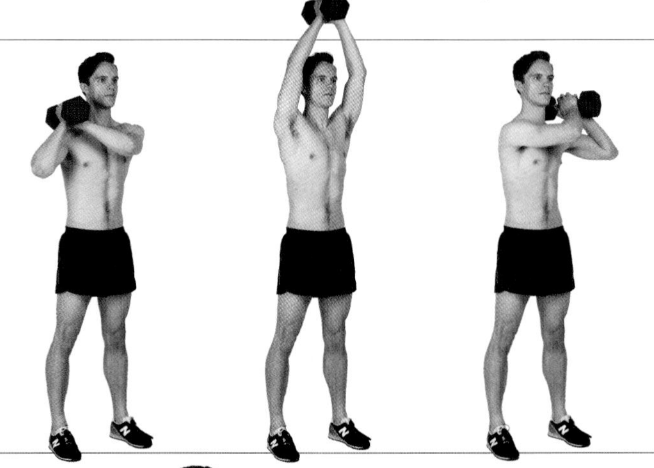

068 Bent-Over Cable Raise

Bend over with the abs fully engaged, the feet shoulder-width apart. With your right hand holding the cable, allow the upper arm to swing open to the side, pulling and raising the cable to shoulder height. Lower with control.

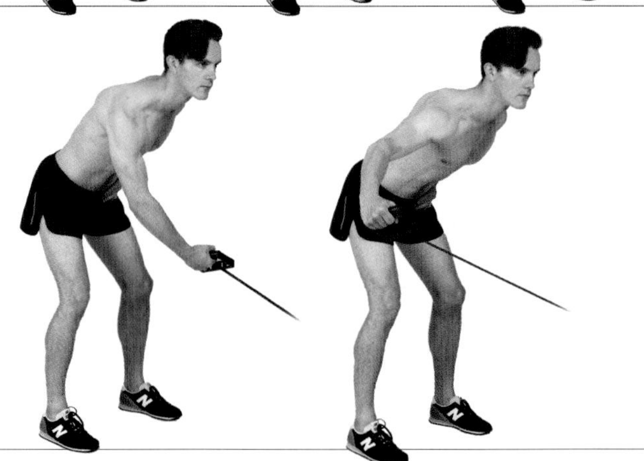

069 Double Kettlebell Snatch

This exercise maximizes strength with quick intervals between moves. Adding an element of plyometrics, using the kettlebells and the bend in the knees, your movement should be explosive and dynamic. The Double Kettlebell Snatch, when performed correctly, will help to stabilize the shoulder joints, as well as enhance overall posture and alignment.

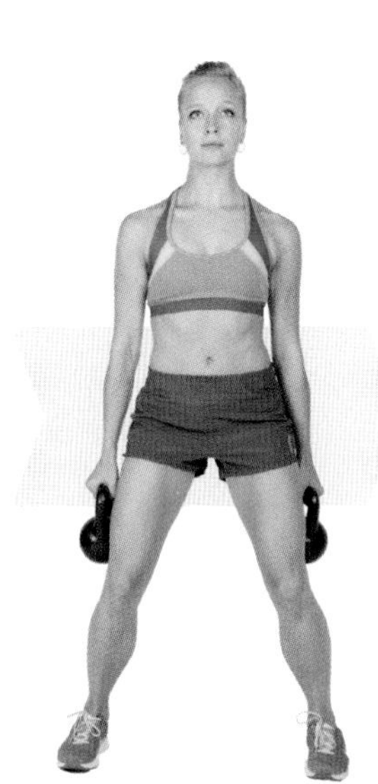
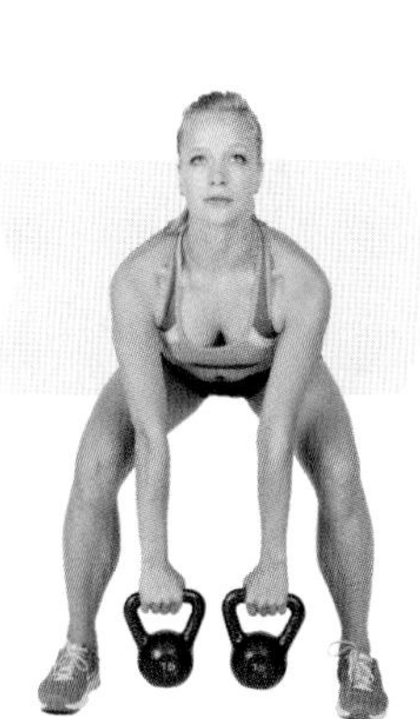
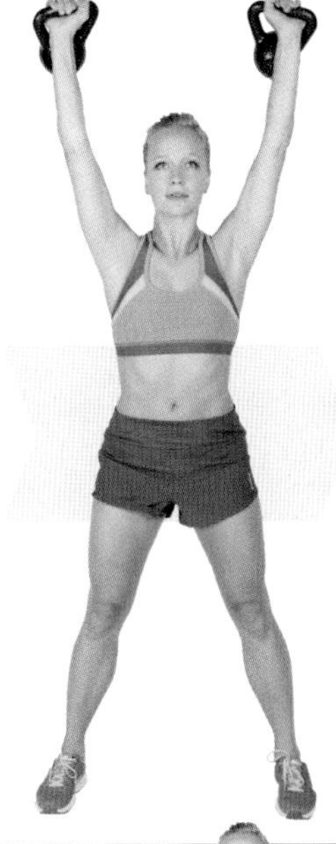

- Start in a wide, open stance, holding the kettlebells in each hand at the sides of the body.
- Bend the knees deeply, swinging the kettlebells together through the inside of the legs.
- In one motion swing the kettlebells up through the legs to end overhead.
- Allow the kettlebells to flip over the backs of your hands.
- Reverse your swing back down, ending with the kettlebells between the legs.

070 Lateral Raise with Resistance Bands

Bring your feet open to about hip-width apart. Fasten the cable under the middle of your feet, horizontally. Keeping your spine long, squeeze the abs into the spine, engage the shoulders, and pull the cable up and out to shoulder height.

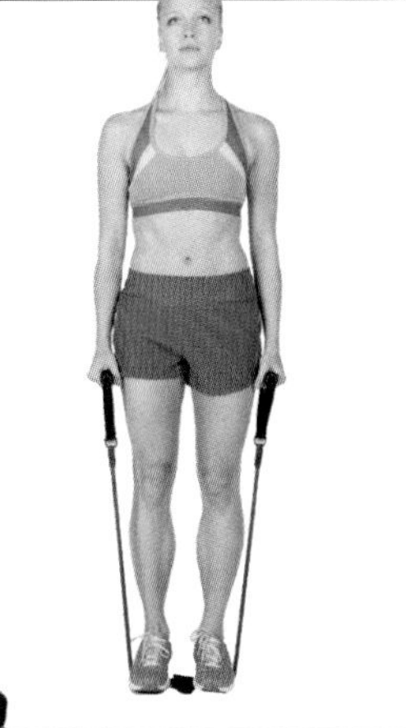
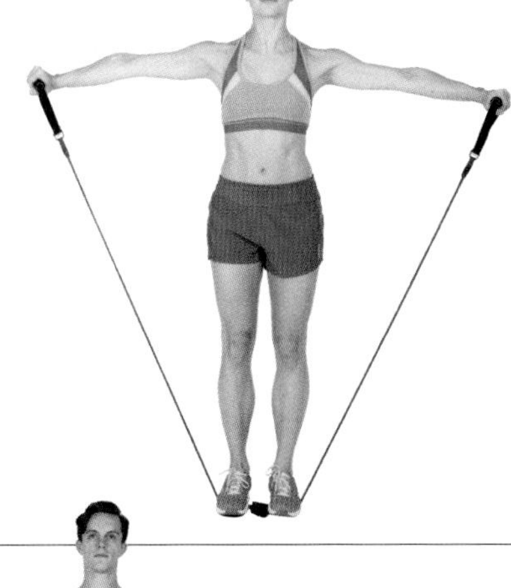

071 Lateral Raise with Cables

With your feet open wide, and keeping your spine long, squeeze the abs into the spine, engage the shoulders, and pull the cables up and out to shoulder height.

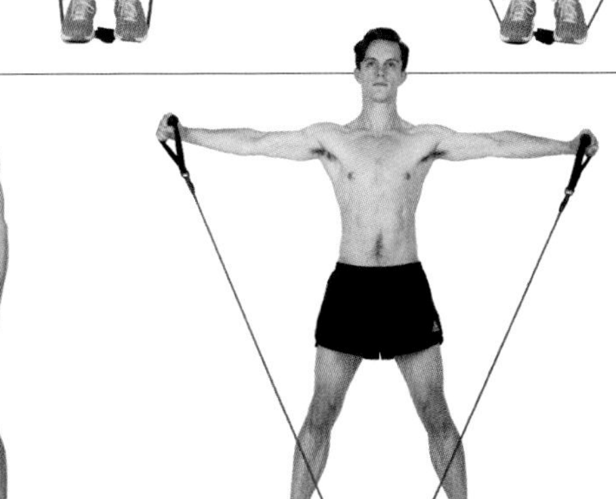

072

Barbell Upright Row

The Barbell Upright Row is another type of Pull-Up. Rowing, primarily, works the back of the upper body, the middle back, and requires lots of abdominal work. Incorporating a barbell, weights, or resistance bands while rowing will help chisel out beautiful trapezius and deltoid muscles, as well as work your forearms.

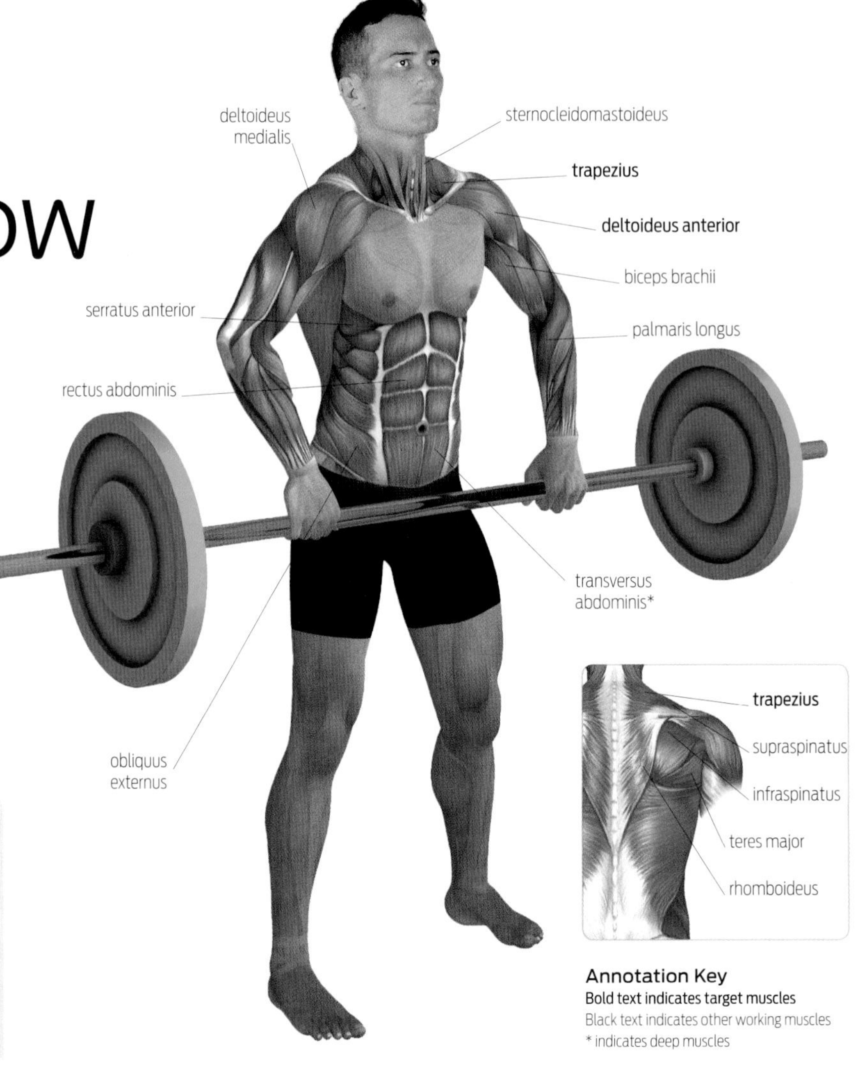

Annotation Key
Bold text indicates target muscles
Black text indicates other working muscles
* indicates deep muscles

Correct form

You will want to engage the shoulders down the back, away from your ears. Imagine that the back of your neck is long and pulling up away from your middle back.

Avoid

Avoid clenching your jaw or squeezing your neck in any way that may put unnecessary tension on your head. This includes lifting the chin too high.

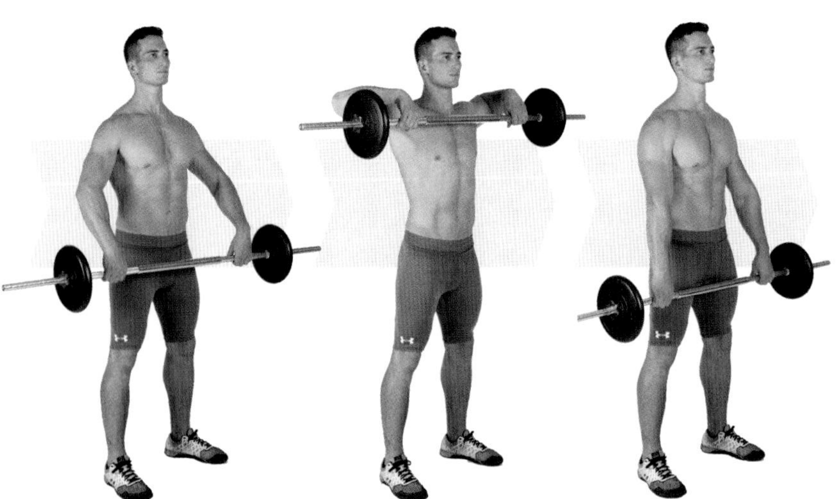

- Stand tall with the chest open, feet shoulder-width apart, and holding the barbell with each hand in a wide grip, palms facing the body.
- Pull the bar up the front of your body, allowing the elbows to open to your sides.
- Once the bar has reached level with your shoulders, lower the bar, and repeat.

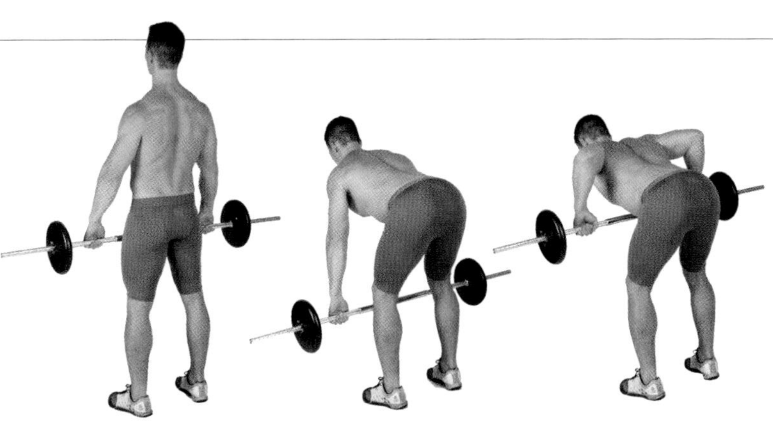

073 Barbell Rows

Holding on tightly to your barbell, hold it straight across the hips. Open the feet wide, take a slight bend in the knees, pitch the torso forward and pull the barbell up into your chest. Make sure your upper body is flat out on the diagonal.

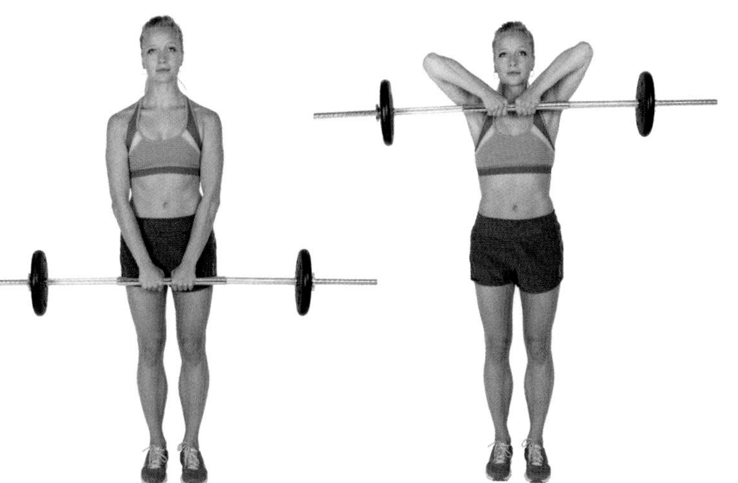

074 Close-Grip Barbell Upright Rows

Firmly gripping the barbell with your hands touching at its center, pull the bar up. Be sure to keep your two hands in line with the center of your body. This grip places more stress on the rotator-cuff muscles. Avoid if you have any shoulder issues.

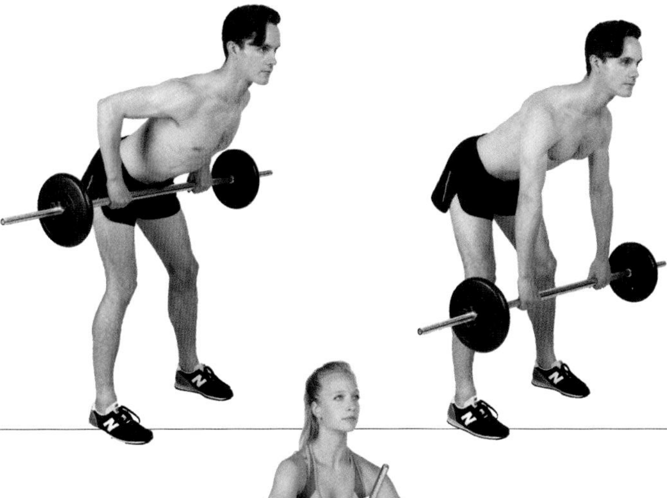

075 Bent-Over Barbell Rows

Holding on tightly to your barbell, open the feet wide. Keeping your legs mostly straight, with a slight bend at the knees, pull the barbell up into your chest. Make sure your upper body is flat out on the diagonal.

076 T-Bar Rows

Stand on either side of a barbell. Open your feet wider than shoulder-width, bend the knees, and reach down to grip the barbell high, just below the top weight. Pull the front of the bar up into your chest.

077 Kettlebell Row

Balance with one leg in front of the other and the body perched over at 90 degrees. Reach down and pick up the kettlebell, with your free hand on your leg. Pull the kettlebell up and into the shoulder, letting the elbow track up high to the back. Switch sides, and repeat.

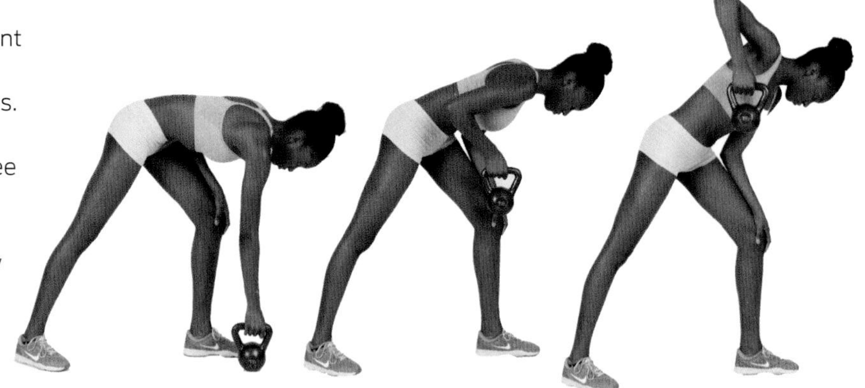

078 Alternating Kettlebell Row

Pull your abdominals in to stabilize your bent-knee stance here. With a kettlebell in each hand, begin your rows, pulling one at a time, up and in toward each shoulder. Allow the chest to open slightly, per side pull.

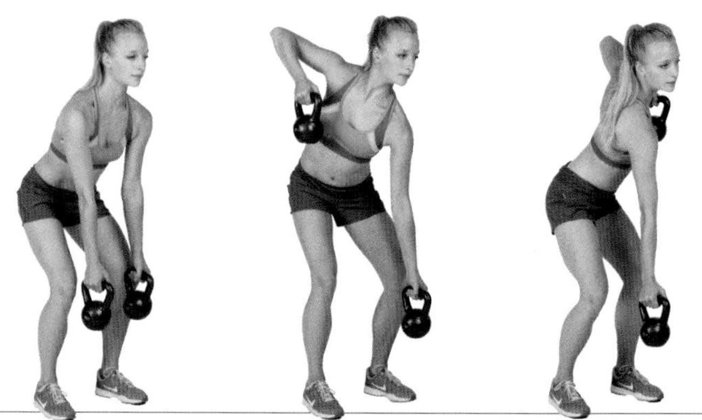

079 Alternating Renegade Row

Holding kettlebells in each hand, get into your best Push-Up position. Make sure your abdominals are pulling strongly up into your back and that your legs are long and strong with the weight on the balls of the feet. With your body parallel to the floor, straighten your arms and pull up your right hand, bringing the kettlebell in line with the side of your body. Bring the kettlebell back down and return to Push-Up position; change sides, and repeat.

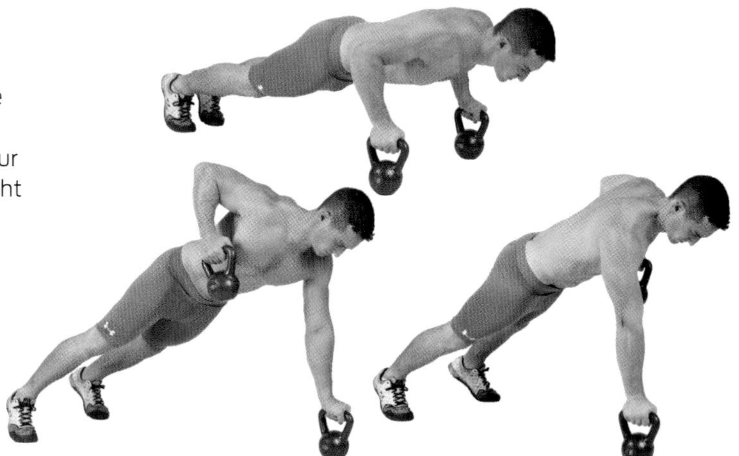

080 Seated Resistance-Band Rows

Sit on the floor with your legs extended out in front of you. Take your resistance band and wrap it around the middle of your feet. Pull the handles of the cable straight up toward your lower ribs. Keep the elbows close to the sides of the body.

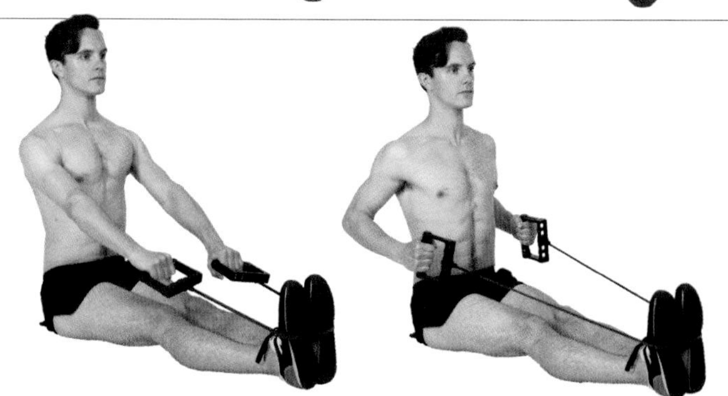

081 Plate Row

The Plate Row focuses on strengthening the back body, specifically, the middle of the back. Utilizing a weighted plate, this Row variation requires that you bend forward at the hips, rowing in a parallel posture. While bent forward you must arch your back slightly so the pressure does not land into the lower-back and tailbone area. This bent forward row position allows you to hyperfocus on engaging the arms, shoulders, and all of the upper back.

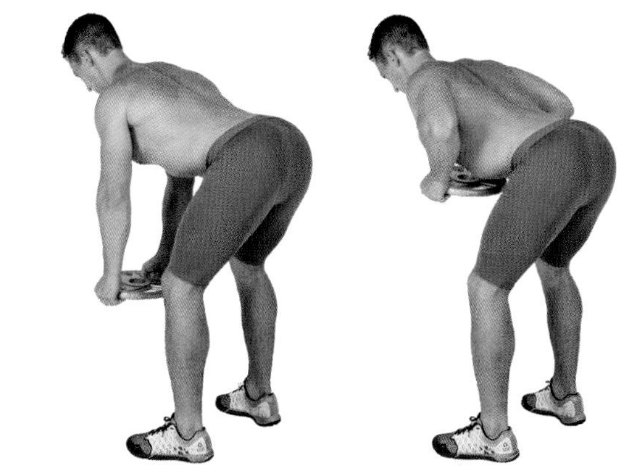

- Bring your feet to shoulder-width apart while holding a weighted plate in front of your chest.
- Bend your knees and hinge forward from the hip, bringing your torso to hover slightly above a 90-degree angle to the floor. Extend the plate down out in front of you.
- Slowly bring the plate back in, keeping the bend in the knees and back out on the diagonal.

082 Incline-Bench Row

Lie with your body extended long against the incline bench. With dumbbells in each hand, loosely hanging on either side of the bench, isolate your upper back and shoulders and pull the weights into your chest on a diagonal.

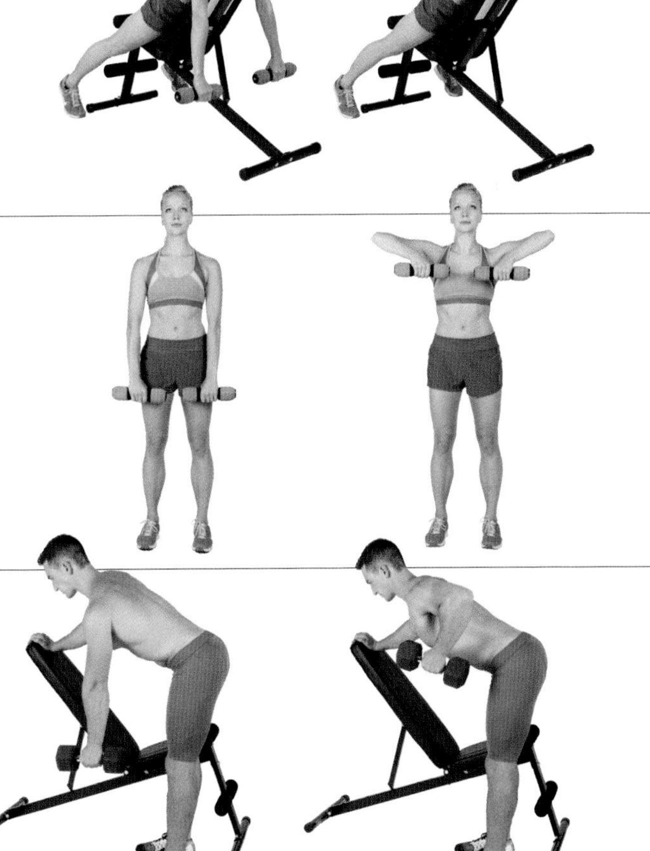

083 Upright Dumbbell Rows

With feet shoulder-width apart, suck your abs up and into the lower back, feeling the middle back long and strong. Holding a dumbbell in each hand, pull them up along the front of the body-tractioning each weight in line with the shoulders. Lower, and repeat.

084 Single-Arm Dumbbell Row

Hold onto the top of an incline bench or a chair with the right hand, holding a dumbbell in the left. Bend the body over so it's just above a 90-degree angle. Using the bench to balance, pull the dumbbell strongly up and in line with your chest.

085 Resistance-Band Rows on Bench

Sit tall on a bench. Secure your resistance band so that it is at chest height. Pull the handles of the resistance straight toward your pecs. Keep the elbows close to the sides of the body.

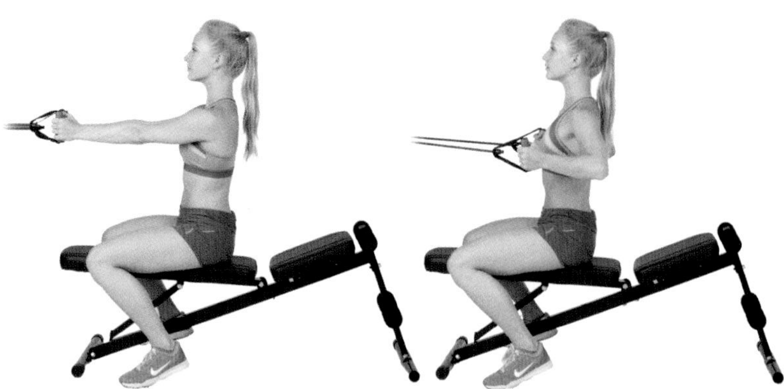

086 Resistance-Band Rows

Stand with the abs fully engaged, the right foot staggered in front of the left. Secure a resistance band under the middle of your right foot. Bend from the elbows and bring your handles up and into the armpits, allowing the upper arms to swing open to the sides.

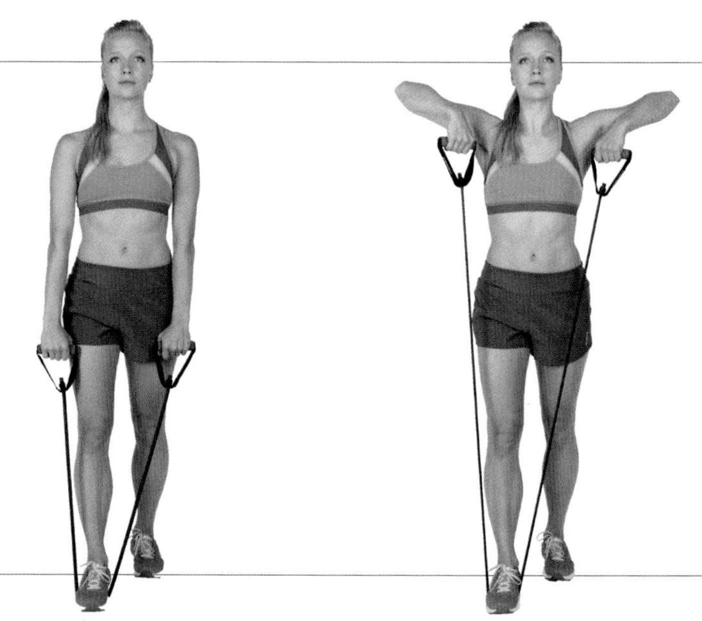

087 Dumbbell Shrug

With a dumbbell in each hand, bring the feet to shoulder-width apart. Squeeze the abs into the lower back and bring your shoulders up to your ears by isolating the trapezius muscles. Lower, and repeat.

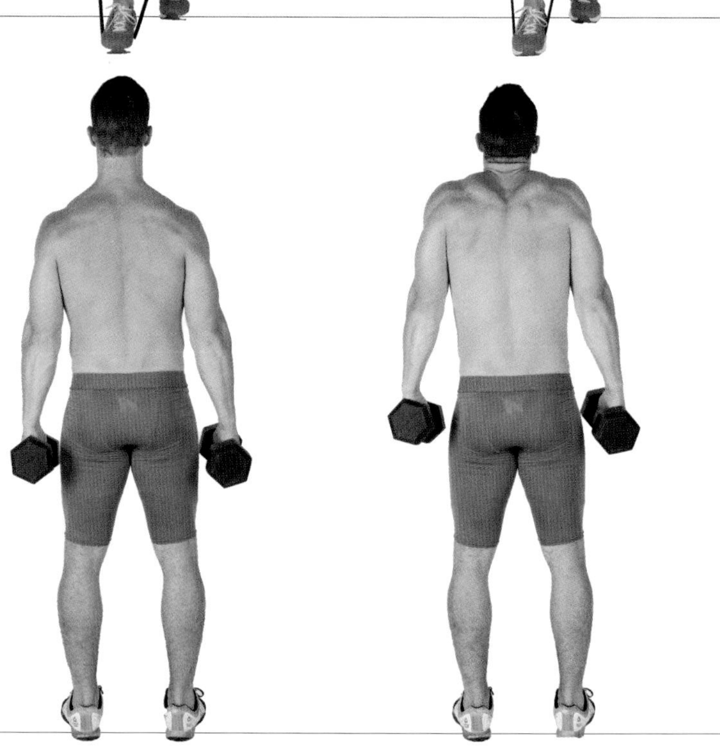

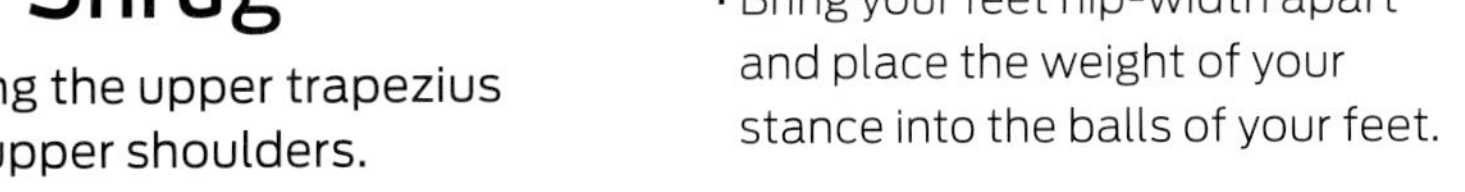

088 Barbell Shoulder Shrug

The Barbell Shoulder Shrug focuses on developing the upper trapezius muscles while also engaging and stabilizing the upper shoulders.

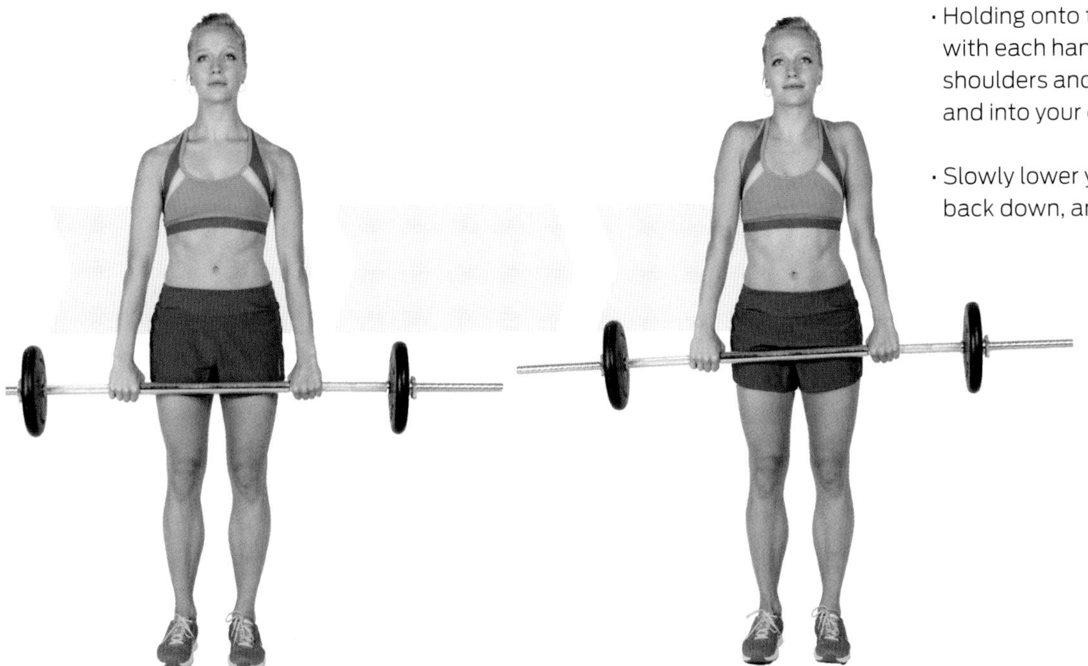

- Bring your feet hip-width apart and place the weight of your stance into the balls of your feet.
- Holding onto the barbell, firmly with each hand, isolate the shoulders and shrug them up and into your ears.
- Slowly lower your shoulders back down, and repeat.

089 Dumbbell Side Push-Out

Stand with a long spine and with your feet shoulder-width apart. Hold the dumbbells at your sides, with your palms facing your body. Squeeze the abs in, engage the upper back, and float the arms out sideways, resisting the weights.

Focus

Be sure to keep targeted areas aligned and engaged the entire time. Try to inhale and exhale freely while performing your workout. Breathing while moving allows the blood to flow organically and the muscles to move with ease.

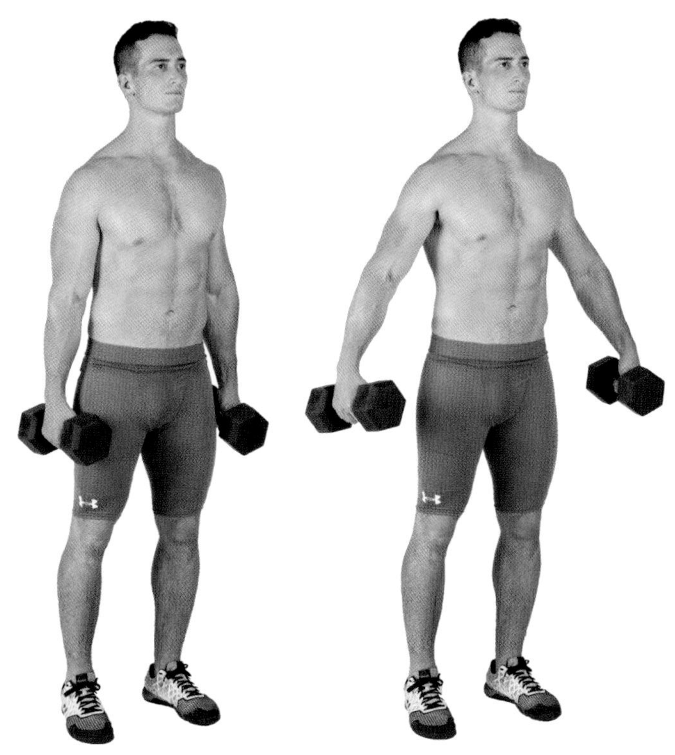

090

Dumbbell Pullover

Isolating the work of the arms while incorporating dumbbells, barbells, or any kind of weight will help define the muscles of the arms and chest. Small movements overhead, also help in stabilizing both large and small muscles throughout the upper body.

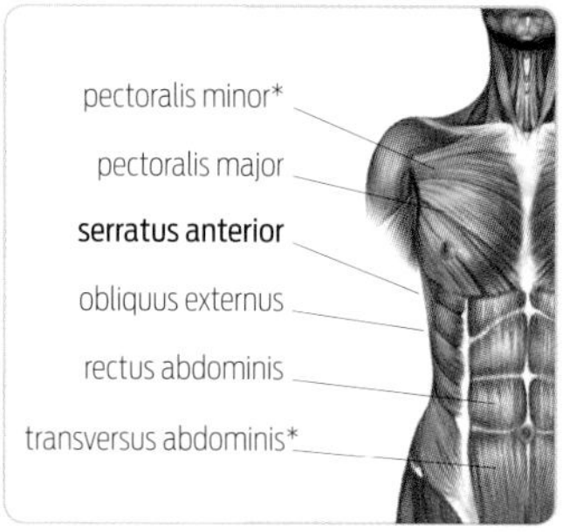

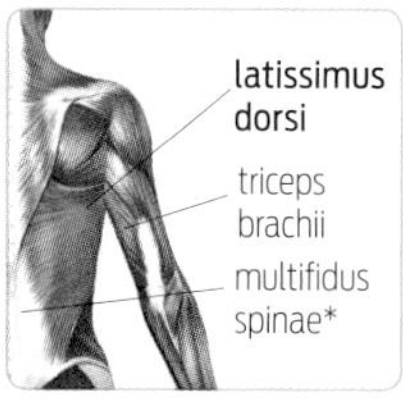

pectoralis minor*
pectoralis major
serratus anterior
obliquus externus
rectus abdominis
transversus abdominis*

latissimus dorsi
triceps brachii
multifidus spinae*

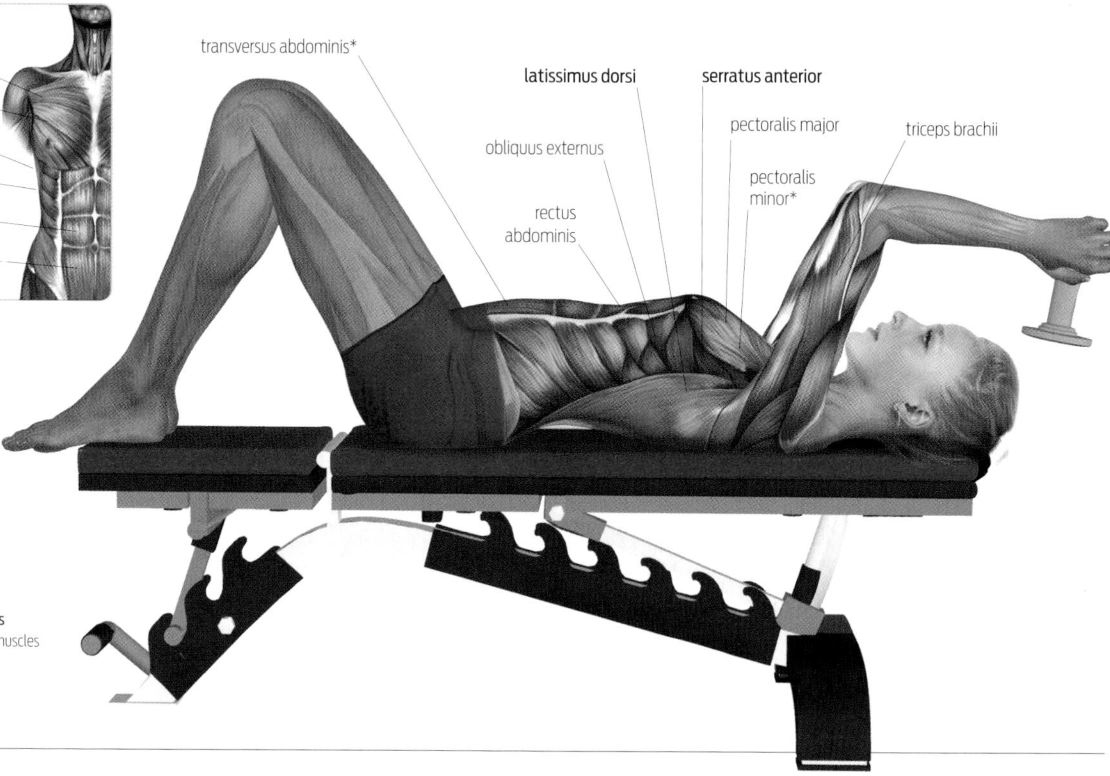

transversus abdominis*
latissimus dorsi
serratus anterior
obliquus externus
pectoralis major
triceps brachii
pectoralis minor*
rectus abdominis

Annotation Key
Bold text indicates target muscles
Black text indicates other working muscles
* indicates deep muscles

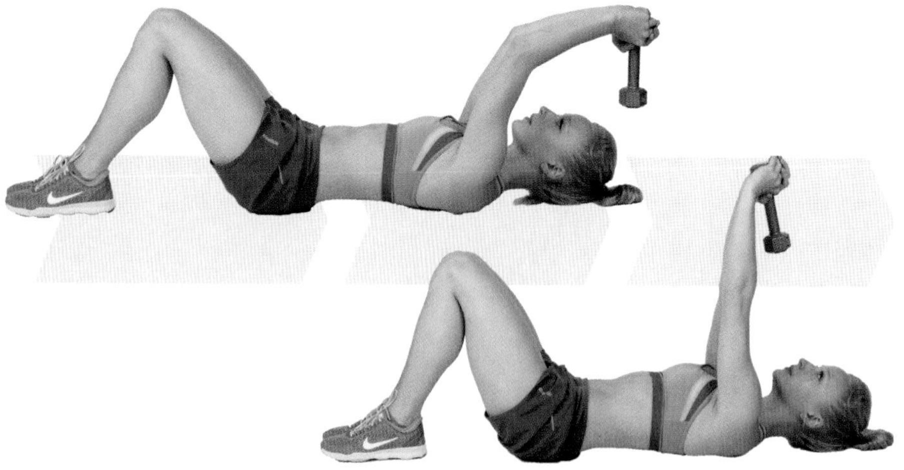

- Lie flat on the floor or a bench with your legs bent together, squeezing the inner thighs in.
- Hold the dumbbell beyond the top of your head with outstretched arms, so that your elbows are above your face. Slowly raise the dumbbell over your head, straightening your arms.

091 Barbell Pullover

This variation of Pull-Over incorporates a heavier barbell overhead. This change will deeply work the pectorals, while also stimulating the shoulder muscles.

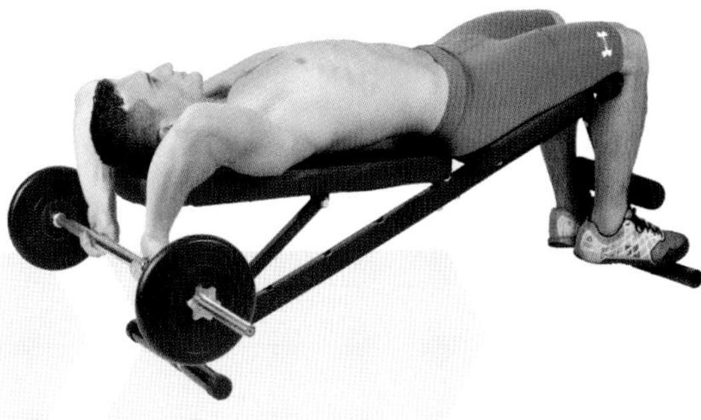

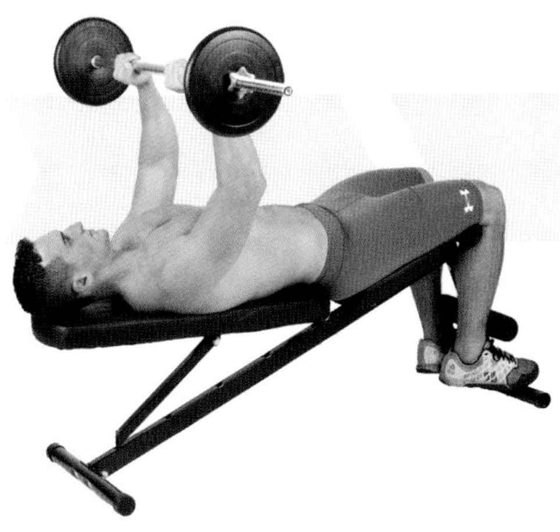

- Lie on a bench with your arms extended above you, holding a barbell, elbows slightly bent.

- Slowly lower the barbell backward in an arc until you feel a stretch in your chest. Bring the barbell back to the starting position, using the same arc.

092 Barbell Pullover with Swiss Ball

Use a Swiss ball in this variation to support your upper back, adding an element of balance while performing your Barbell Pullover. Be sure to keep your hips in line with your knees and back.

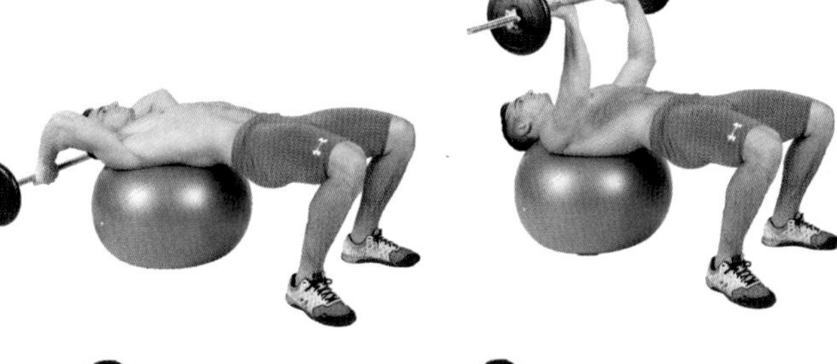

093 Incline-Bench Pull

Lie with your body extended long against the incline bench. Holding onto the barbell with each hand, isolate your upper back and shoulders and pull the bar into your chest on a diagonal.

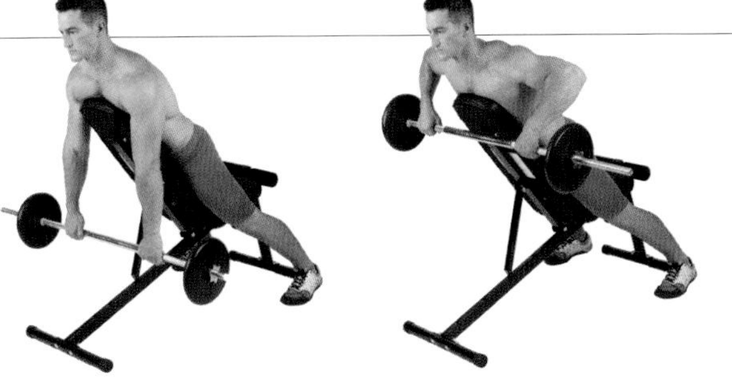

094 Dumbbell Bench Press

Lie back on a bench turned sideways so that only your upper back and head are in contact with the bench. Your feet should be flat on the ground and your knees bent at a 90-degree angle. With your abs and thighs engaged, use both hands to slowly raise and lower a dumbbell above your chest.

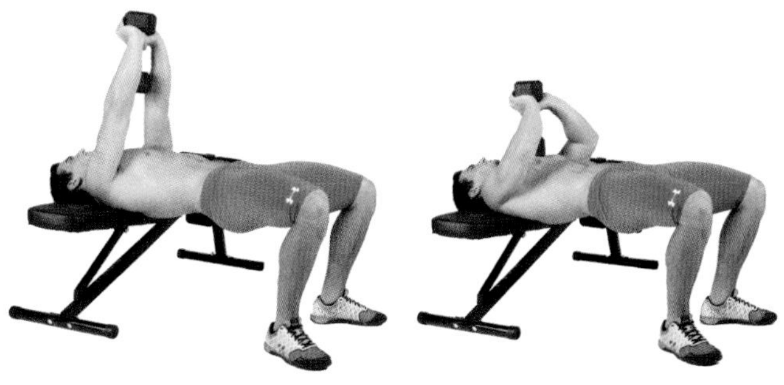

095

Barbell Bench Press

The classic Barbell Bench Press is one of the most effective exercises for building and strengthening the pectoral (chest) muscles on the front of the body. If you are looking to define and chisel out this section, mastering the bench press will do exactly that for you!

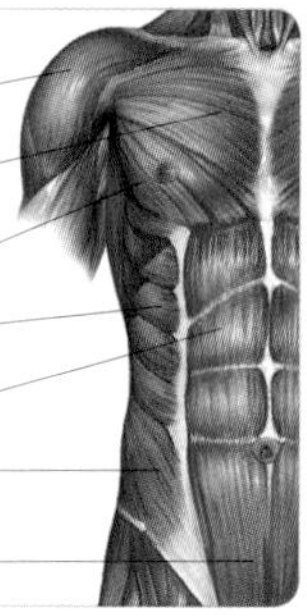

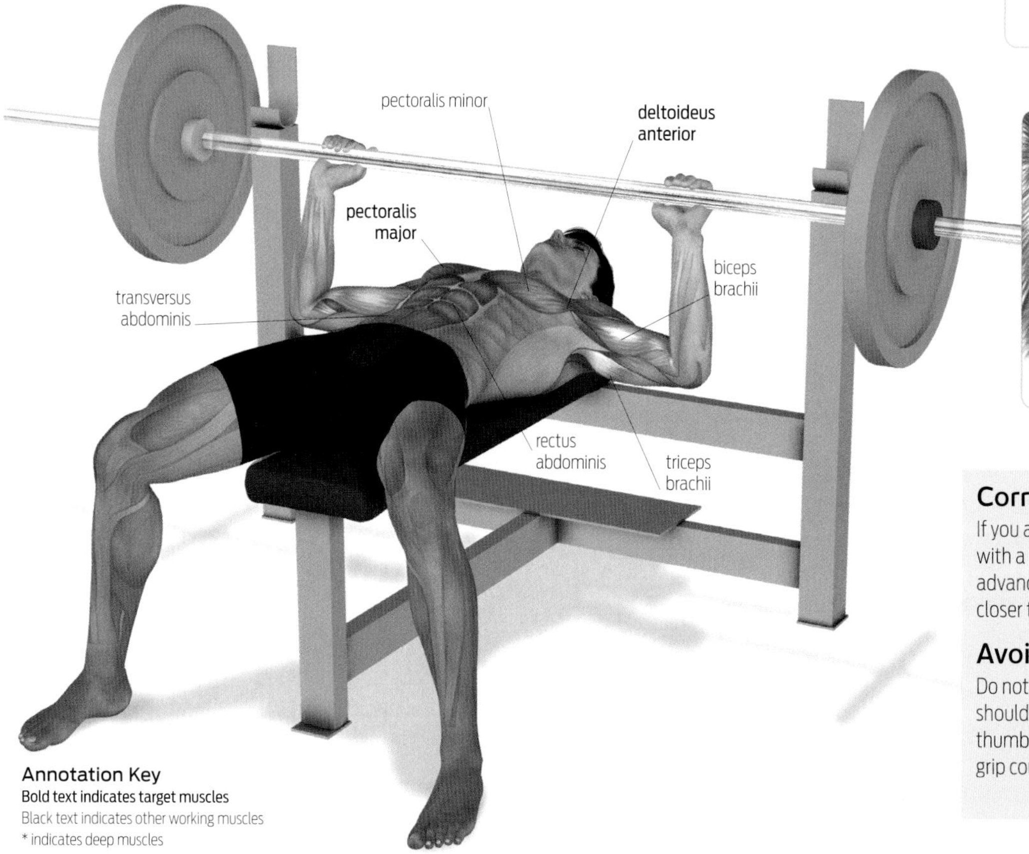

deltoideus anterior
pectoralis minor*
pectoralis major
obliquus externus
rectus abdominis
obliquus internus
transversus abdominis*

pectoralis minor
deltoideus anterior
pectoralis major
biceps brachii
transversus abdominis
rectus abdominis
triceps brachii

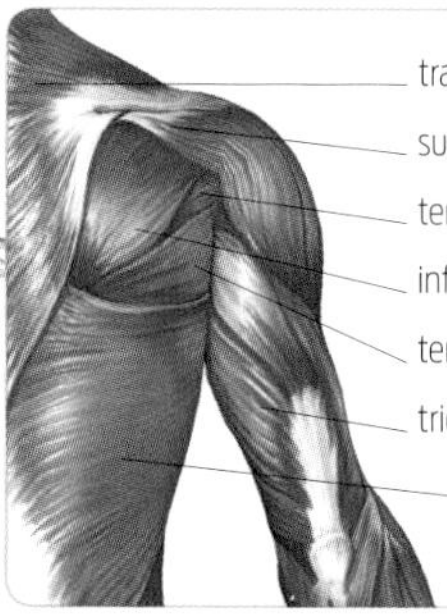

trapezius
supraspinatus
teres minor
infraspinatus*
teres major
triceps brachii
latissimus dorsi

Correct form

If you are a beginner, holding the barbell with a wider grip is best for you. As you advance, you can move your hands in closer together for an added challenge.

Avoid

Do not grip the bar incorrectly. The fingers should be on one side of the bar while the thumb holds onto the other. An incorrect grip could be very dangerous!

Annotation Key
Bold text indicates target muscles
Black text indicates other working muscles
* indicates deep muscles

- Lie on an exercise bench, facing upward.
- Position your hands wide on the barbell. If using a rack, push the barbell up slightly, then bring it forward so it's directly over the center of your chest.
- Slowly lower the barbell to your chest, but do not touch it to your body, then return.

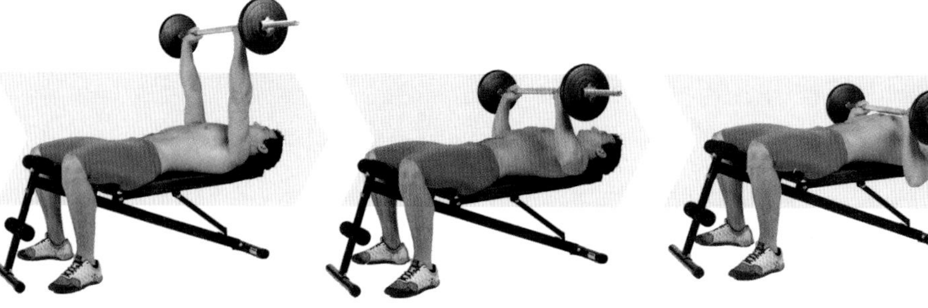

096 Seated Arnold Press

The Seated Arnold Press is a great exercise that focuses the work on the deltoids (shoulders). Because this press shifts through three different planes of movement, it targets all of the parts of the deltoid muscles.

- Sit with the arms extended long at your sides, a dumbbell in each hand.
- Isolate the elbows and pull the dumbbell up into your shoulders. Hold there.
- Next, open your arms so that both are at 90-degree angles.
- Then, push the dumbbells up overhead.

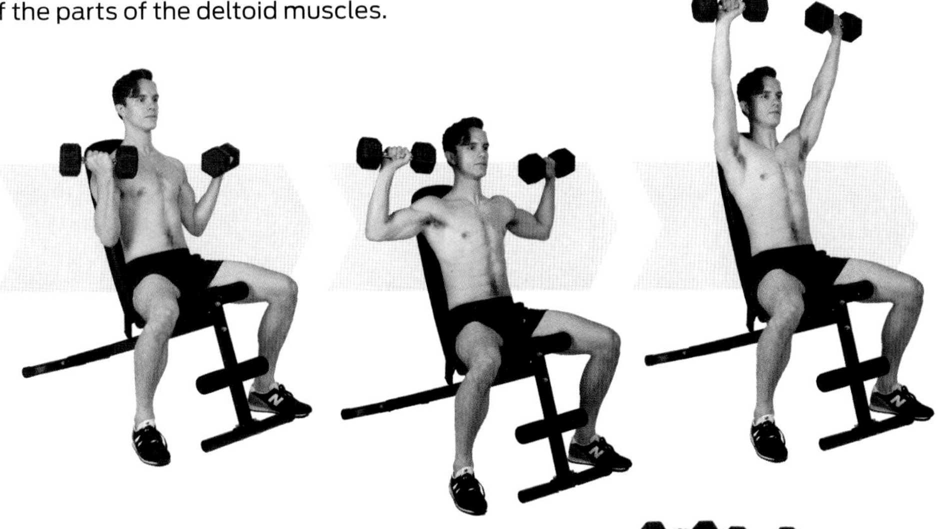

097 Seated Dumbbell Shoulder Press

Sit with the arms extended long at your sides, a dumbbell in each hand, with your palms facing to the front. Bring the arms open to 90-degree angles at your shoulders. Isolate the elbows and push the dumbbells up overhead. Slowly lower back down, and repeat.

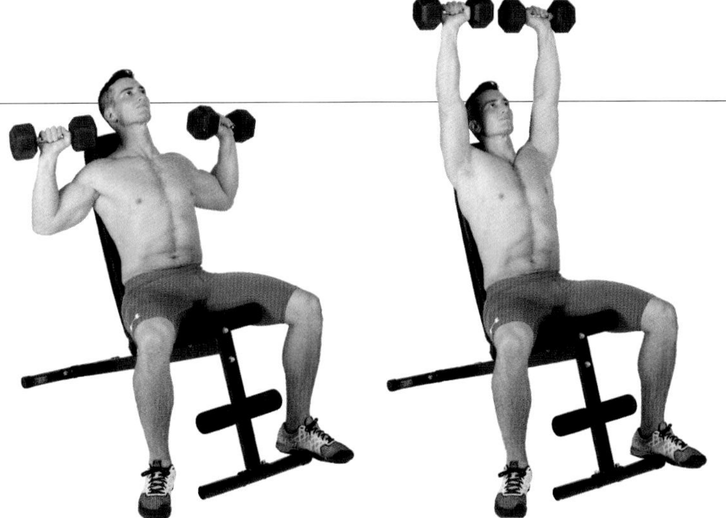

098 Standing Dumbbell Shoulder Press

Stand with the arms extended long at your sides, a dumbbell in each hand, with your palms facing front. Open the arms to 90-degree angles from your shoulders. Isolate the elbows and push the dumbbells up overhead. Slowly, lower back down, and repeat.

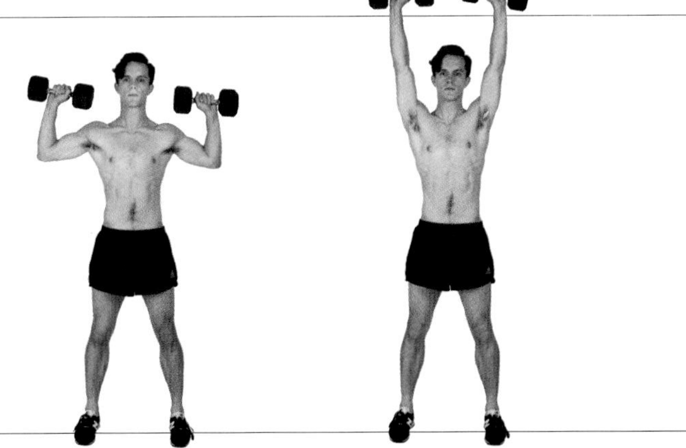

099 Aerobic-Step Bridge with Leg Lift and Chest Press

Lie on your back on the floor with your knees bent, and your feet flat on an aerobic step, while holding a dumbbell in each hand at your sides. Lift your butt up into a high bridge, and slowly raise your right leg to point it straight up; at the same time raise both dumbbells until both arms are pointing straight up—your elbows and right knee should be locked. Lower to start the position and repeat on the other side.

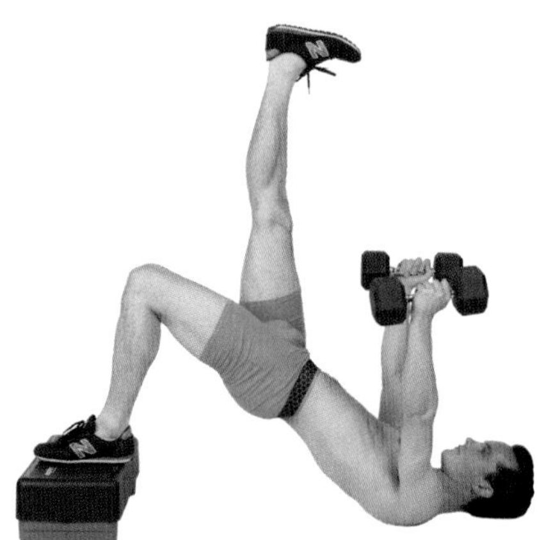

100 Military Press

From standing, engage your deltoids and bring your weights up, directly over the shoulders. Next, stabilize the shoulders and abdominals and press the weights up alongside your ears. Lower, and repeat.

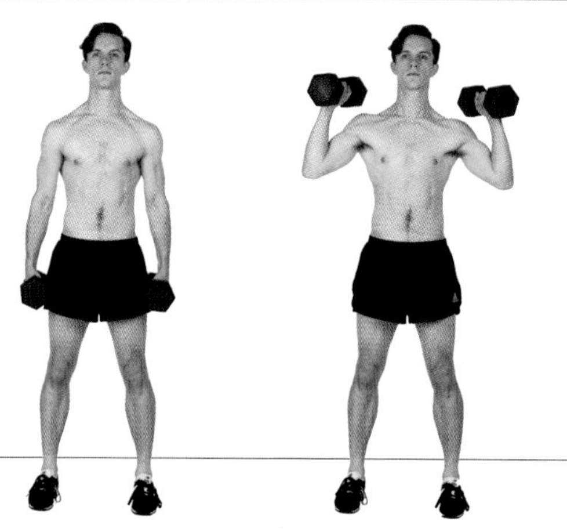

101 Dumbbell Shoulder Press

Start by standing with dumbbells in each hand, the palms facing toward the body. Engage your deltoids and pull the dumbbells up along the body, bringing the hands to the chest. From there, push out directly from the chest with straight arms. Bend the elbows and rotate them open to right angles. Push the weights overhead, bend the elbows, and lower back down.

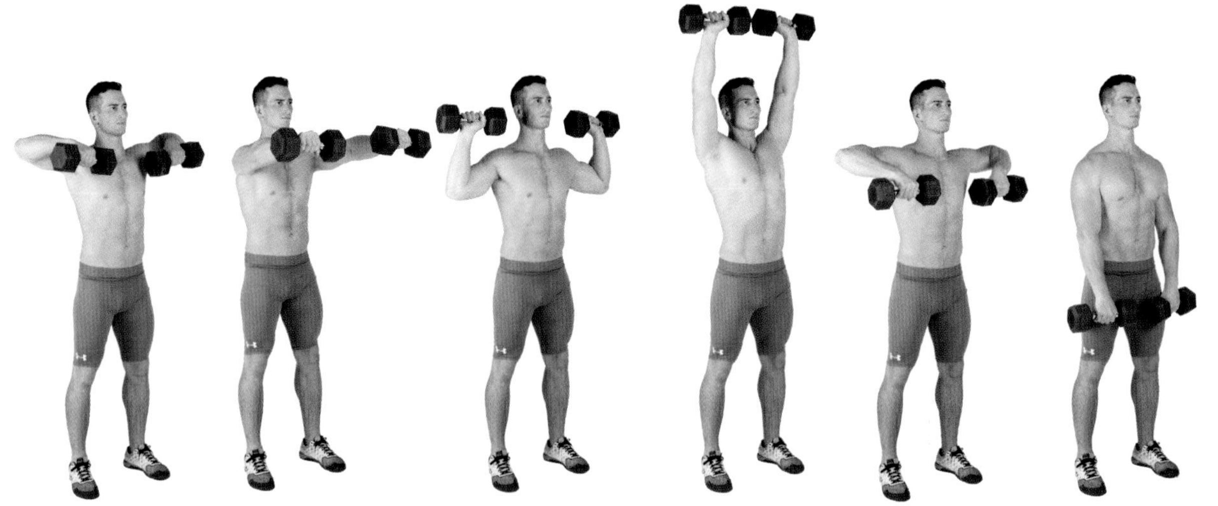

102 Overhead Band Press

Stand with the abs fully engaged, with the right foot staggered in front of the left. Secure a band under the middle of your right foot. Bend from the elbows and pull the band up and into 90-degree angles from the armpits. Next, extend directly up overhead along the sides of your body.

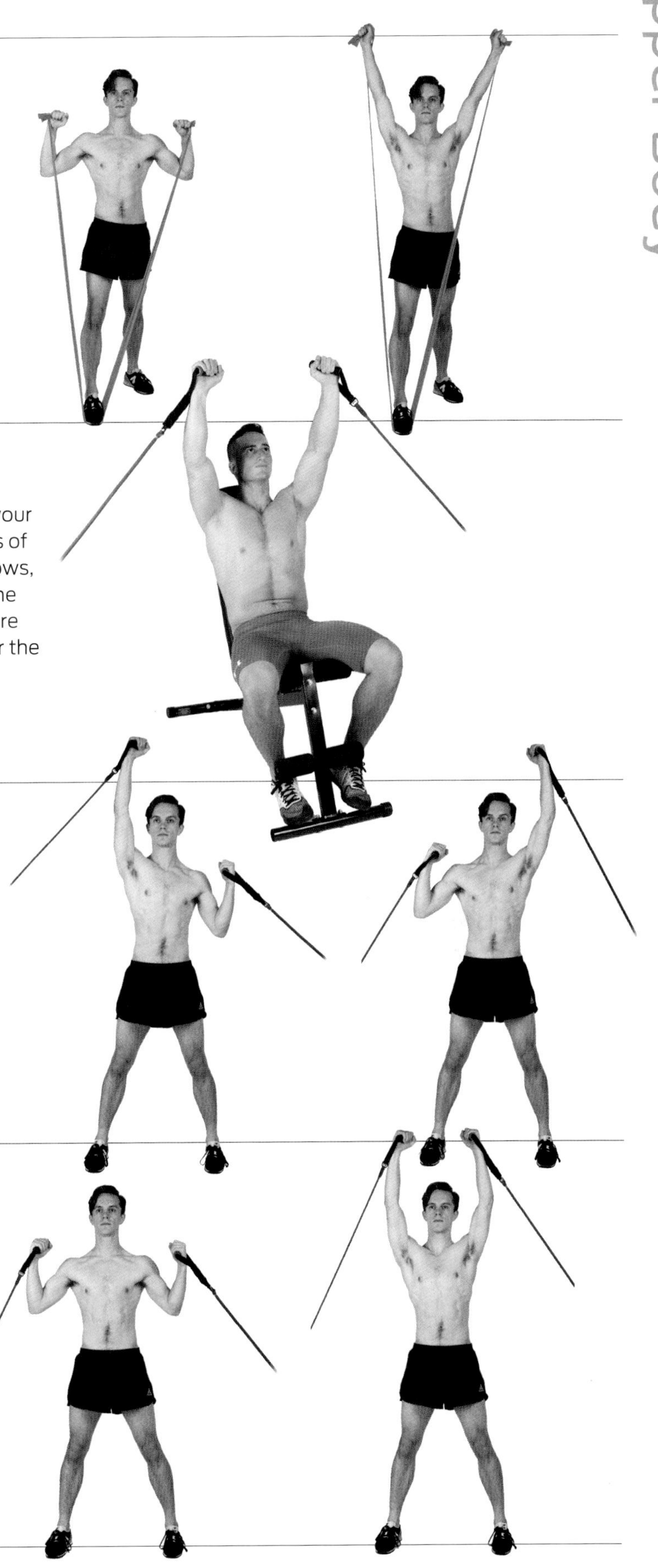

103 Overhead Cable Press

Sitting up in a supported chair, secure your cable handles in each hand at the sides of the body. With a slight bend of the elbows, engage the shoulders, and pull up on the cable. The motion should be as if you are trying to bring your hands together over the top of your head.

104 Alternating Cable Shoulder Press

Stand with the back engaged and the feet wider than shoulder-width apart. Bring both elbows to right angles, and pull up on one cable with a straight arm while leaving the other bent. Alternate each arm from bent to straight.

105 Pyramid Cable Press

Secure your cable handles in each hand at the sides of the body. With a slight bend of the elbows, engage the shoulders, and pull up on the cable ends. The motion should be as if you are trying to bring your hands together over the top of your head to form a pyramid shape.

106 Hammer Grip Press

Executing the Hammer Grip Press is another of the best presses for building and expanding the pectoral muscles on the front of the body. Unlike the Barbell Bench Press, the Hammer Grip Press allows you to hold separate weights in each hand. This gives you a wider range of motion and mobility.

- Start by sitting with your back up, a dumbbell in each hand.
- Slowly, lower yourself down to lie along the incline bench. Pin the elbows in toward your sides and hold the weights at your shoulders.
- With straight arms, press the dumbbells directly up over your chest, and bring your hands to meet in the middle over your chest.

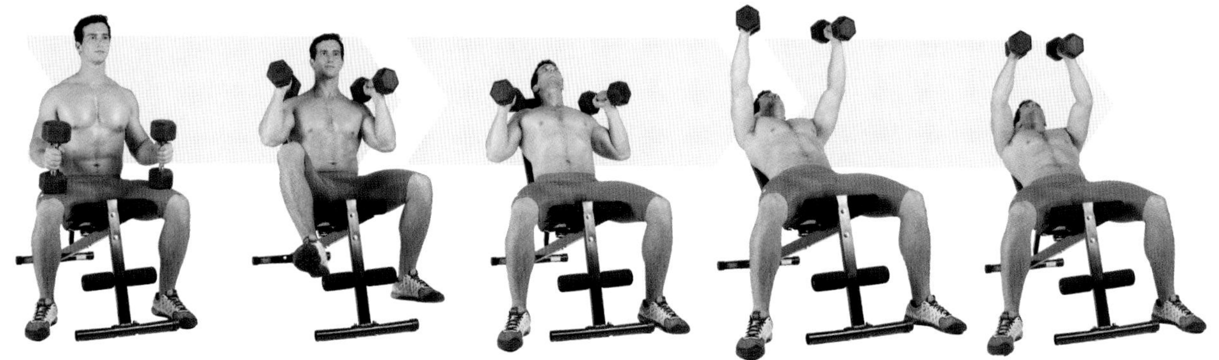

107 Reverse-Grip Incline Bench Press

Change your grip from the previous Hammer Grip Press workout and perform your press. This reverse grip will focus on developing the top of the pectoral muscles.

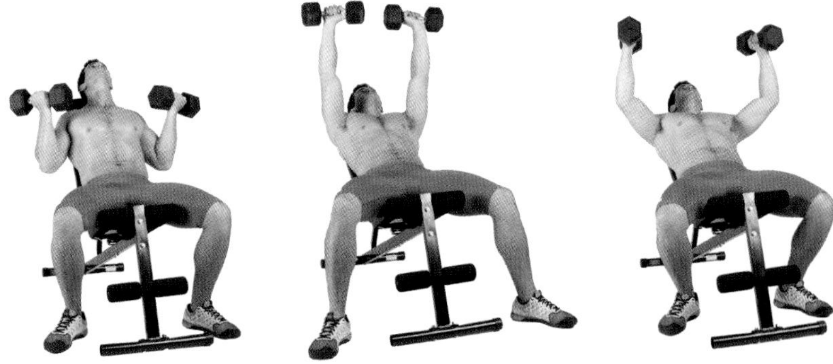

108 Swiss Ball Flat Dumbbell Press

Using the Swiss ball to support your upper back, take a dumbbell in each hand, and press up over the chest. Be sure to keep your hips in line with your knees and back.

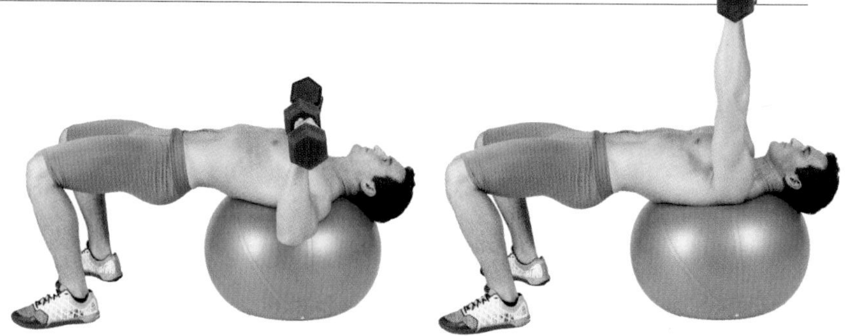

109 Decline Barbell Press

Lie on an exercise bench set to a decline position. Secure your feet around the base of the bench. Position your hands wide on the barbell. If using a rack, push the barbell up slightly, then bring it forward so it's directly over the center of your chest. Slowly lower the barbell to your chest, then return.

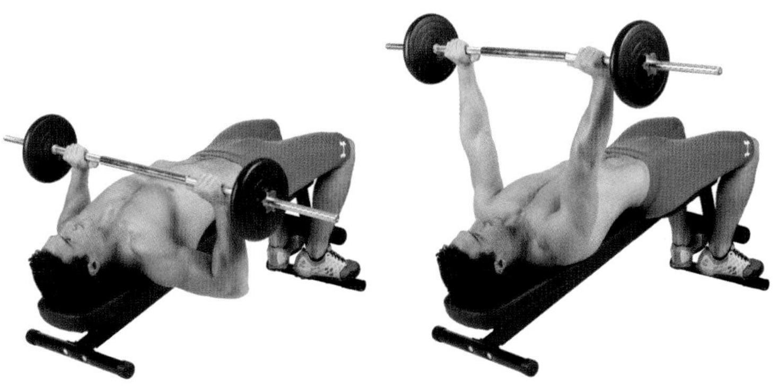

110 Skull Crushers

This exercise is not intended to crush the skull at all but, rather, to crush your arms! More specifically, executing this move will increase the overall strength and definition of your triceps. By giving the elbows a wide range of flexion and extension, you will have your triceps activated through and through. Begin by sitting with the barbell on your legs. Lie back and bring the barbell to your chest. Extend the bar straight up over your chest and then lower it toward your forehead. Re-extend your straight arms back over the chest. Repeat.

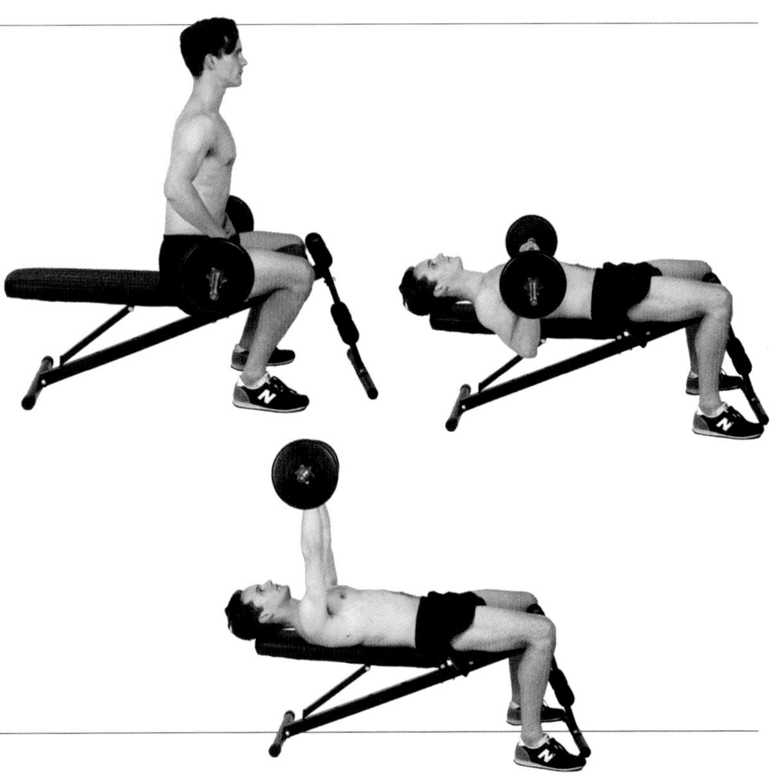

111 Band Skull Crushers

With a band secured to each end of your bench, grip the band with each hand. Push out and up on the band, away from your chest, until the arms straighten.

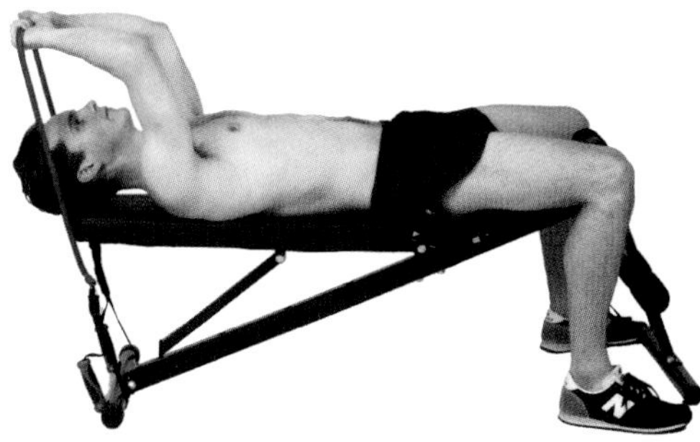

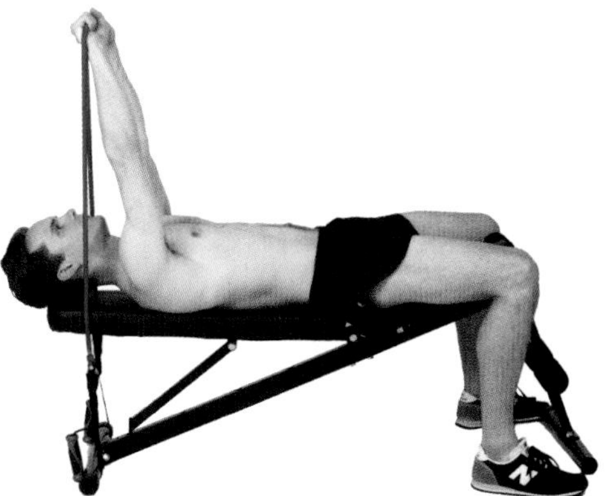

112

Cable Fly

The Cable Fly is another great exercise that employs the use of resistance bands or cables to strengthen the pectoral muscle group. Working the muscles, both deeply and superficially, performing any version of Fly engages the chest and core via the basic elements of pulling and pushing.

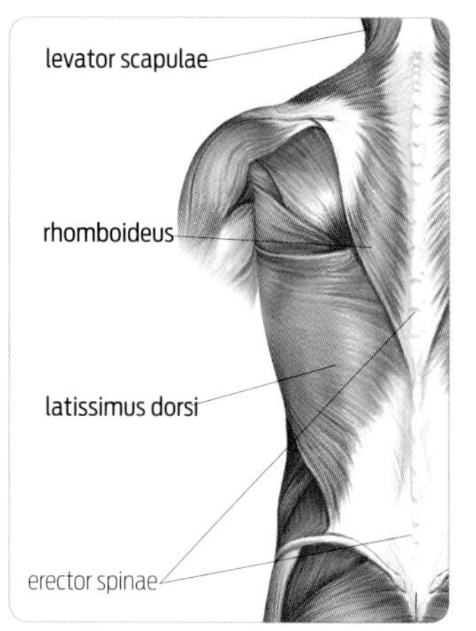

Correct form

Be sure to keep the elbows slightly bent the entire time you are pulling on the cables.

Avoid

Do not move quickly with the Cable Fly movement. Moving slowly will ensure that you are working correctly and with steady resistance.

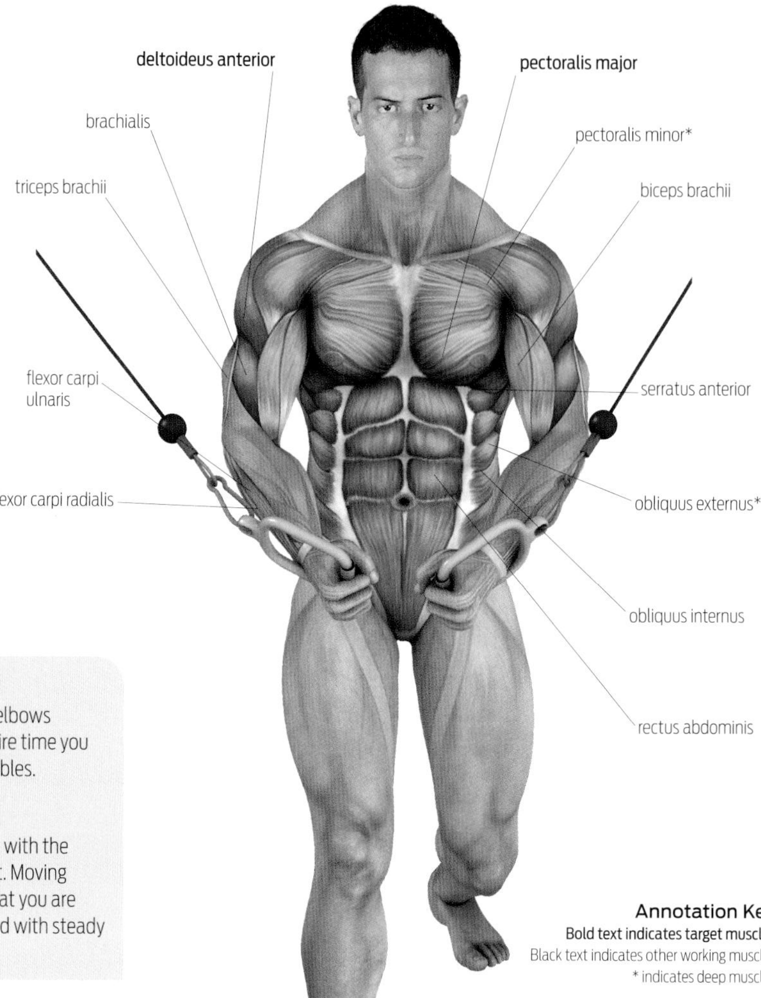

Annotation Key
Bold text indicates target muscles
Black text indicates other working muscles
* indicates deep muscles

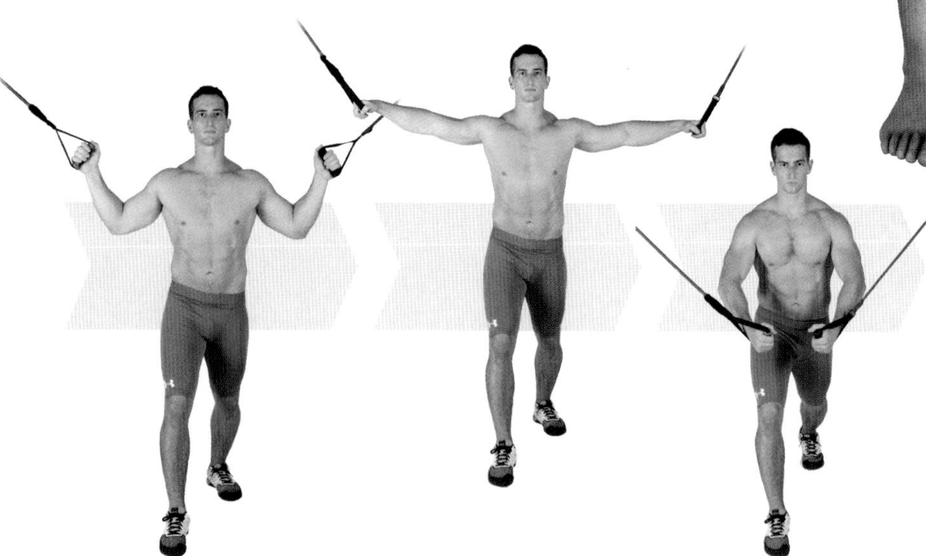

- With the right foot staggered in front of the left foot, securely hold the cable handles in each hand. Start with the arms open wide to the sides.
- Bend the right knee and use the weight of your body to move you forward in space.
- Pull down on the handles, bringing both hands together in front of the pelvis.
- With control, open the arms back out.

113 Reverse Fly

When performing the Reverse Fly, you are pinpointing the work along the back of the shoulders. Doing this creates strength in the deltoids and trapezius, mainly. In theory, you are actually just reversing the movement of the traditional Fly.

- Stand against a supported incline bench with dumbbells hanging at your sides.
- Press your abs into the lower back and engage your upper back. Open the dumbbells out to each side, keeping a slight bend in the elbows.
- Hold the arms open for a moment, then lower back down.

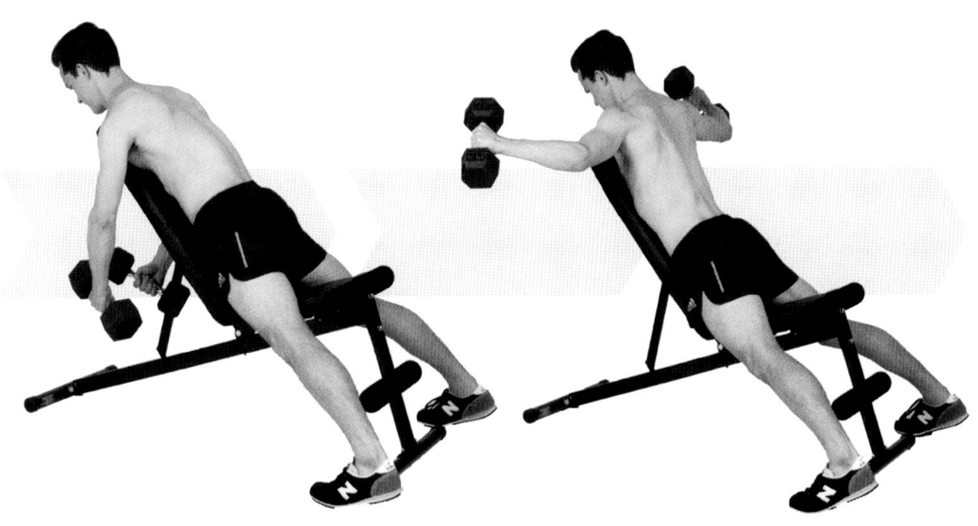

114 Swiss Ball Reverse Fly

Lie with a Swiss ball under your upper torso. Extend your legs long and balance on the balls of your feet. Squeeze your abs deeply to help you balance and open your arms to the sides, with dumbbells in your hands. Hold open, then lower.

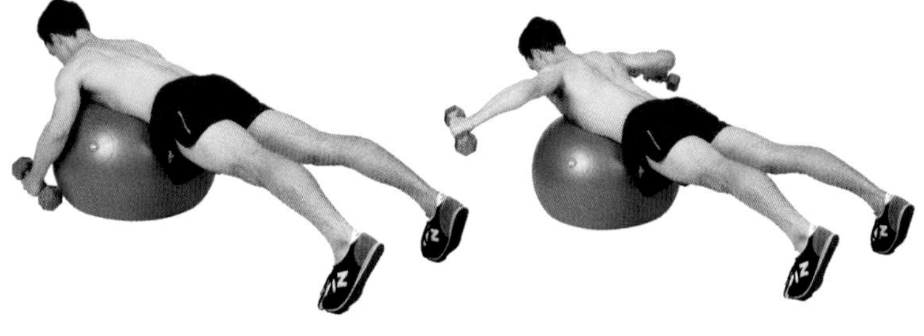

115 Alternating Resistance-Band Crossover

Stand with your band secured behind you, holding the handles firmly in each hand. With your feet wider than shoulder-width, take turns alternating pulling the cable across your body. Control the cable by resisting with the core and chest.

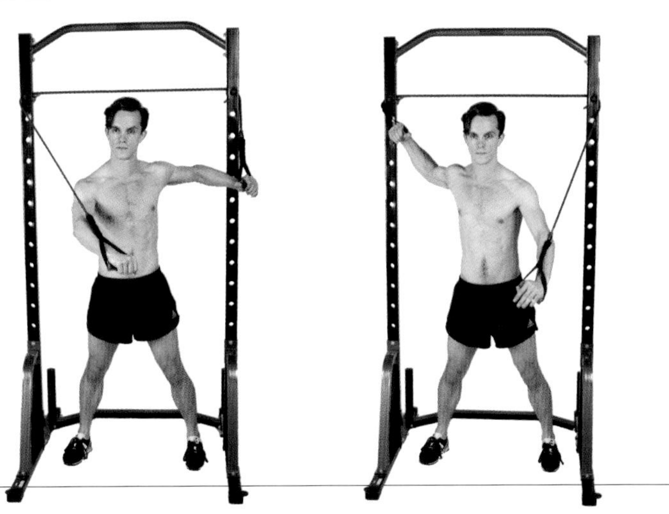

116 Resistance-Band Decline Raise

Working with a surface, cable, or machine on the decline means that you will be enhancing your exercise by including the element of gravity. Pulling or pushing down or up against an added amount of gravity creates more strength, balance, and stability in the muscle.

- Stand with your cable secured below your midsection, behind you.
- Hold the handles of your cable wide, with an open chest.
- Pull up on the cable, raising the handles up and into your center.
- With control, lower back down.

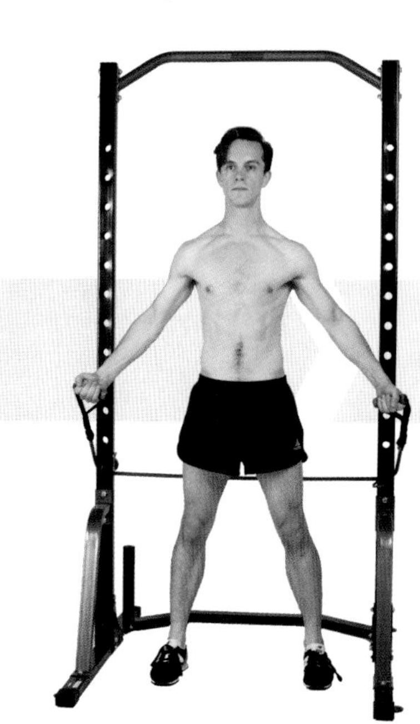

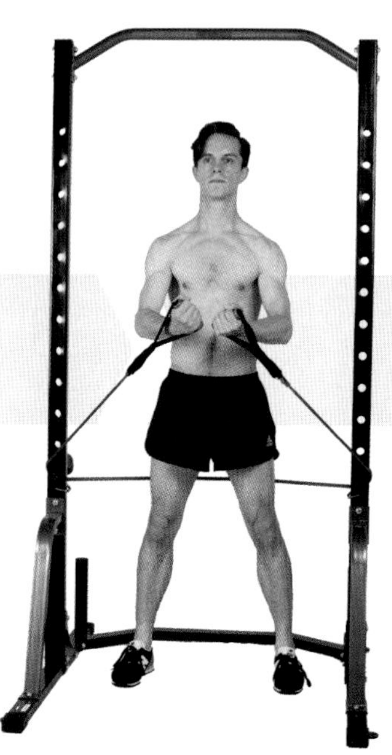

117 Resistance-Band Crossover Fly

Lie on an incline bench positioned in a lifting rack. Your cable should be looped behind the incline pad and around the uprights of the lifting rack. Keeping the elbows bent slightly, grasp the handles and pull up on them, reaching the hands together over the center of the chest.

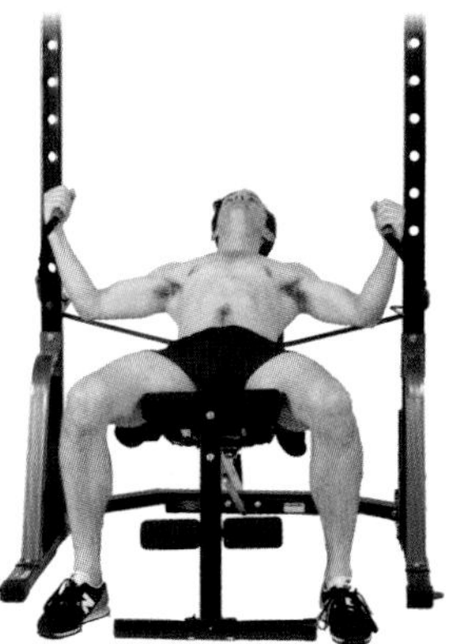

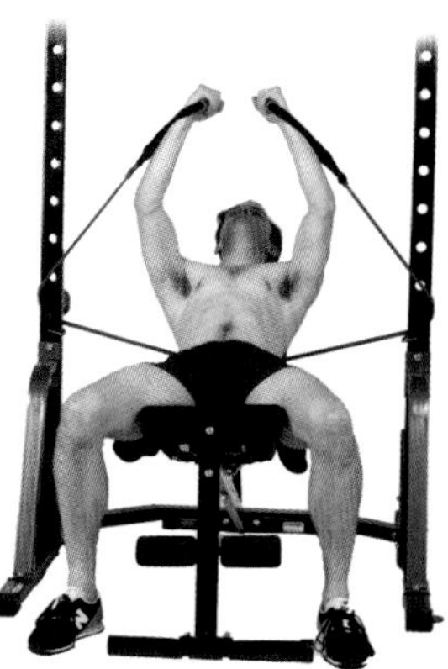

118 Resistance-Band Decline Fly

Stand with your cable secured above your head, behind you. Hold the handles of the cable wide, with an open chest. Pull down on the cable, bringing the handles into your center, in front of your hips. With control, lower back down.

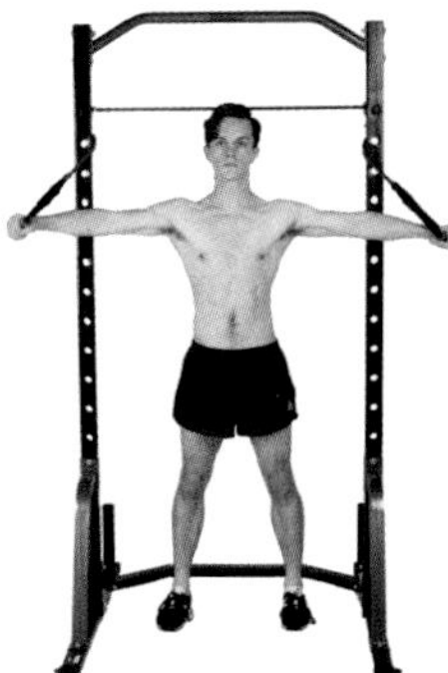

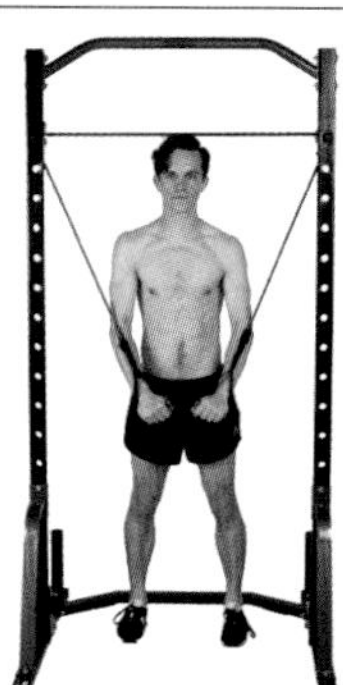

119 Dumbbell Fly

The Dumbbell Fly also employs the use of weights to strengthen the pectoral muscle group. Incorporating a change in level, by lying down, this version of Fly increases the amount of gravitational pull on the weights, increasing the work in the chest and core via the basic elements of pulling and pushing.

- Begin by sitting with the dumbbells on your legs.
- Lie back, bend your elbows, and bring the weights to the sides of your chest.
- Extend the arms straight up over your chest.
- Open your arms out to the sides. Close the arms, and repeat.

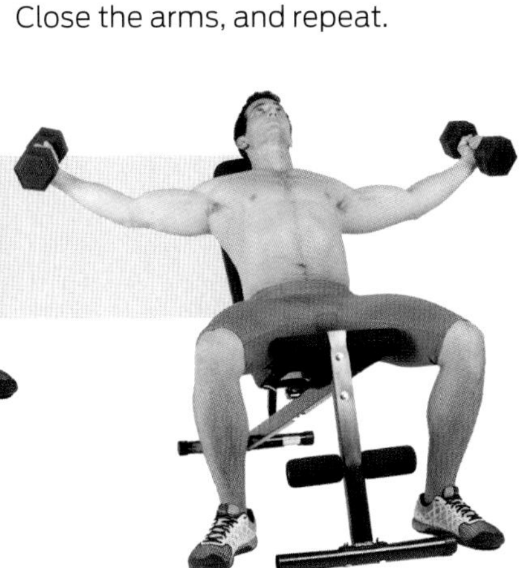

120 Decline Fly with Dumbbells

Lie with your bench on the decline. Keeping the elbows bent slightly, grasp the handles of your dumbbells and pull up on them, reaching the hands together over the center of the chest. Open slowly, and repeat.

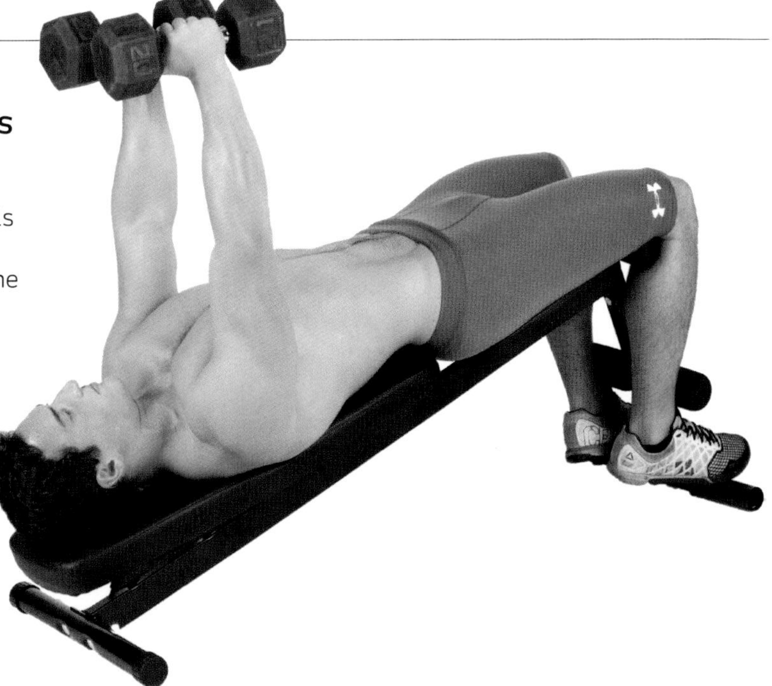

121

Rope Crunch

When you execute the Rope Crunch, whether with a machine or with cables, you are working your abdominal wall.

Annotation Key
Bold text indicates target muscles
Black text indicates other working muscles
* indicates deep muscles

Correct form

Make sure to pull strongly on the rope as you bend forward from the hips. The pull should initiate the whole movement.

Avoid

Avoid sitting the hips too far back. You do not want to feel like you are sitting on your heels at all.

- Begin by kneeling with the knees and feet together.
- Grasp the rope handles, bend at the hips, pull in your abs, and pull down on the handles. Each end of the rope handles should frame either side of your head.
- With resistance, uncurl the spine and raise your body upright to kneel again.

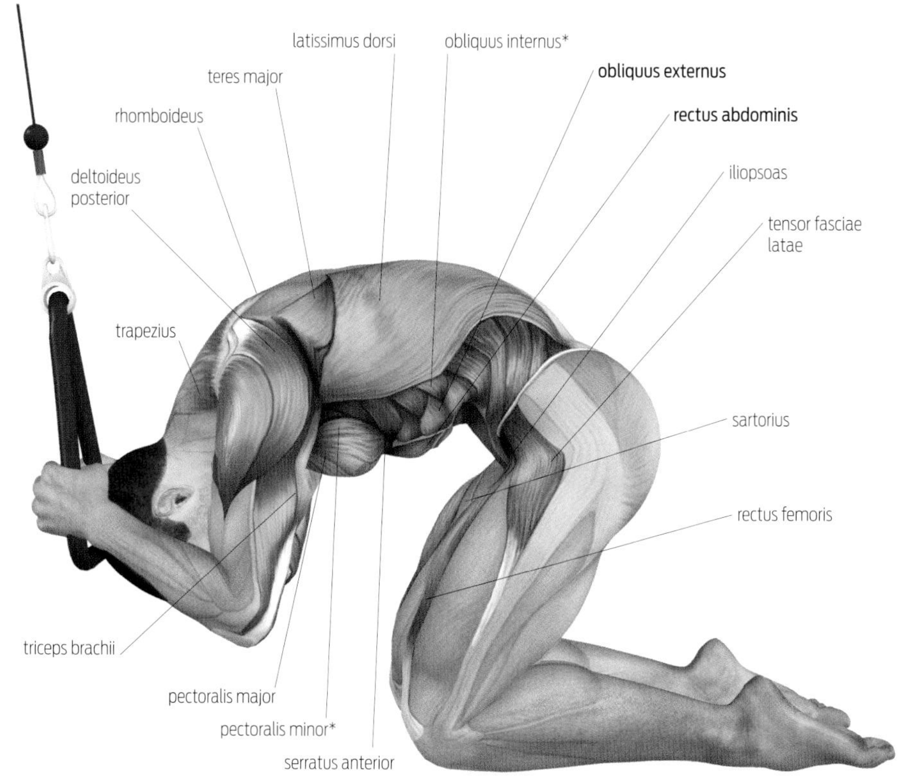

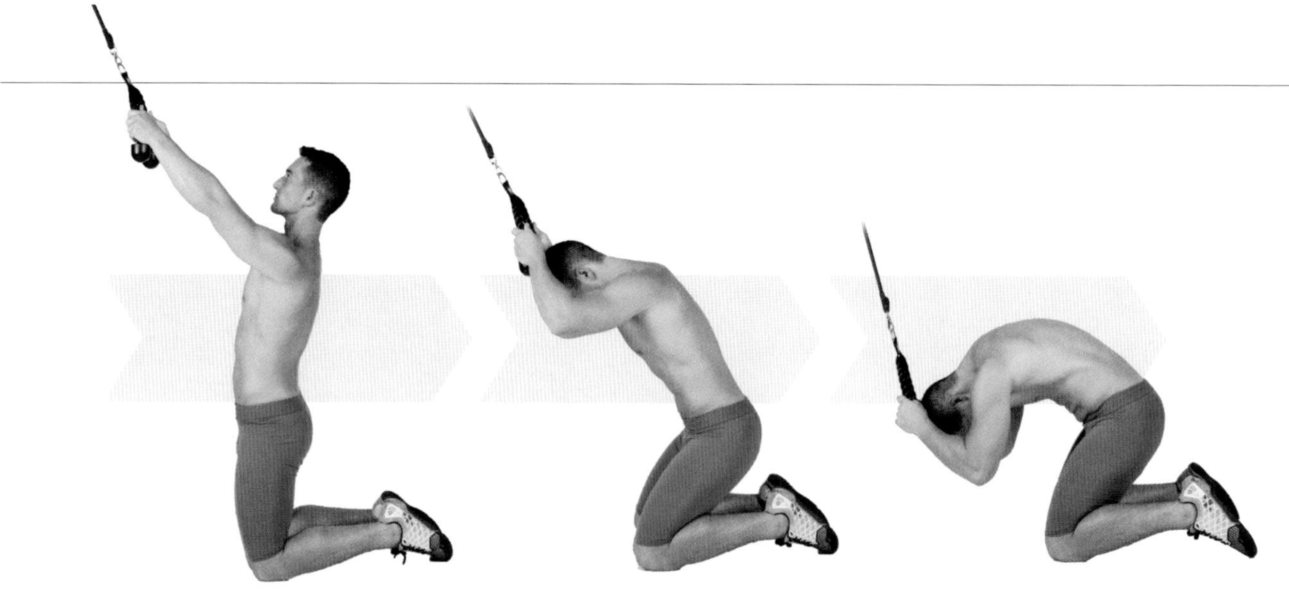

122 Double Resistance-Band Lean-Over

This movement will give you a dual workout for both the side abdominal muscles and the arms. Any exercise that incorporates the use of resistance cables or bands allows you to strengthen while working with your own body weight.

- Take a wide, open stance in the legs with a band secured under the center of each foot.
- Holding the handles of the band in your hands, pull open the cable wide at your sides.
- Keeping your arms where they are, bend from the waist, to the right, then to the left.

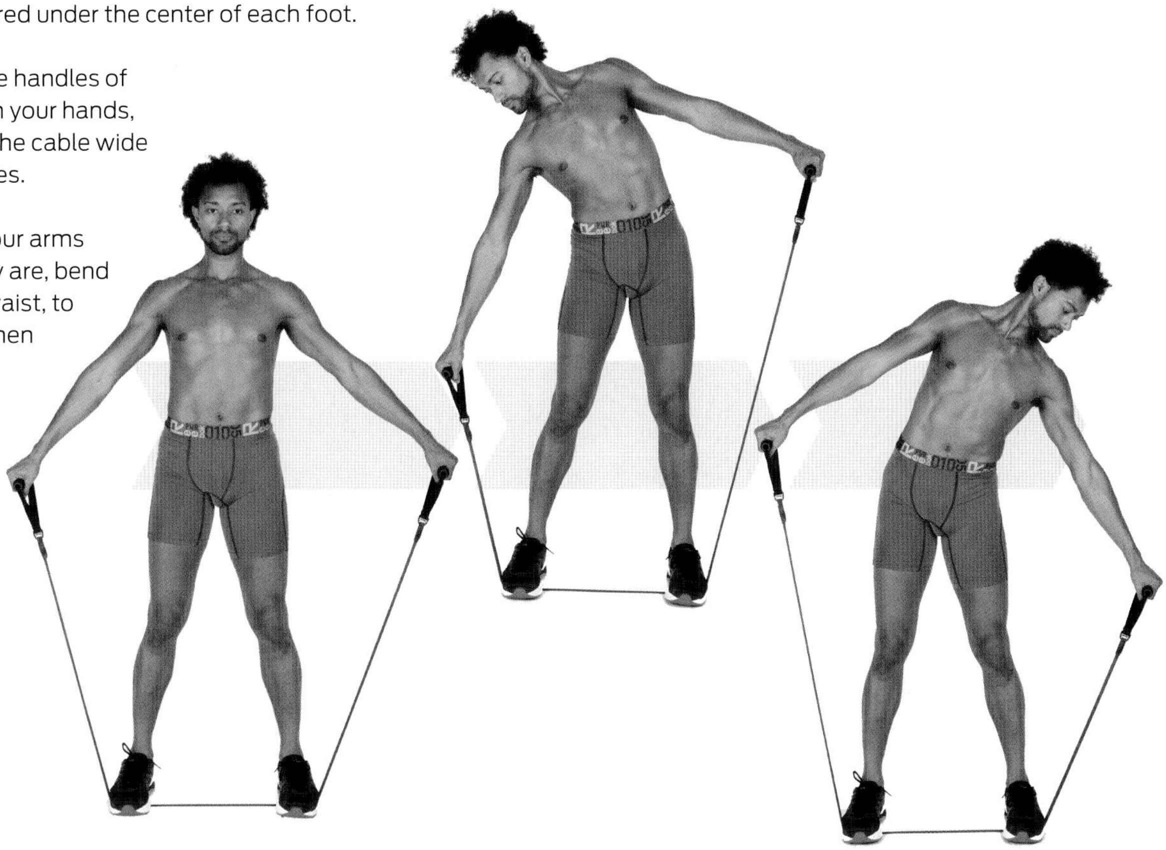

123 Lat Pulldown with Resistance Bands

Start by standing, holding onto each end of a resistance band, with crossed arms in front of the body. Firmly, take the arms from being crossed to being open, pulling down on the bands, framing the chest.

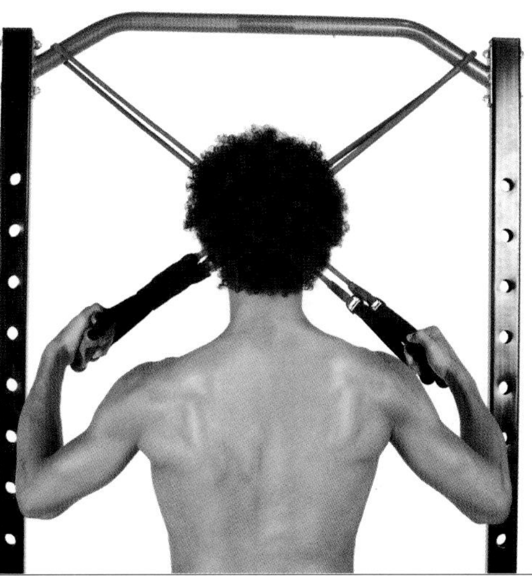

124

Cable Wood Chop

Simulating chopping wood (but without the wood or the axe), this exercise will challenge your core as well as ask you to engage the back-of-the-arm muscle groups. Utilizing the cable as your prop, you will enhance the upper body's side-to-side rotation, bringing the cable back and forth across the body.

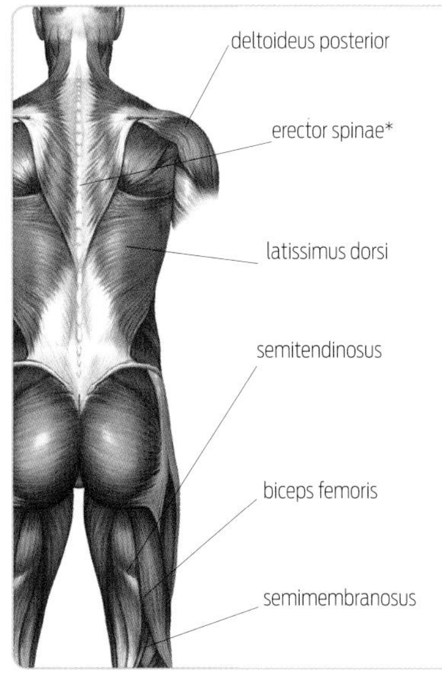

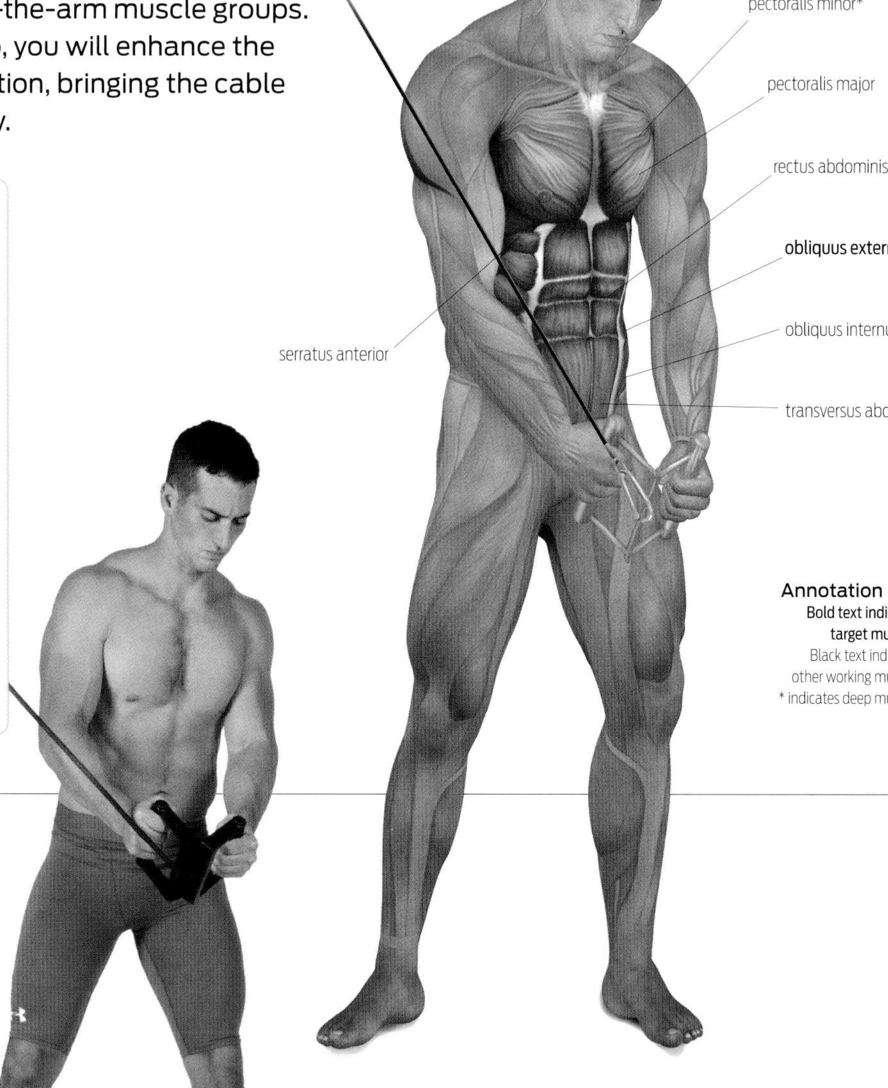

Annotation Key
Bold text indicates target muscles
Black text indicates other working muscles
* indicates deep muscles

- Holding the cable handle with each hand, stand with the legs straight.
- With the cable off to your right, allow the arms to reach up into the cable resistance.
- Firmly, engage the abdominals, and pull the cable down across the body to the left hip.

Correct form

Keep both feet flat on the floor and the shoulders over the hips, facing frontward. The rotational movement of the cable should not disrupt the facing of your body.

Avoid

Do not pull the cable too far across the body. You only need to rotate enough to bring the cable right outside of the opposite hip.

125 Power Cross Chop

Being able to twist from side to side with this Power Cross Chop while keeping the lower extremities still and solid is indeed a great challenge, but will certainly reap huge benefits! Correct execution of this move will not only create deep stabilization of the hips and pelvis, it will also fire up and stimulate all of your back and core muscle groups, inside and out.

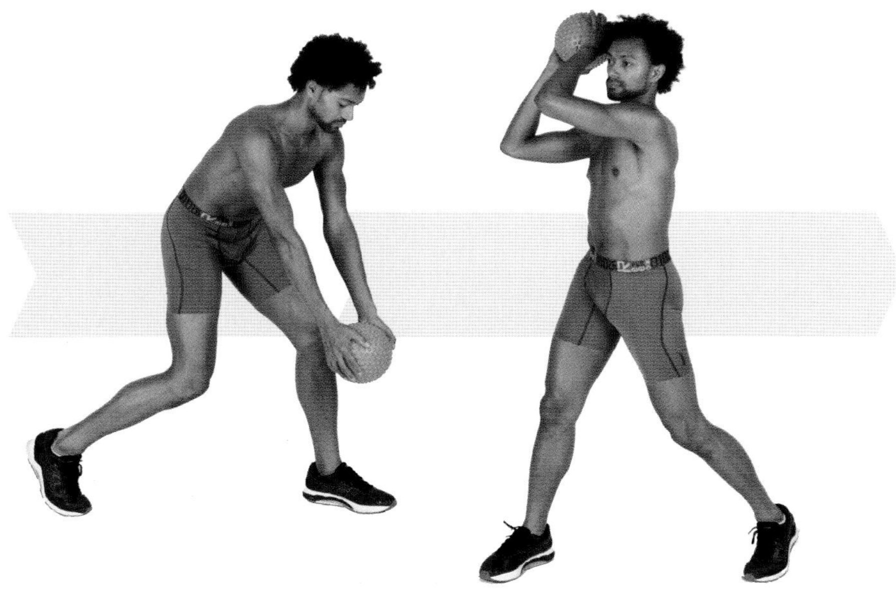

- Start with both feet wide, holding a weighted ball in your hands.
- Twist your body to the left with the ball low, knees slightly bent, and thrust, rotating the ball strongly to the right corner behind you, bending the arms and pivoting the legs.
- Switch sides, and repeat.

126 Weighted Ball Wood Chop

With wide legs, hold the weighted ball out to the side. Take a deep lunge, swinging the ball over your left knee. Then, stand, thrusting the ball right, up behind your shoulder, with straight legs.

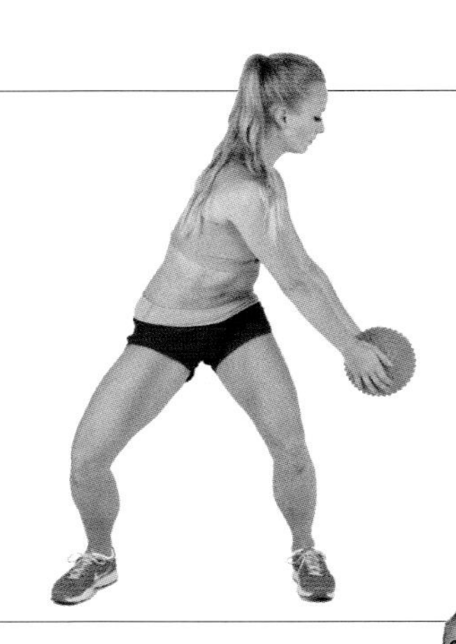

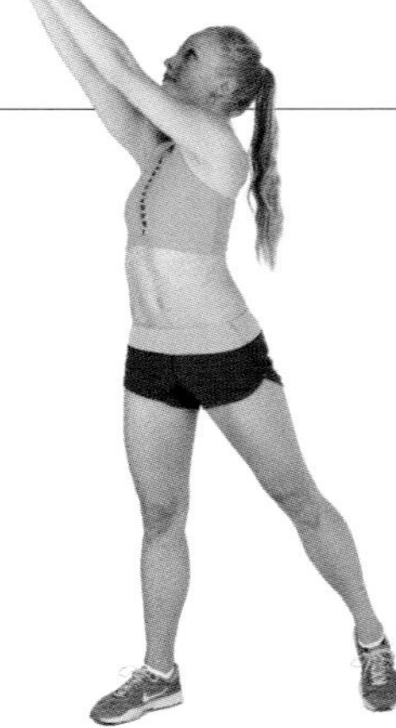

127 Shoulder-Height Wood Chop

Holding the cable handles with each hand, stand with your legs straight. Have the cable off to your right, at shoulder height. Allow the arms to reach out with the cable pull. Firmly, engage the abdominals, and pull the cable directly across the body to the left shoulder.

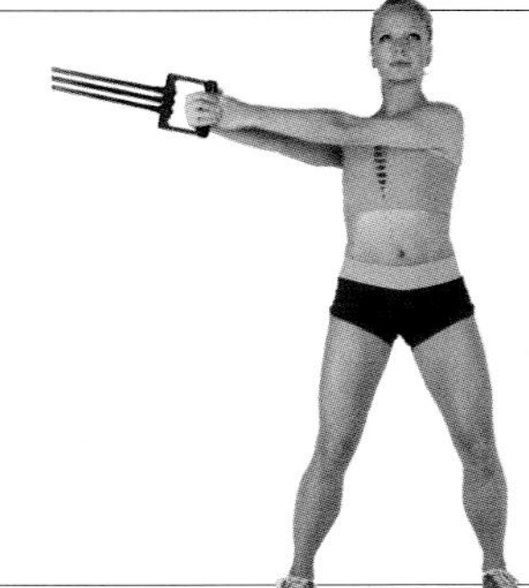

128

Medicine Ball Throw

The Medicine Ball Throw takes a real-world movement—throwing—and adds the explosive power of a Medicine ball to provide rotational drive that can help you build stamina and core stability. It can be performed alone or with an exercise buddy. Any kind of weighted ball will work for all of the exercises in this section.

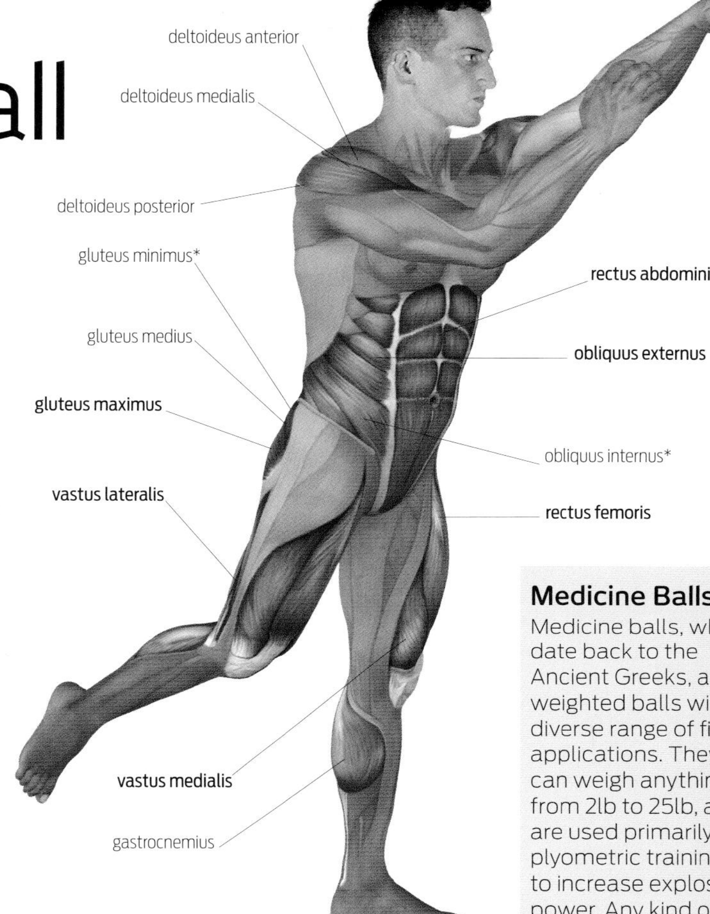

Correct form

You want to throw the Medicine ball from your center. The abdominals should be engaged from start to finish, initiating the throw.

Avoid

Do not shift your weight back into your heels. When performing throws and tosses, always keep the weight forward in your feet.

Annotation Key
Bold text indicates target muscles
Black text indicates other working muscles
* indicates deep muscles

Medicine Balls

Medicine balls, which date back to the Ancient Greeks, are weighted balls with a diverse range of fitness applications. They can weigh anything from 2lb to 25lb, and are used primarily in plyometric training to increase explosive power. Any kind of weighted ball can be used for exercises in this book where a Medicine ball or weighted ball is referenced.

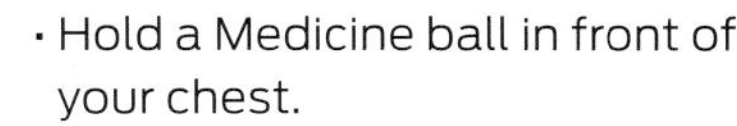

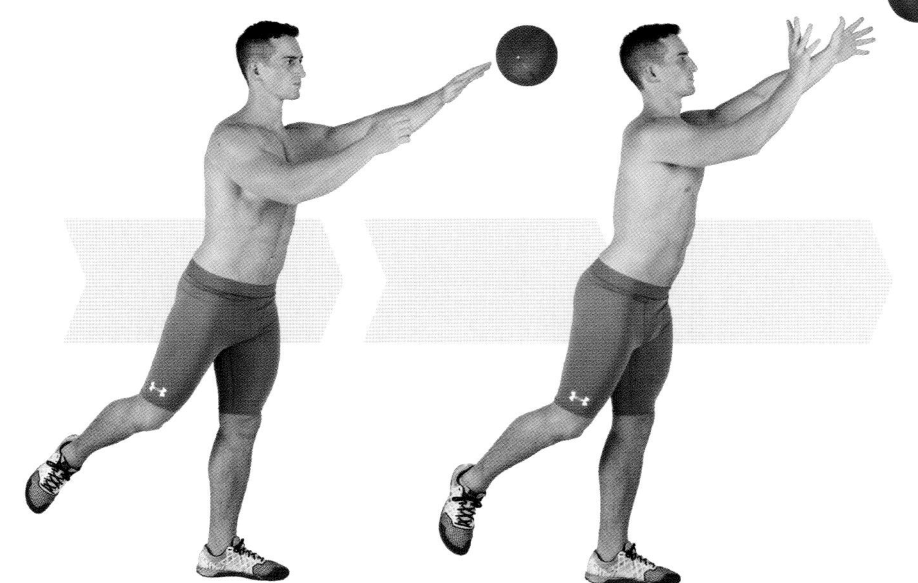

- Hold a Medicine ball in front of your chest.
- Position your left foot behind you, heel raised, and, keeping your torso stable, raise the ball above your right shoulder.
- Bend the knee of your back leg, lifting your foot off the floor as you throw the ball forward.
- Retrieve the ball and repeat on the opposite side.

129 Weighted Ball Wall Ball

Using the surface of a wall, you can work on explosive lunges, squats, and jumps with your weighted ball, tossing it onto the wall and catching it on the rebound.

- Bend the knees deeply, holding the ball in both hands.
- Explosively, extend the legs up out of your squat, onto the balls of your feet, tossing the ball against the wall.
- As the ball bounces back off the wall, catch it, and lower again.

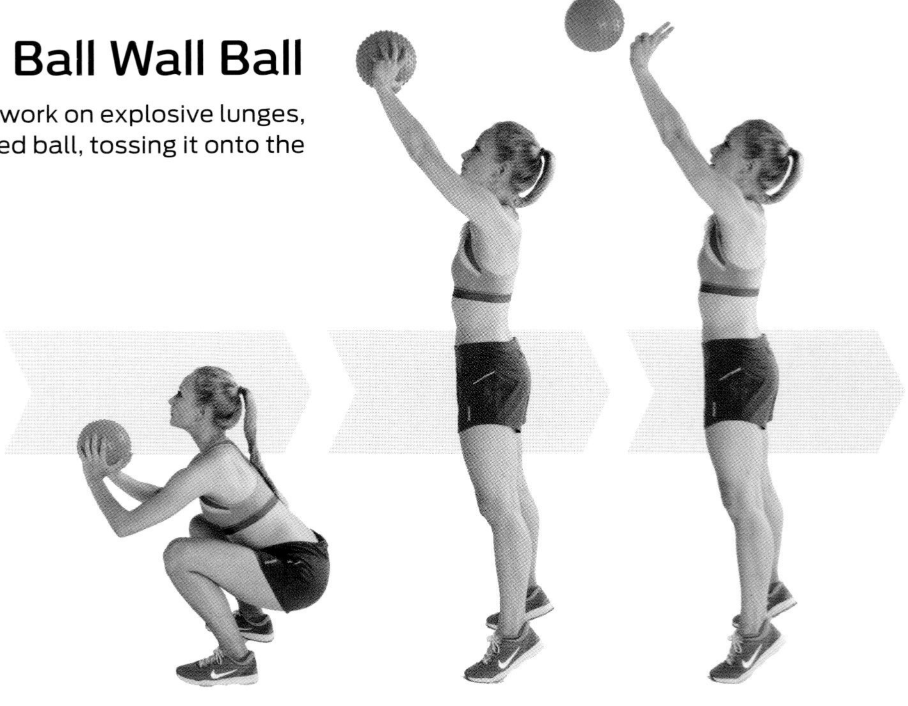

130 Weighted Ball Throw and Catch

With a partner, practice tossing a weighted ball back and forth. Be sure to use your core muscles to launch the ball from your hands to theirs. Also, use the bend in your knees to help with stabilizing the balance in your legs.

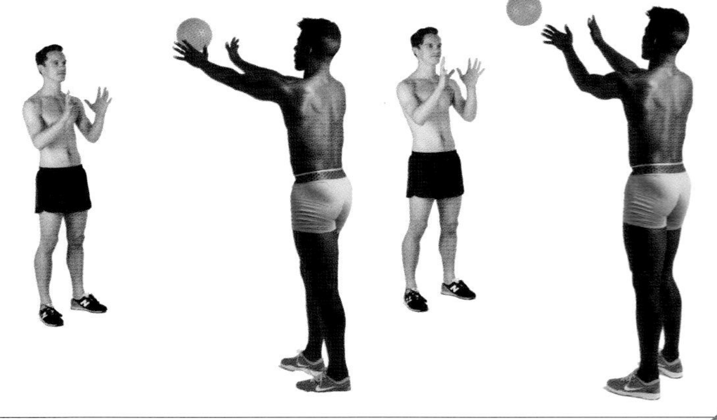

131 Over-the-Shoulder Throw

Either with a partner or on your own, try tossing a Medicine ball over your shoulder. Start with slightly bent knees. Swing the Medicine ball to the right, and then throw it over your left shoulder.

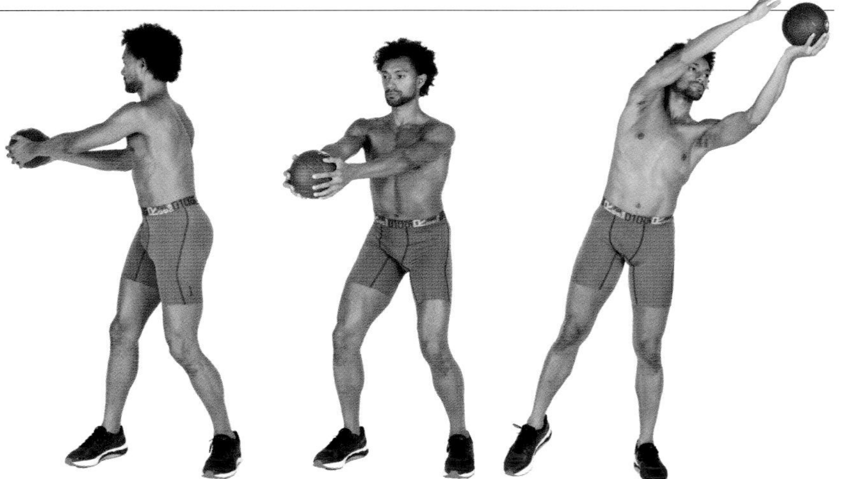

132 Weighted Ball Slam

Weighted ball Slams, believe it or not, help in stretching the back and increasing strength in the abdominals. The act of quickly lifting the arms up while holding a ball, and then slamming it into the ground, is an isometric movement that develops explosive dynamic power.

- Start with your legs slightly bent, with the ball up toward the right.
- Quickly swing the ball across your middle down to the left, explosively slamming the ball into the floor.

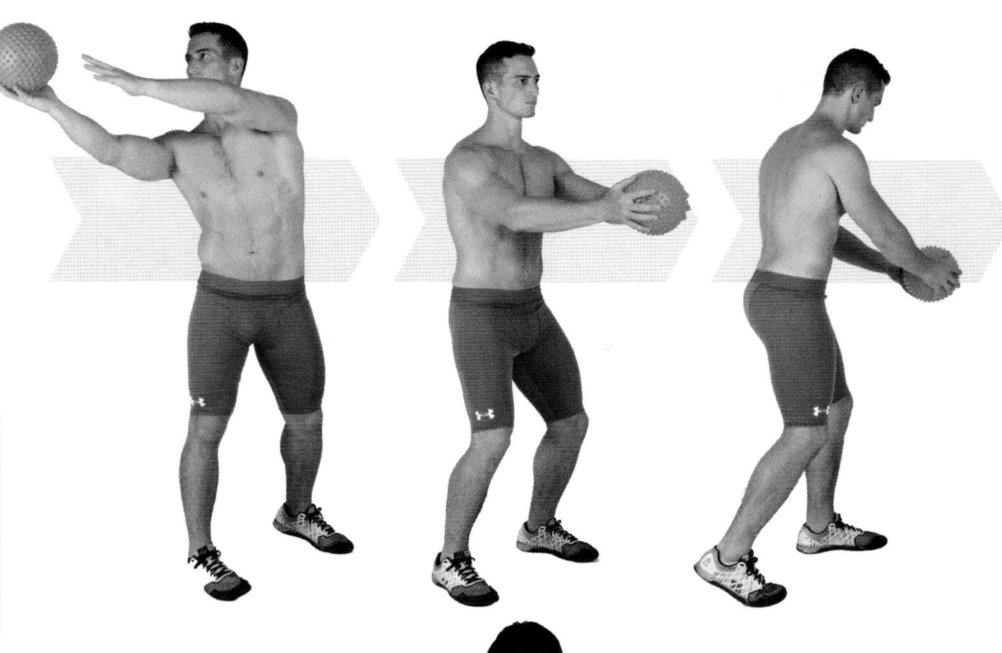

Benefits
Weighted ball throws and tosses are a great way to enhance dynamic power, rotational flexibility, and balance, as well as work on the nervous system's cross-circuiting.

133 Medicine Ball Big Circles

Holding your Medicine ball with both hands, open the legs wide. Circle the ball around yourself, starting to the right, then low to the ground for center, then to the left, then overhead.

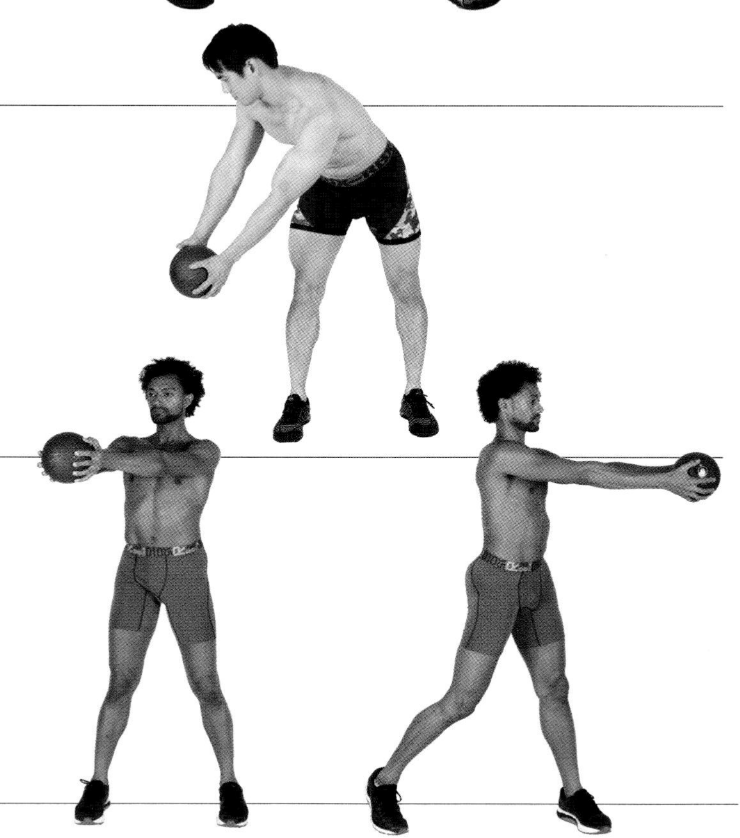

134 Standing Russian Twist

Start with both feet wide, holding a Medicine ball in your hands. Twist your body to the right, knees slightly bent, and then to the left, rotating the ball strongly each way, twisting and rotating the core and the legs.

135 Figure 8 Scoop

Stand with wide legs, holding the ball toward your left hip. In one move, sweep the ball across the body up to the right corner. Making this sequence quickly develops lateral core and glute power.

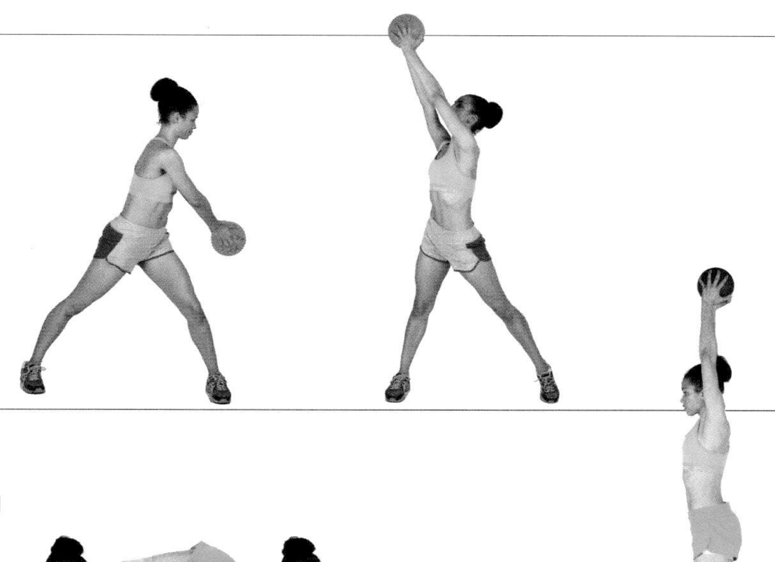

136 Medicine Ball Burpees

Take a Medicine ball and firmly hold it in your hands. Squat down and put the ball on the ground between your legs. Engage your abs and jump the legs back into a Plank Push-Up position (#213), balancing on the ball and your feet. Jump the legs back into a squat, swing the arms up to the sky, and jump.

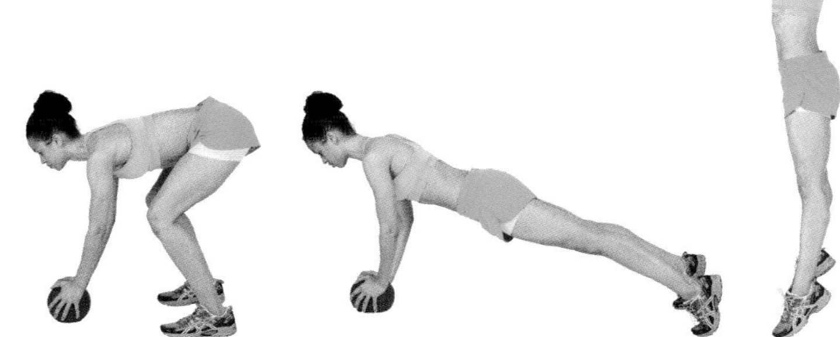

137 Reverse Swing

The movement of the Reverse Swing creates length in the spine while, simultaneously, enhancing balance and stretching the lower back, hamstrings, and shoulders. This is also a great exercise to do if you are working on strengthening your legs via a squat routine.

- Stand in a large open-legged stance.
- Bend forward with both legs bent, swinging the weighted ball quickly through the legs.
- Come to a stand, swinging the ball up and behind the head.
- Then, using the arms, slam the ball down into the floor.

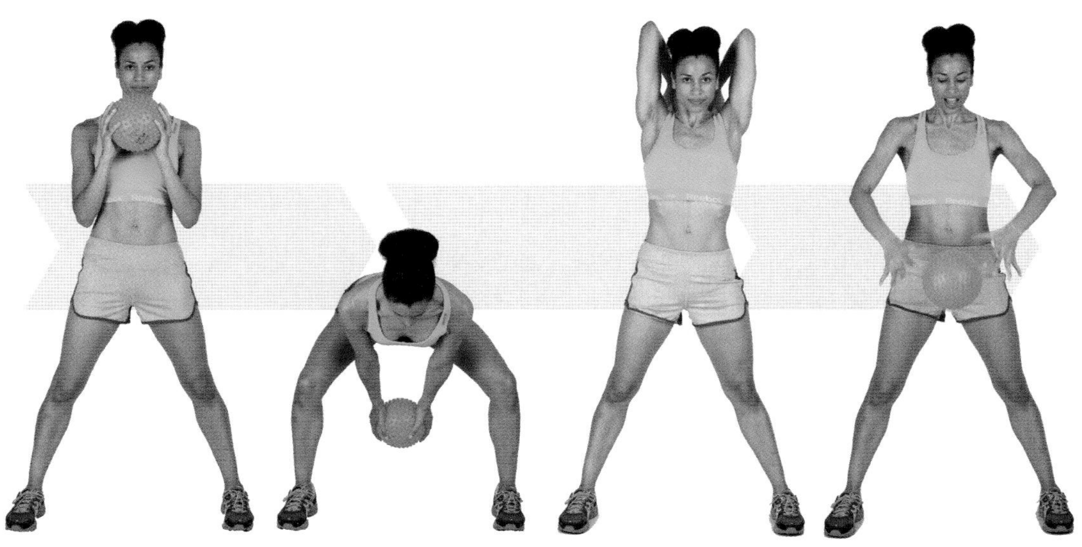

138 Around the World

Using the weighted ball as a light weight to stretch the arms, back, abs, and hips is an easy way to create more mobility in the spine! Moving in a wide, circular movement in this exercise will keep you open and limber.

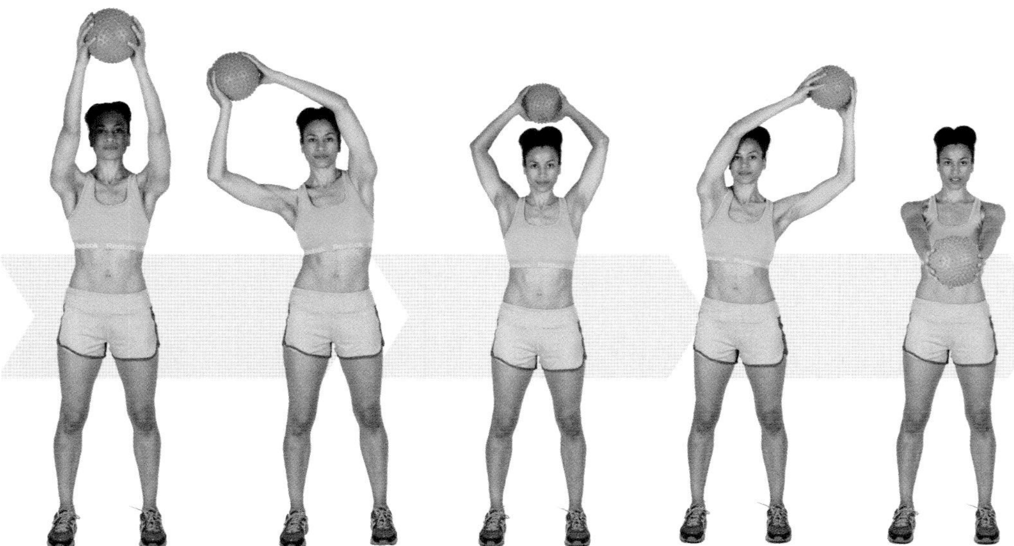

- Start with the feet shoulder-width apart, holding a weighted ball overhead.
- Circle the ball to the right.
- Circle the ball back behind your head.
- Circle the ball to the left.
- Then, finally, bring the ball forward. Repeat as much as you like.

139 Overhead Slam

Start with your legs slightly bent, with the ball up overhead. Quickly swing the ball down through your center, explosively, slamming the ball into the floor.

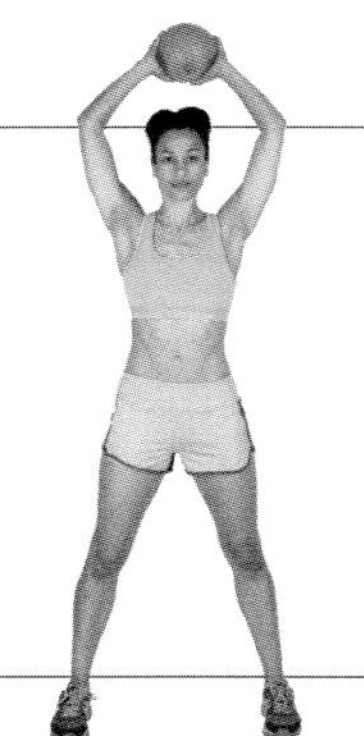

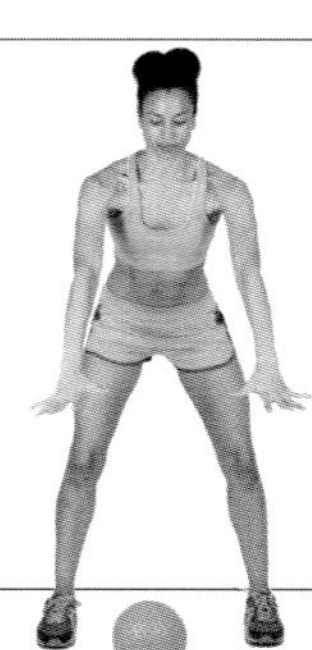

140 Figure 8

Stand tall with your feet under your shoulders. Hold a weighted ball in your hands, at the base of your abdominals. Raise your arms and the ball on a diagonal, up toward your right shoulder, keeping your hips forward, but letting your left foot turn slightly. Look up toward the ball. Bring the ball and your arms back down along the same diagonal line into your center and repeat to the left.

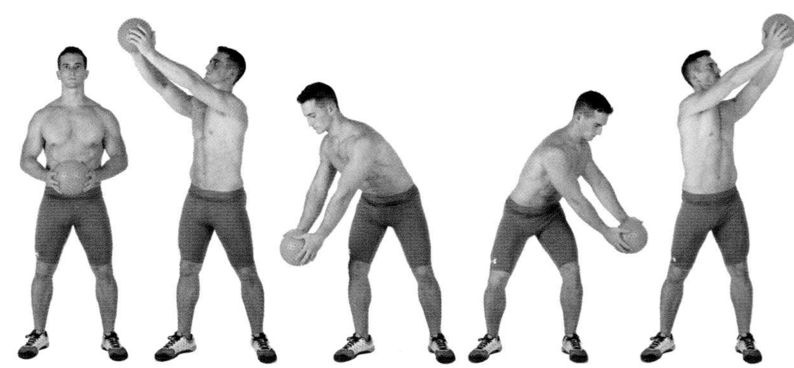

141 Wall Pass

Bend the knees gently, holding the weighted ball in both hands. Engage the abs and leg muscles, and toss the ball against the wall. As the ball bounces back off the wall, catch it, and start again.

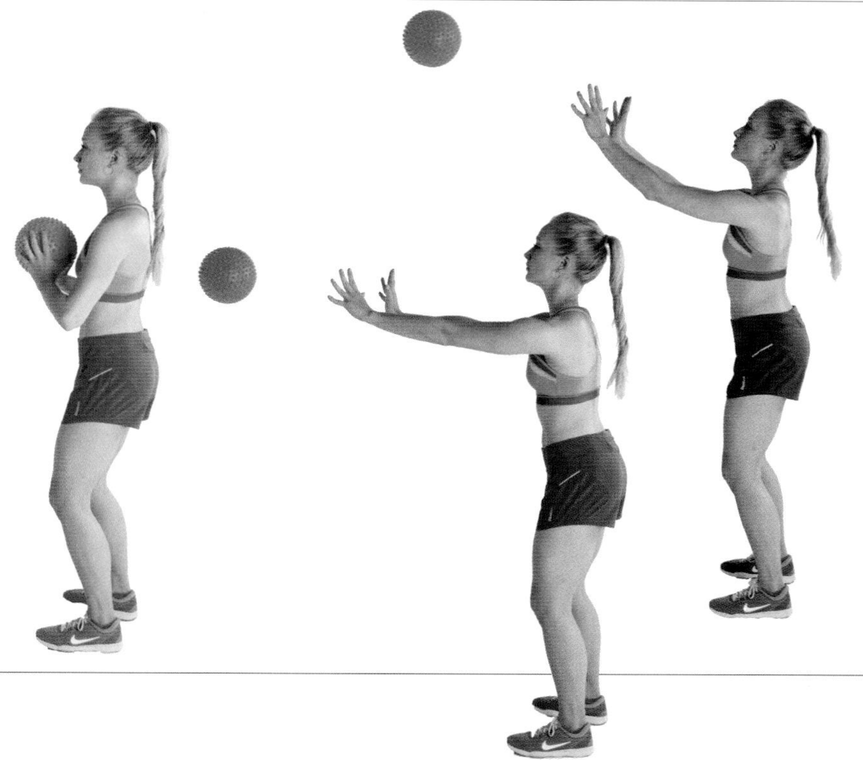

142 Weighted Ball Sit-Up and Throw

This throw is a variation of the traditional Sit-Up (#210). We all know the Sit-Up engages the abdominals, lower back, and, basically, the entire core section. When you incorporate a weighted ball into the Sit-Up—throwing the ball at the top of the movement—you are working the body with isometrics. In addition, you are giving the back and arms a good stretch by launching the ball with the core.

- Start by lying down with a weighted ball extended overhead.
- As you engage your abs and sit up, toss the ball.

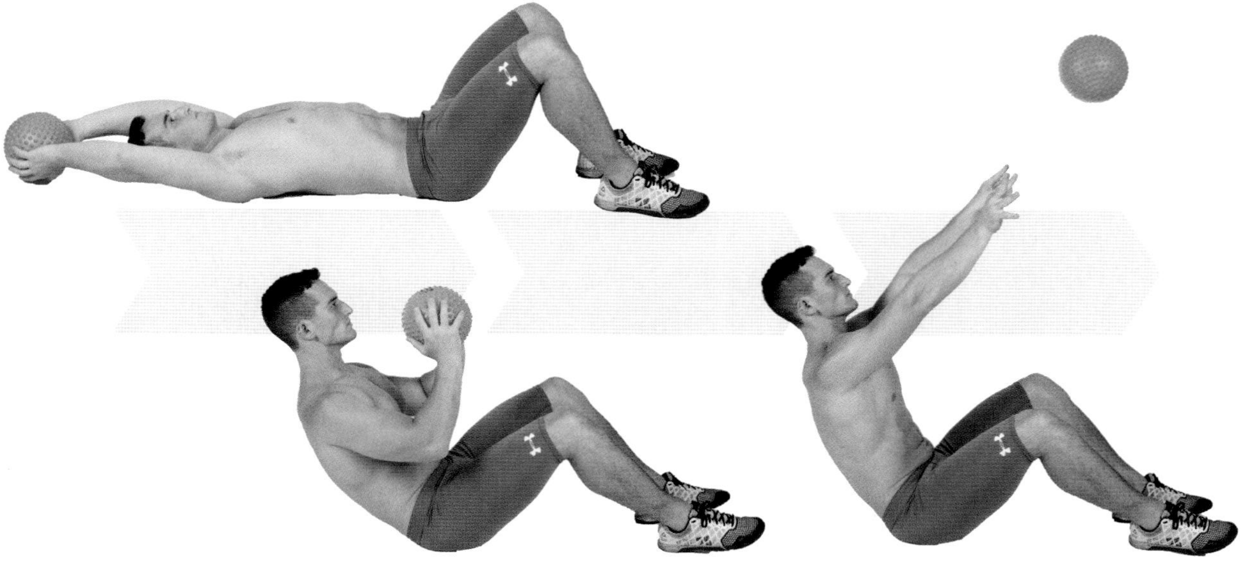

143 Rock and Roll Sit-Up

Start in your Sit-Up (#210) position with the weighted ball overhead. Engaging your abdominals, explosively rock your body forward through the Sit-Up position into a squat, with your arms holding the ball out in front of you. Bring your arms up overhead and stand up tall and long, keeping your abdominals strong and engaged.

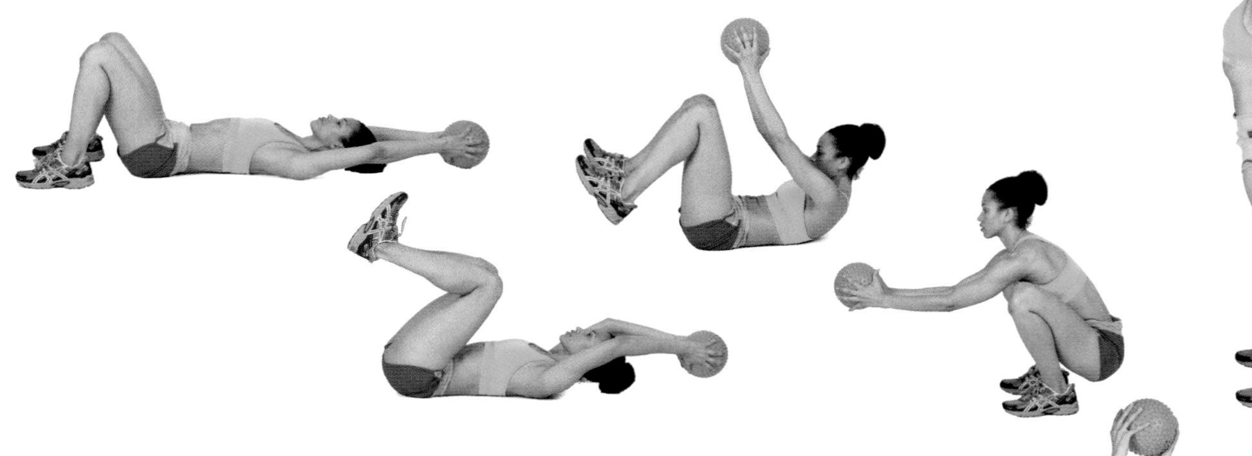

144 Hay Bailer

With a weighted ball suspended at your front, take a staggered stance. Kneel onto the right knee with the left leg forward. Swing the ball from your right hip, up into the sky toward the left. Quickly recover back to the right.

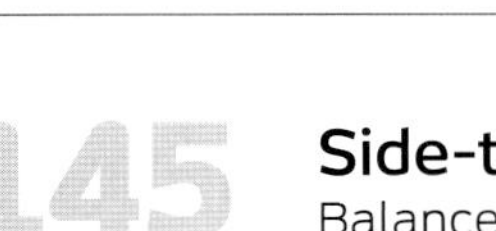

145 Side-to-Side Slam

Balance with the legs bent together, hovering off the floor. Pull up out of the hips, with the arms reaching to the front, holding your weighted ball. Rotate the upper body to each side, twisting as far as you can while keeping the legs still and slamming the ball into the floor each way.

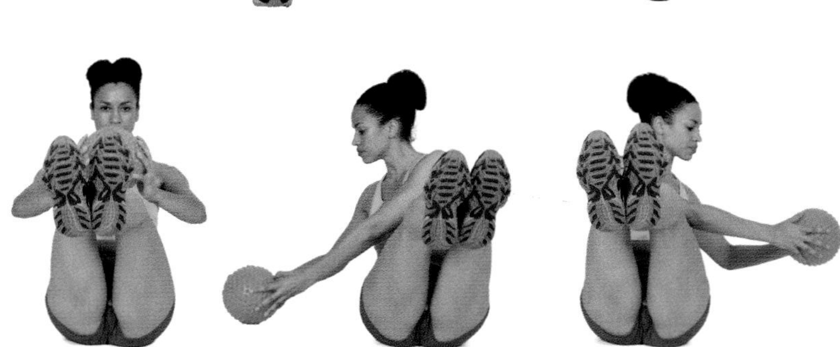

146 Weighted Boat-Rock

Start by sitting with a weighted ball between your knees. Scoop the lower abdominals a lot and stabilize the hips. Raise your legs up and sway them to the right, and then to the left. Breathe, and use your arms to sway in the opposite direction of your legs.

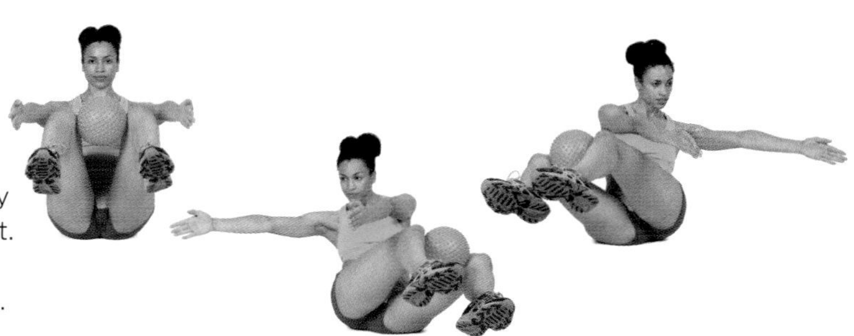

147 45-Degree Twist

Come to balance with the legs bent together, hovering off the floor. With your torso long, pull up out of the hips, arms reaching to the front with your weighted ball, then rotate the upper body to each side. Twist as far as you can while keeping the legs still.

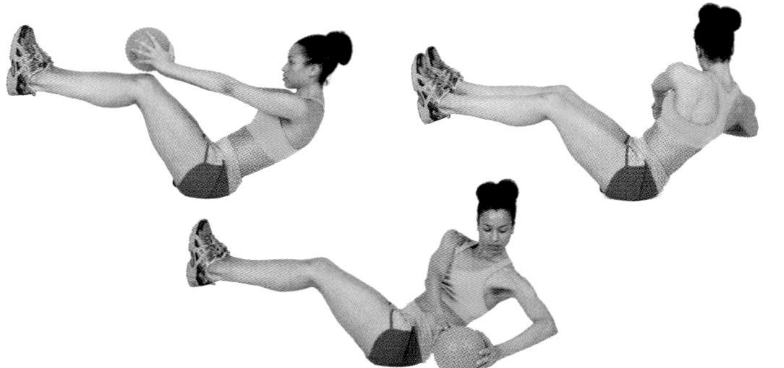

148 Rocky Solo

Sit with your legs long, and feet apart. With your torso tall, pull up out of the hips, hands holding a Medicine ball. Take a rotation to each side. Twist as far as you can while keeping the legs still, and drop the ball onto the floor. Pick up the ball, twist back to the middle, and repeat on the other side.

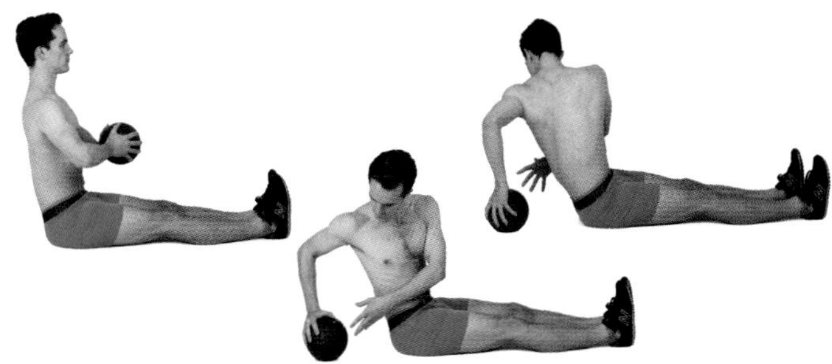

149 Medicine Ball Front Raise

Stand tall with the Medicine ball low in front of your hips. Squeeze the abdominals into the low back, lengthen the spine, and lift the Medicine ball up to chest height. Hold a moment, and lower again.

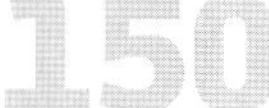

150 Foam-Roller Twist

Sit comfortably on a foam roller with the legs slightly bent out in front of you. With your abdominals engaged, lift the weighted ball to chest height, and take turns twisting the ball to either side of the body.

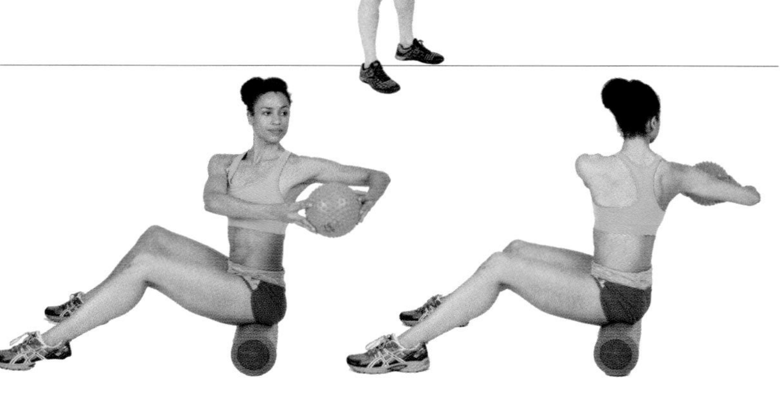

151

Battle-Rope Side-to-Side Swings

Annotation Key
Bold text indicates target muscles
Black text indicates other working muscles
* indicates deep muscles

If you are looking to have a full-body strengthening session and also up your cardio, battle ropes will give you this and more! Battle ropes, because of their wide range of movement, are able to give you a more dynamic workout, achieving and reaching far more angles than the basic weights. Your core works a ton when using battle ropes, and your cardio kicks up to a high level.

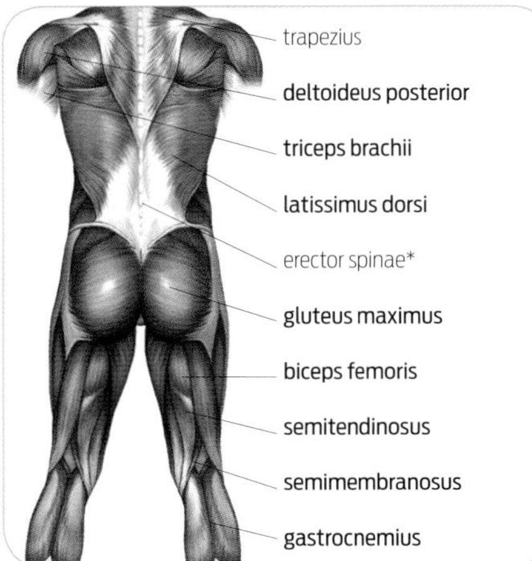

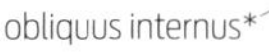

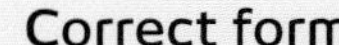

Correct form

Keep a firm, strong grasp on your battle ropes as they are very heavy and can easily slip out of your hands.

Avoid

Avoid having a loose core. Your abs need to be very engaged so as to keep your lower back protected from forceful impact.

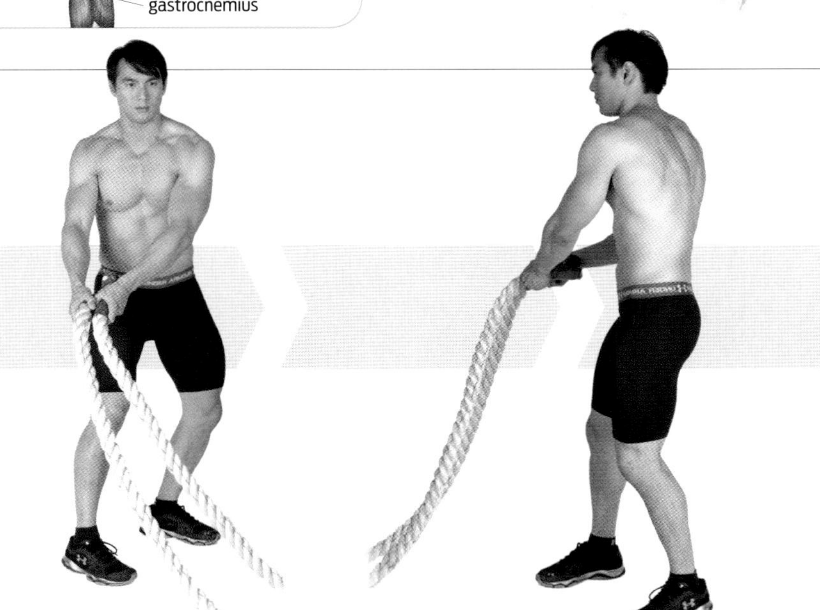

- Stand with your legs open, knees bent for balance and range.
- Take the ropes in each hand and swing them to the right.
- Then, swing them to the left, rotating your upper torso against your hips and legs.

152 Battle-Rope Alternating Waves

The Battle-Rope Alternating Waves are probably the most common pattern of wave used today in workout routines. Creating alternating waves focuses the work through the body, and really works the biceps too.

- Stand with your feet shoulder-width apart, holding onto the ropes firmly in each hand.
- Take a bend in the knees and begin with one arm tossing the rope up into the air, making a wave.
- Next, toss the opposite arm up.
- Keep alternating arms, making waves, until you have achieved a consistent rhythm with the ropes.

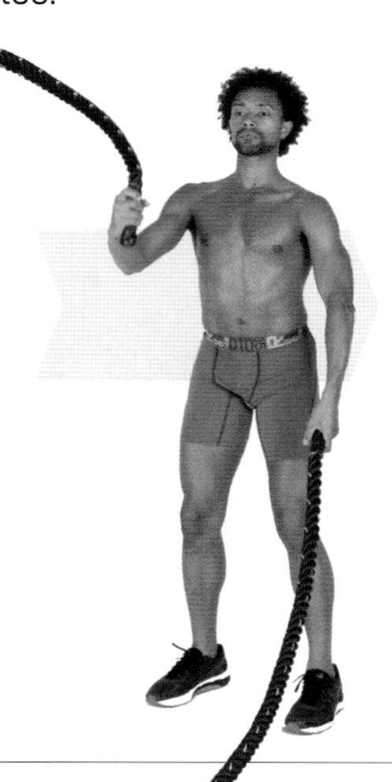

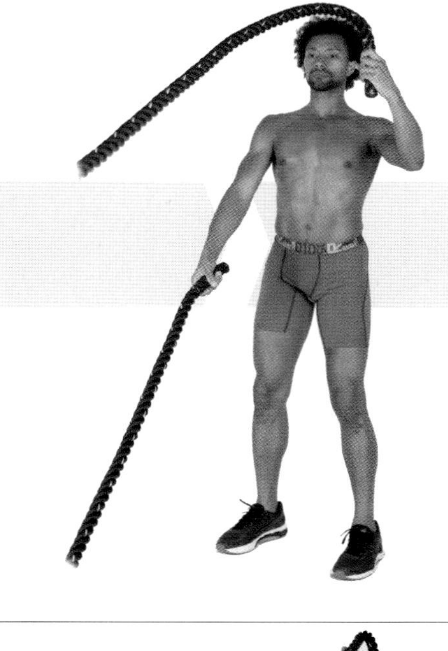

153 Battle-Rope Full-Squat Alternating Waves

With the battle ropes in your hands, come into a deep squat. Once at the bottom of your squat, hold there by engaging the core and leg muscles. Begin flinging your ropes up and down, slamming the ropes as you go.

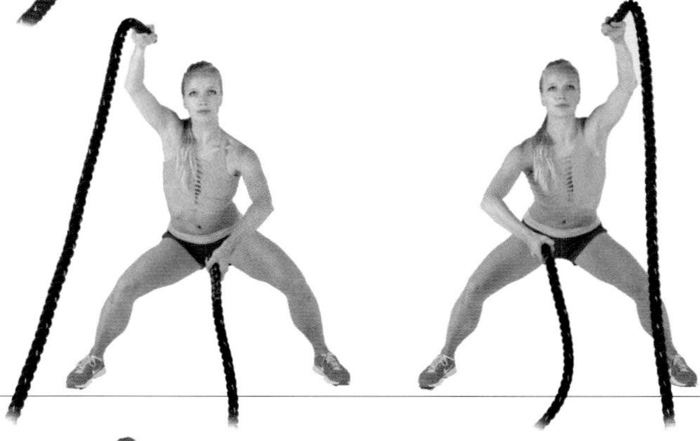

154 Battle-Rope Jump Squat and Slam

With the battle ropes in your hands, stand with your feet hip-width apart. Lower to a squat and, once at the bottom of your bend, explode up into a jump with straight legs, flinging your ropes up, and slam back down into a squat.

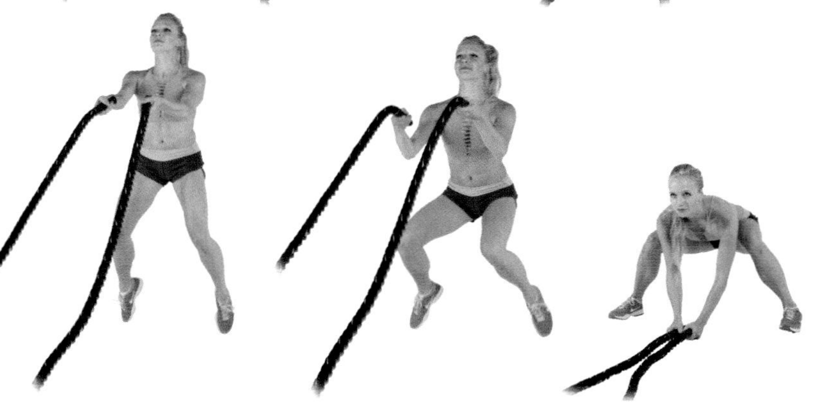

155 **Battle-Rope Crossover Slam**

Stand with your knees slightly bent, with the end of a battle rope in each hand. Bring the hands together and move the ends of the rope in an arc above your head, lifting them to your right before slamming them down hard to your left. Repeat, alternating sides.

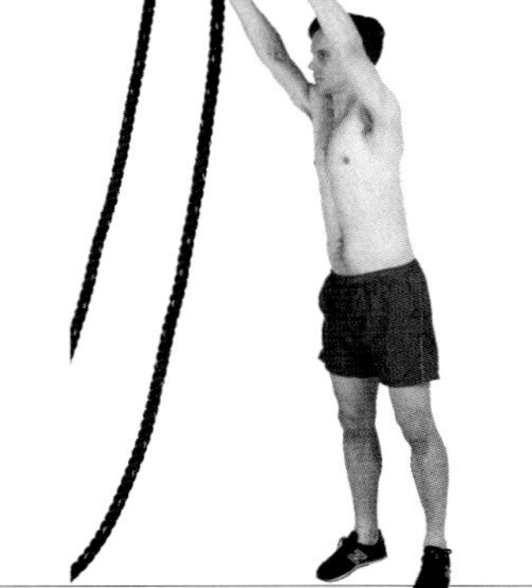

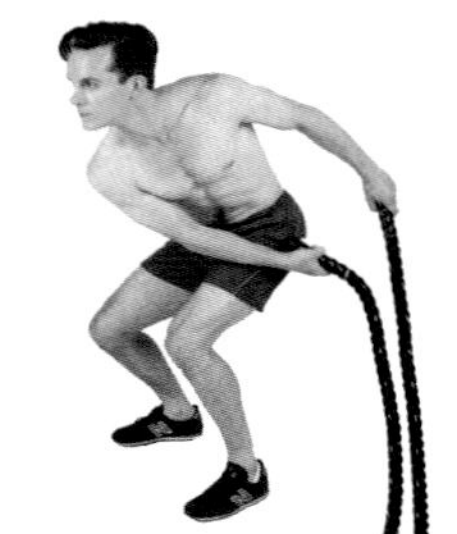

156 **Battle-Rope External Rotation Spirals**

Stand with your legs securely shoulder-width apart. Holding onto your battle ropes, begin by strongly swinging the ropes out away from each other, allowing the ropes to cross, and creating spirals that rotate out away from your body.

157 **Battle-Rope Claps**

Stand with your legs securely shoulder-width apart. Holding onto your battle ropes, begin by strongly swinging the ropes far out away from your center line. Bring the ropes back in to strike each other, making a clapping movement.

158 **Battle-Rope Battle Jacks**

For this challenging variation with the battle ropes, perform a standard jumping jack while holding the ropes in your hands. Jump the feet open wide while bringing the arms together overhead into a jumping jack.

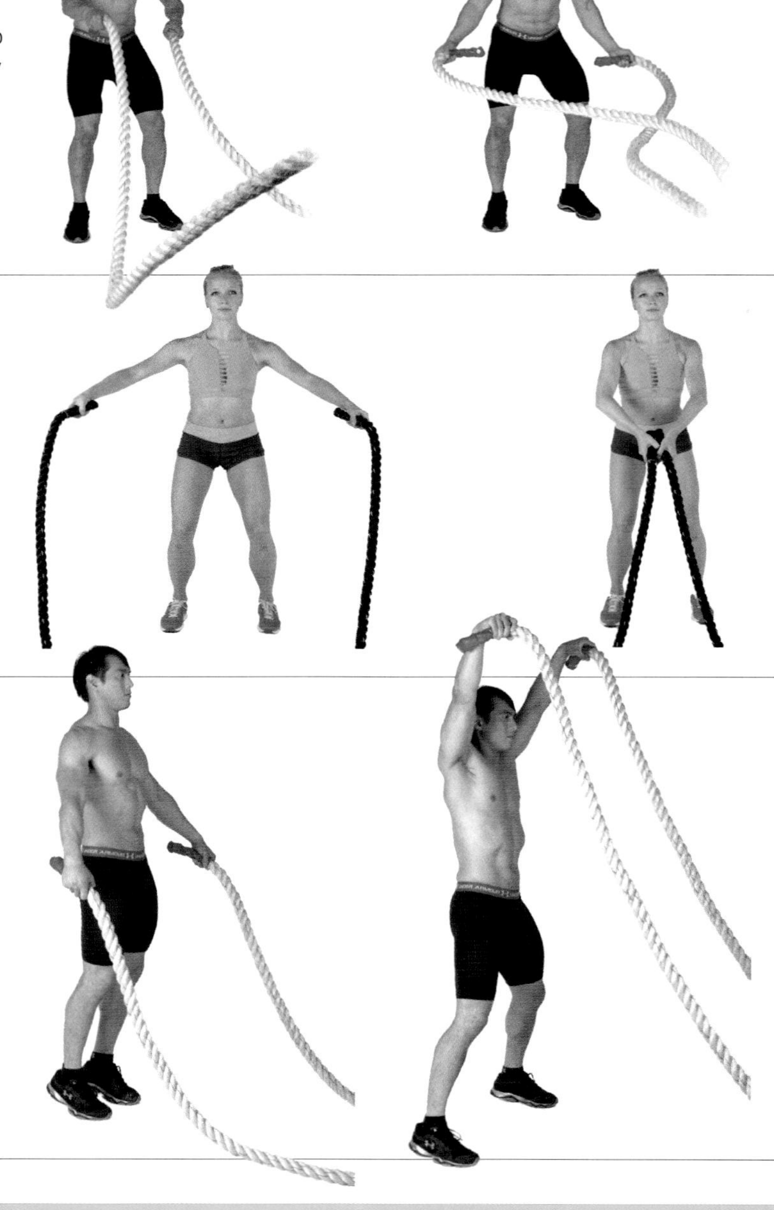

159 Battle-Rope Double-Arm Wave

Take a shoulder-width stance and begin with both arms tossing the ropes up into the air, together, making two large waves. Keep thrusting the ropes up, making waves, until you have achieved a consistent rhythm with the ropes. As you move the ropes more, feel free to bend the knees as much as you need to in order to keep your balance and support the rope movement.

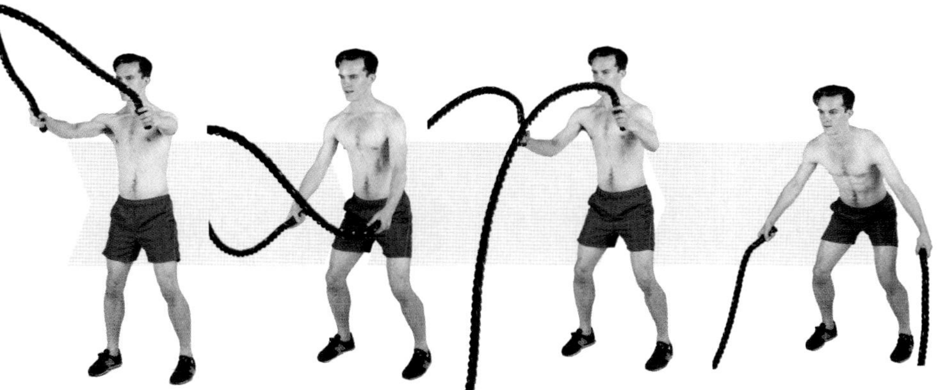

- While waving your battle ropes, maintain a secure grip on the rope ends, working the lower portion of the arms.
- For an added challenge, experiment with how much force you put into waving your ropes.
- Try to move the ropes by engaging the core and legs only. Every time you make a wave, you should feel your abdominals squeeze into your center.

160 Battle-Rope Double-Arm Slam

Open the legs wide and take a bend in the knees, coming into an easy squat. With one big movement and a lot of force on the rope, fling the battle ropes up into the sky and slam them down strongly against the ground.

161 Battle-Rope Snakes

Stand with your legs securely shoulder-width apart. Holding onto your battle ropes close to your feet, begin by strongly swinging the ropes in toward each other, crossing the ropes, and creating snake shapes across the ground with the body of the ropes.

162 Battle-Rope Grappler Throws

Stand with your legs open, knees bent for balance and range. Take the ropes in each hand and swing them to the right, under the side of the body, with a rounded core. Then swing them to the left, rotating your upper torso side to side, while pivoting the feet.

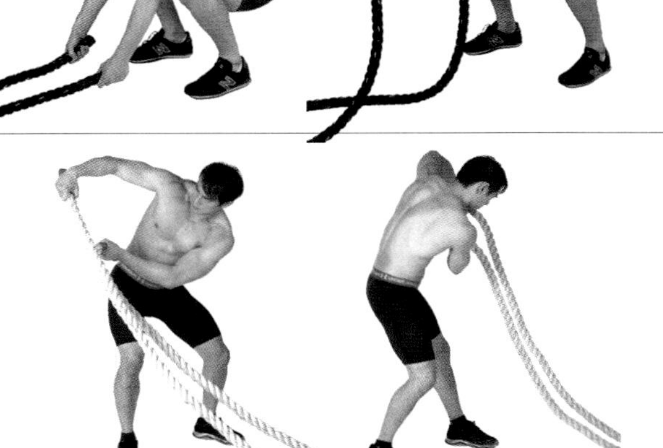

163

Dips

Adding Dips into your upper-body workout routine will enhance the power developing in the chest and triceps. By isolating the elbows and using them as a sort of vector, you will place the weight of this exercise into your upper arms for the lowering portion, and into the chest for the lift part. A healthy dose of Dips will keep your upper body balanced and strong.

Correct form

The Dip is a challenging move. If you can maintain a still body posture while allowing the elbows to bend and straighten freely, you are off to a good start.

Avoid

Avoid letting the elbows bend past 90 degrees on the bar. Doing this adds too much stress on the shoulders and elbow joints.

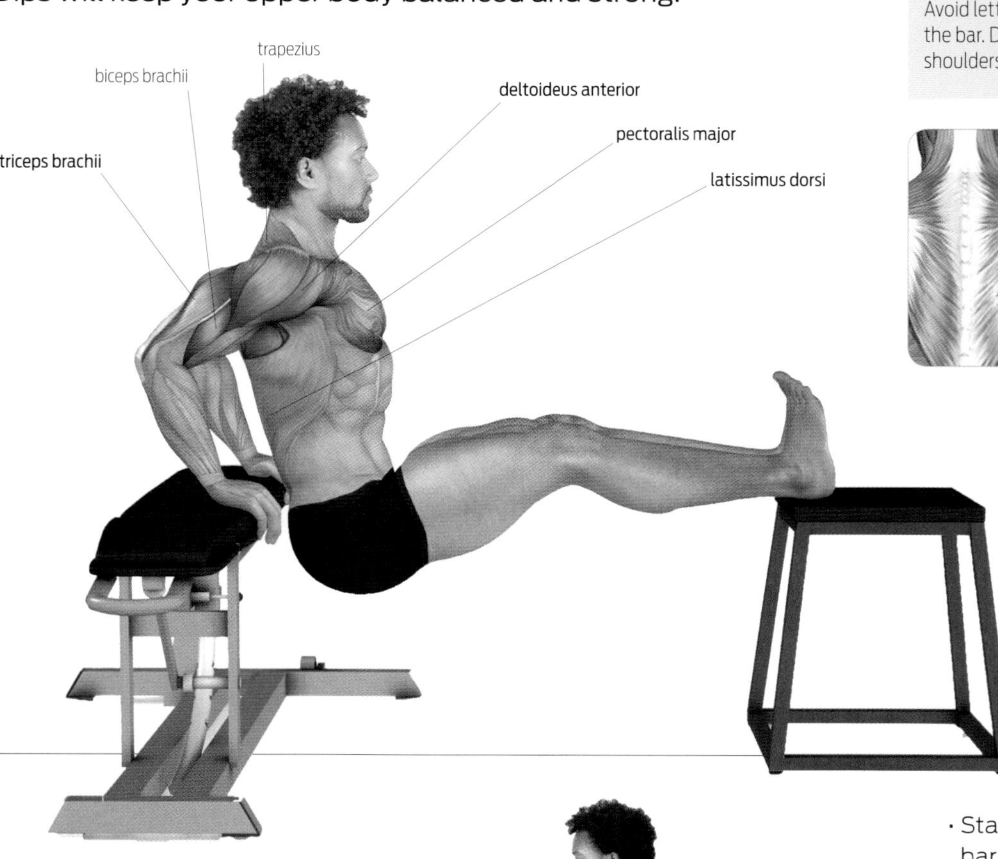

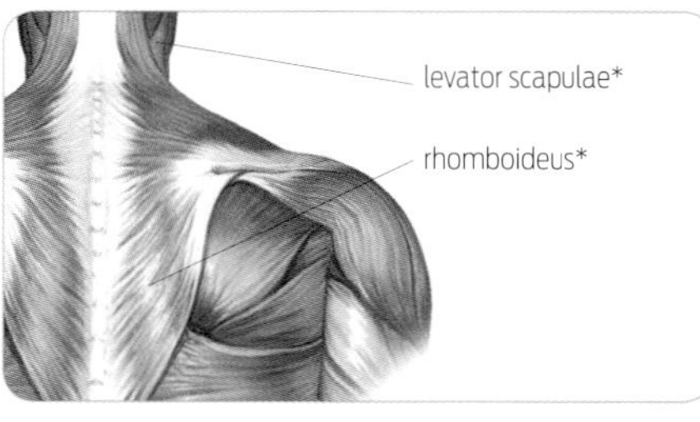

Annotation Key
Bold text indicates target muscles
Black text indicates other working muscles
* indicates deep muscles

- Start with a strong grip on your dip bar, with your arms straight.
- Bring the ankles together to touch.
- Slowly lower your body down, bending only at the elbows, until the arms reach a right angle.
- Push down against the bar, and lift your body back up, straightening the arms.

164 Weighted Dips

Start with a strong grip on your dip bar, with your arms straight. Place a weighted ball between your upper legs. Slowly lower the body down, bending only at the elbows, until the arms reach a right angle. Push down against the bar, and lift your body back up, straightening the arms.

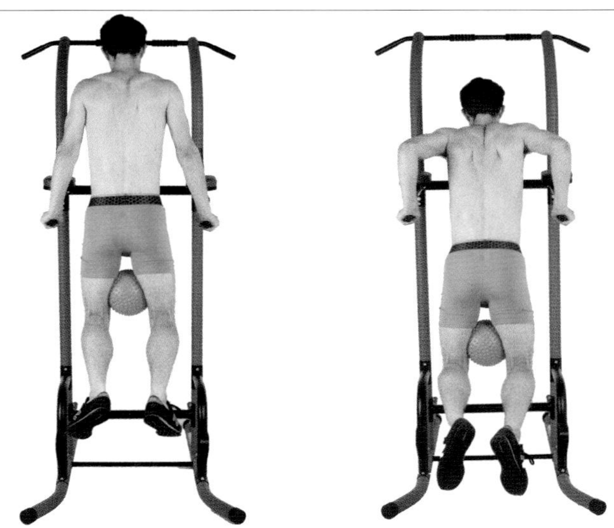

165 Assisted Dips

If you are seeking a little assistance with your Dips, try this option. Secure an elastic band, cable, or yoga strap to your dip bar and allow it to hang with some tension. When going for your Dips, use the band to support your knees.

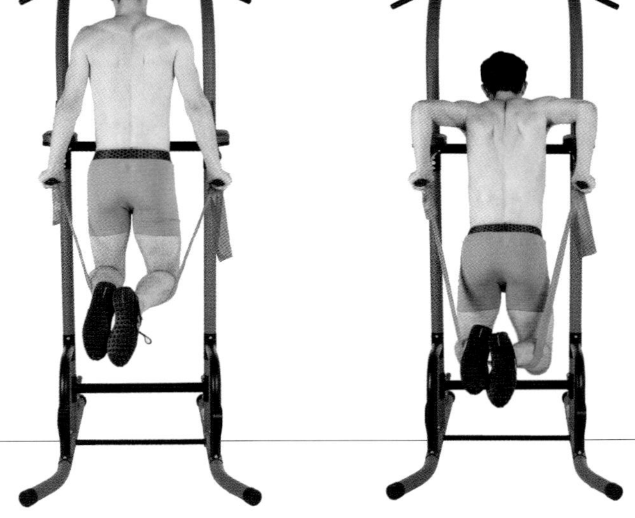

166 Triceps Bench Dips

For this variation, position your hands on a low bench or surface, and then prop your feet up onto an adjacent surface. Go for your Dip in this position. This is an excellent choice for beginners. Make sure both of your surface choices are sturdy and stable.

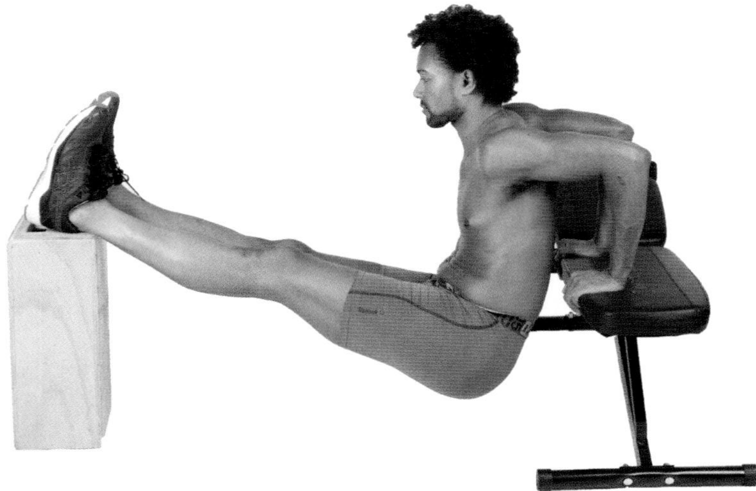

167

Basic Crunch

You can find the basic Crunch mixed in alongside many other Sit-Up-type workouts. Performing a Crunch is, essentially, the beginning part of the full Sit-Up. With the Crunch, you do not bring your full torso up into flexion. Instead, you squeeze the abs into the lower back, keeping the front and back sides of the body long and strong against the floor. This shortening of the abdominal wall deeply strengthens the many layers that make up your core.

sternocleidomastoideus
splenius
scalenus
trapezius
deltoideus anterior
pectoralis minor*
pectoralis major
biceps brachii

Annotation Key
Bold text indicates target muscles
Black text indicates other working muscles
* indicates deep muscles

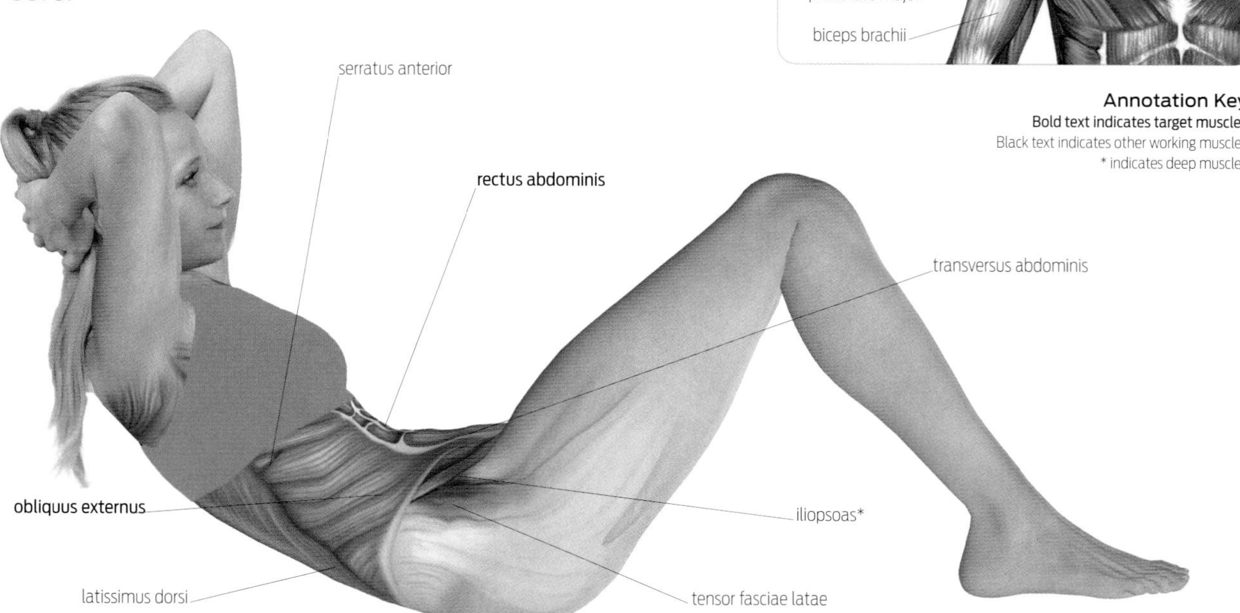

- Lie down on your back and bring your feet in, along the floor, toward your hips about 2 feet (60 centimeters).
- Stack your hands behind your the lower part of your head.
- Engage your abs, tuck your chin into your chest, and curl your body up just until your upper back comes off the floor.

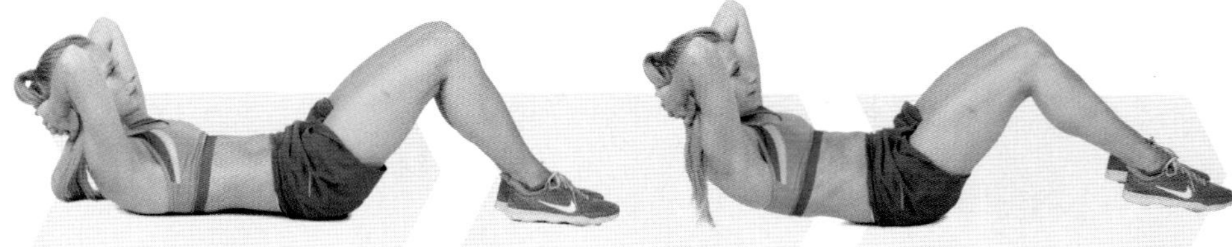

Correct form

Keep your lower back long on the floor and try not to arch your spine away from the ground under you.

Avoid

Do not crunch the neck into your chest. You want to keep the neck long, even if you cannot bring your body far up off the floor.

168 Crossover Crunch

Incorporating some opposition into your Sit-Up and Crunch routine is a great way to keep your nervous system sharp, as well as develop the cross-sections of muscles that run from your back body to the front. The abdominals and upper-back muscles will become more stable when you bring this Crossover Crunch variation into your workouts.

- Bend your legs and bring them together at a 90-degree angle from your hips.
- Come up into your Crunch position and hold there.
- Extend your right leg out and twist the upper body toward the left raised leg. Alternate sides, and repeat.

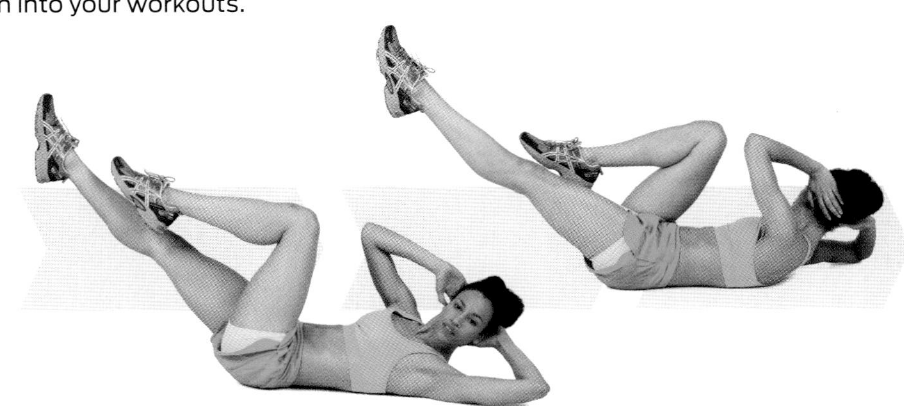

169 Abdominal Kick

Lie flat on the floor. Curl up into your abdominal Crunch and bend the right leg. Reach for the bent knee with both hands, switch, and bend your left knee. Alternate sides, and repeat.

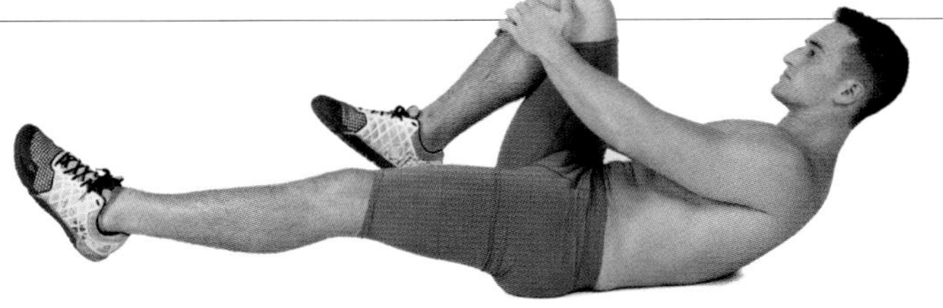

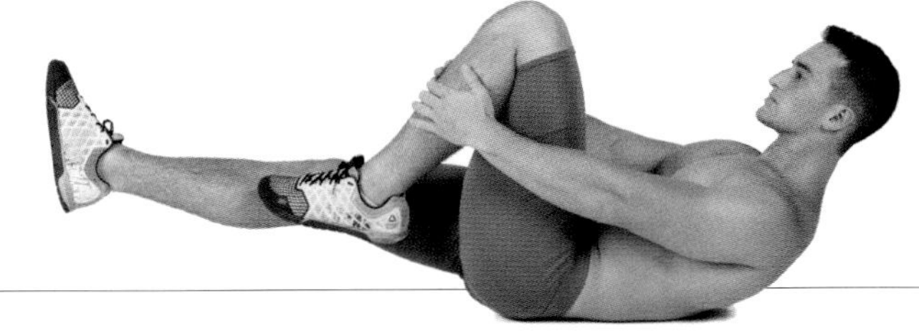

170 Lemon Squeezer

Begin with your body flat on the floor. Place your hands behind your lower back and bend your left leg in. Engage your lower abdominals deeply and come up into a Crunch. Take care to not push yourself up with your hands—only let the core do the work.

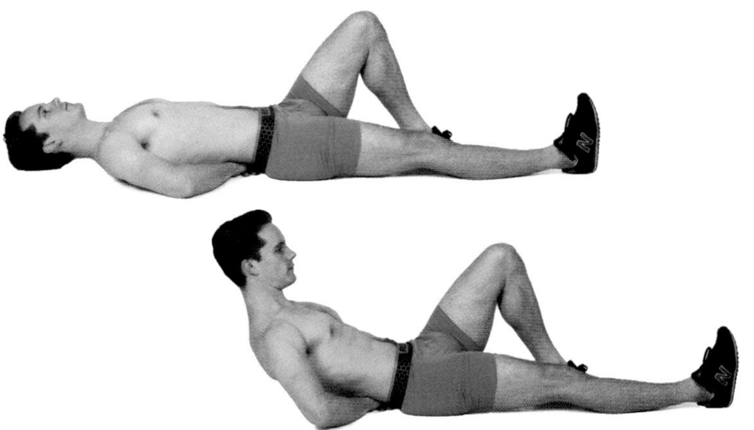

171 Russian Twist

Come up into your Crunch with your arms long out in front of you. Twisting side to side, let the knees be still each time you switch sides. Keep your torso on an angle, challenging the core.

172 Standing Knee Crunch

Stand with your feet staggered. Bring your arms up onto the diagonal, and explosively pull your left knee up into your chest, while swinging your arms down and back behind your body. This move is great for overall coordination and balance control.

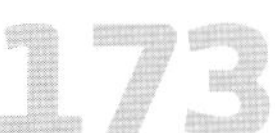

173 McGill Curl-Up

Begin with your body flat on the floor. Place your hands behind your lower back, and bend your left leg in. Engage your lower abdominals deeply and come up into a Crunch. Keep the neck long and the eyes gazing far out beyond your bent knee.

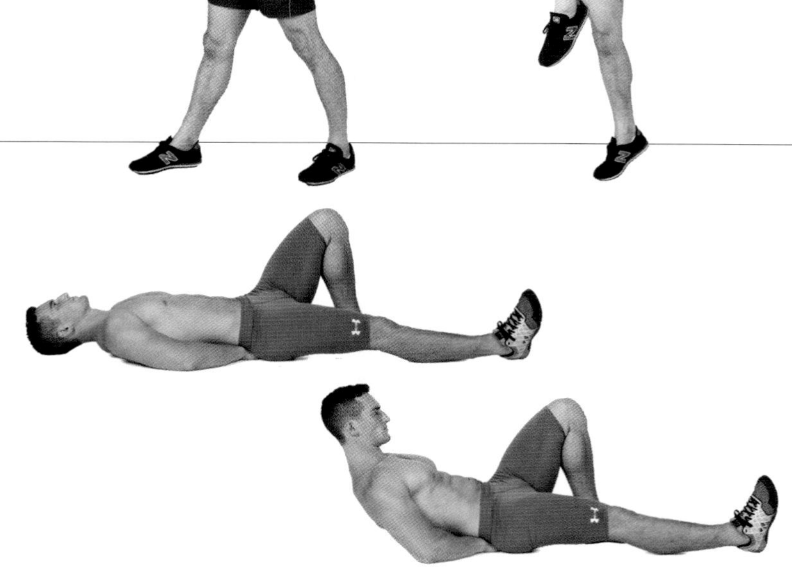

174 Alternating Crunch

Bend your legs and bring them together, crossing the right foot over the left knee. Come up into your Crunch position and hold there. Twist the upper body toward the left side, lower down, then crunch up, and twist the body to the right. Alternate legs, and repeat.

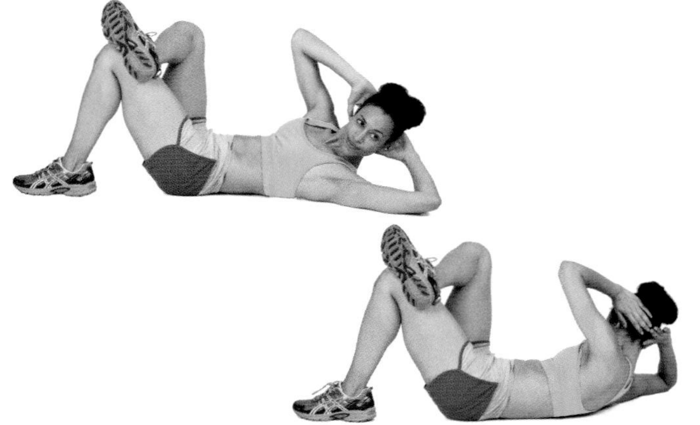

175 Side Raised-Legs Crunch

Begin lying on the left side of your body. Place your left hand behind your head and your right hand on your core. With the feet flexed, bend the knees into a 90-degree angle. Squeeze the abs in, lift the legs, and crunch into the right side of your abdominals. Lower, and repeat.

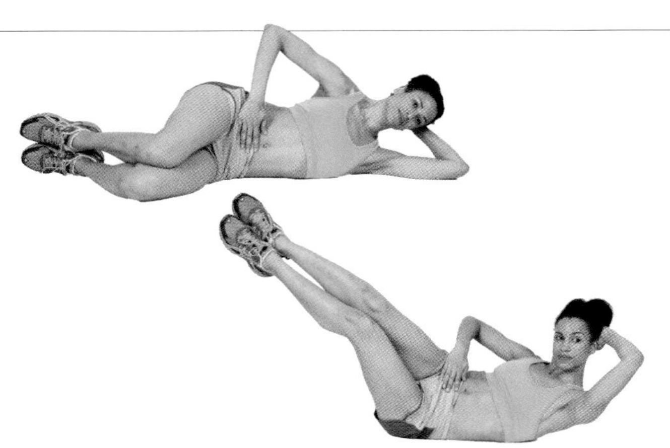

176 Bicycle Crunch

Bend your legs and bring them together at a 90-degree angle from your hips. Come up into your Crunch position and hold there. Extend your right leg out and twist the upper body toward the left raised leg, bringing your right knee into your chest.

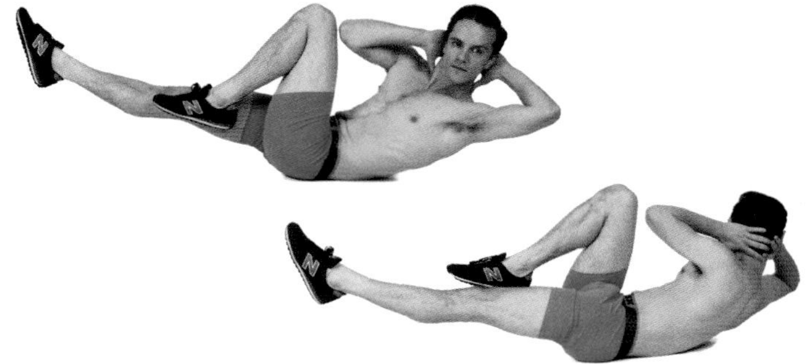

177 Swiss Ball Weighted Ab Curl

Lie with your lower back supported by a Swiss ball. Holding a weighted ball overhead, slowly curl your torso forward, contracting your abdominal muscles.

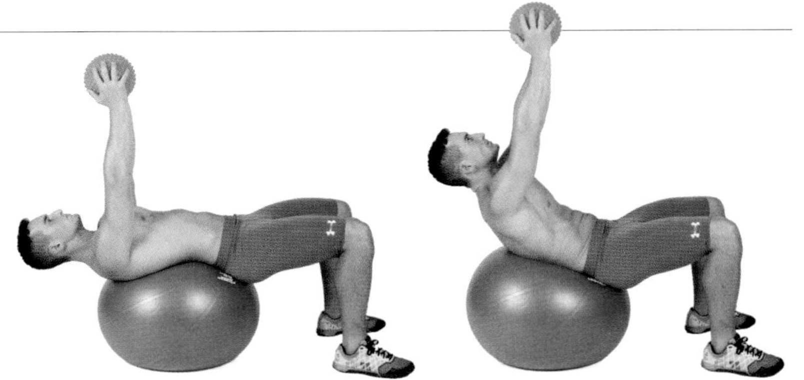

178 Hundred I

The Hundred is a movement that originates from Pilates workouts. This version is the simplest version. Begin by lying down in your standard Crunch position. Bring your legs together and your arms to your sides. Squeeze your lower abdominals into your back, reach your arms forward and off the floor, and come into your Crunch.

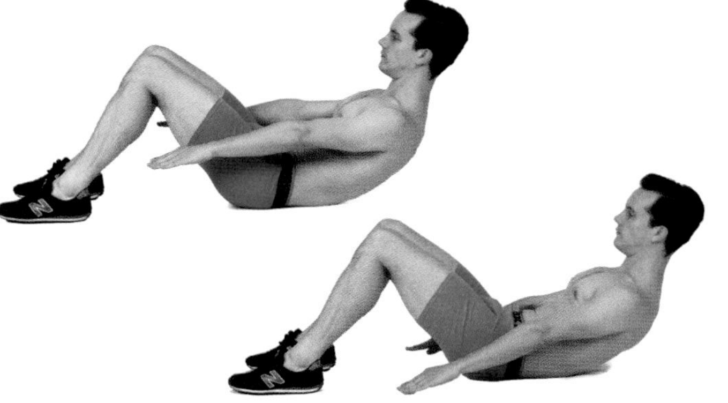

179 Hundred II

Start in your standard Crunch position. Bring your legs together and your arms to your sides. Engage the core muscles and levitate your legs off the floor into a right angle. Reach your arms forward and off the floor and crunch into your abs.

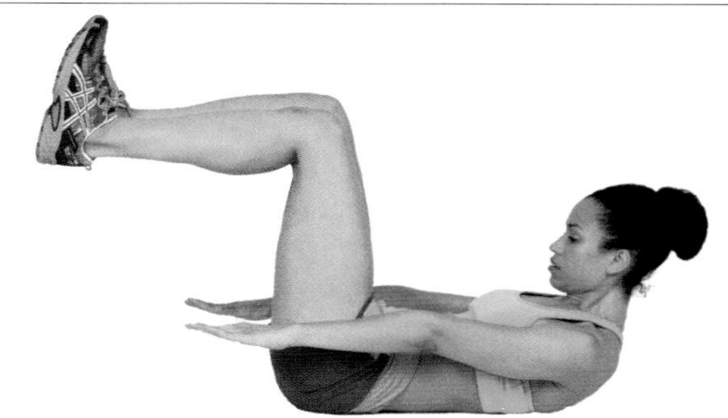

180 Thigh Rock Back

Come to a kneeling position with the legs slightly apart. Rest your arms at your sides and squeeze the core and back of your legs. Pull your abs strongly into your lower back and press your hips forward while you lean back from the knees. Keep your torso in one line.

181 Reverse Crunch

Bring your legs together and your arms to your sides. Engage the core muscles and levitate your legs off the floor into a right angle. Press your arms into the floor and squeeze your legs into your chest for a Reverse Crunch.

182 Swiss Ball Vertical Leg Crunch

Bring your legs straight up into the air with a Swiss ball between your ankles. Place your hands behind your head, squeeze the abs, and curl up into your Crunch. Hold in your Crunch position while you lower and lift your legs.

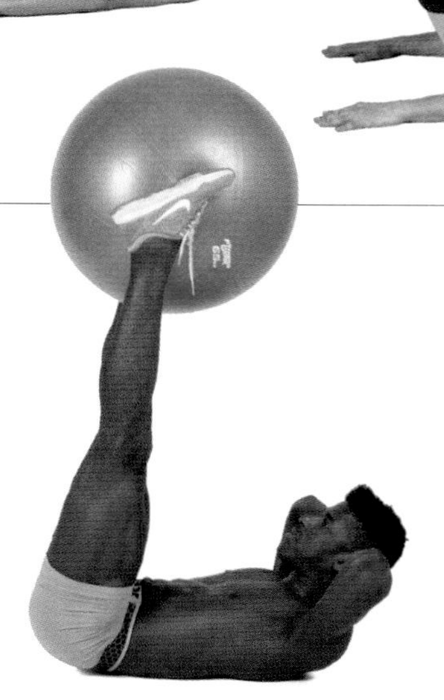

183 Alternating Heel Touches

Performing these heel touches is a great way to strengthen your overall core, and, more specifically, your side abdominal walls. You can do them slowly to work on stability, or quicken your touch tempo to add a little bit of cardio into your Crunch routine. Either way, it is a good way to warm up the core before any workout.

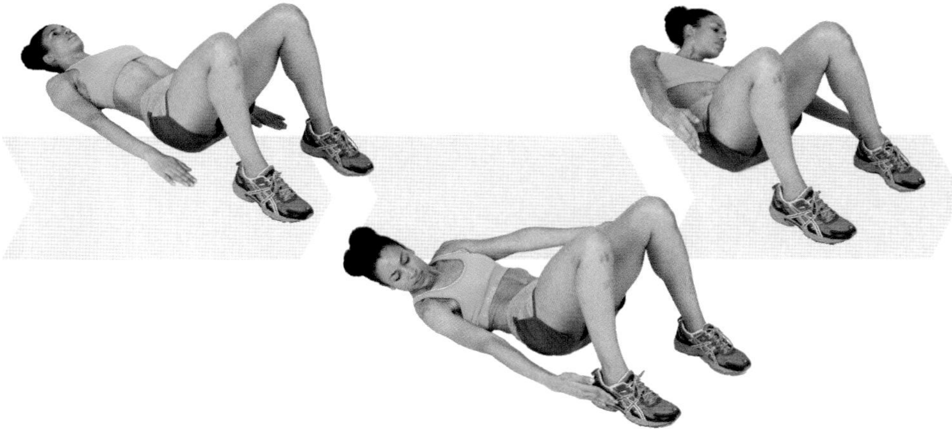

- Begin lying down in your standard Crunch position.
- Bring your legs close together and your arms to your sides.
- Squeeze your lower abdominals into your back and reach your arms forward and off the floor.
- Come into your Crunch and alternate tapping the outside of your right heel, and then the left heel.

184 Swiss Ball Crunch

Lie with your legs up, supported by a Swiss ball. Place your hands behind your head and dig your heels into the ball. Squeeze the abs, down and into the floor, and curl up into your Crunch.

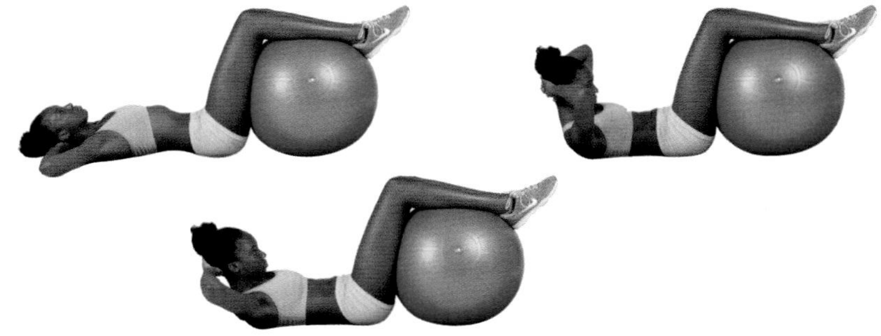

185 Chair Ab Crunch

Sit on a sturdy chair and hold the sides of it firmly with each hand. Scoot your hips to the front of the chair. Engage your lower abdominals and core muscles and pull your knees up into your chest. Hold for a moment, and lower the legs. Repeat.

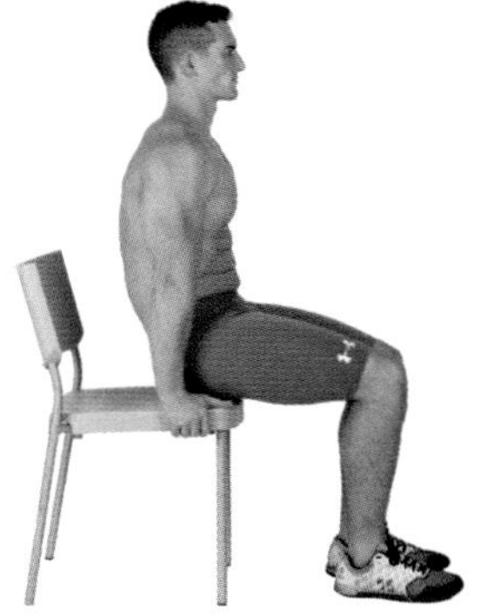

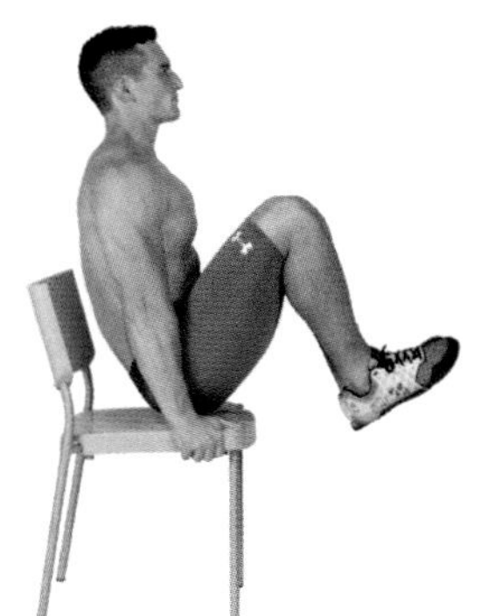

186 Balance Ball Crunch

Working with the balance ball in this Crunch variation provides an unstable, soft surface for the lower back and core to stabilize on. Giving you an element of instability, the balance ball will help you to develop balance in the core and lower back, as well as, work deeper into your abdominals.

- Lie down on a balance ball with the flat side flush on the floor.
- Press into the balance ball and put your hands behind your head.
- Raise your torso up into a Crunch.

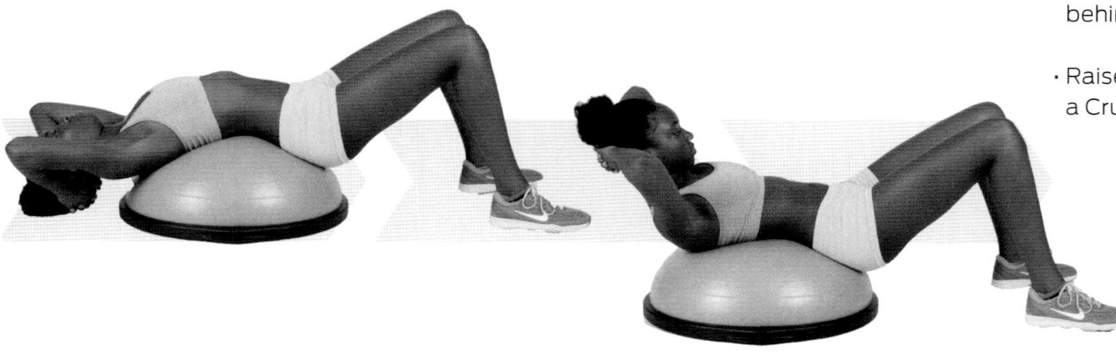

187 Balance Ball Bicycle Crunch

Lie with the balance ball supporting your upper back. Bend your legs and bring them together at a 90-degree angle from your hips. Come up into your Crunch position and hold there. Contracting your abs, raise your left leg toward you, then extend your right leg out and twist the upper body toward the left raised leg. Alternate sides, and repeat.

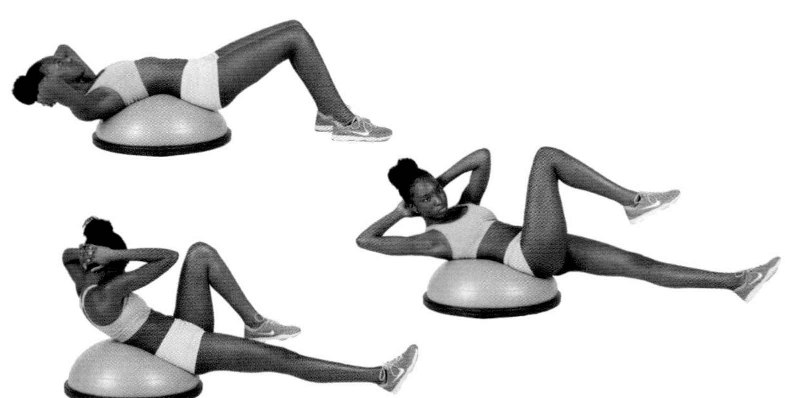

188 Balance Ball Oblique Crunch

Cross your arms over your chest and come to sit at the edge of the balance ball. Lie back, keeping your knees bent. Come into a Sit-Up position, engage the obliques deep along the front body, sit up tall, and rotate the torso to the right. Alternate sides, and repeat.

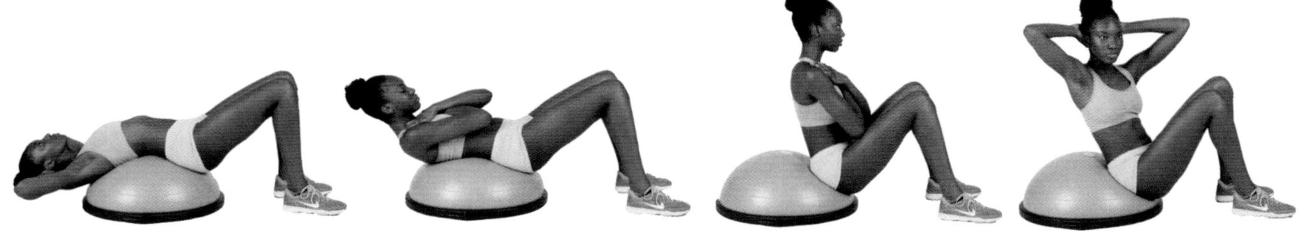

189 **Balance Ball Single-Leg Ab Extension**

Lying back on the balance ball with the arms behind your head, extend your right leg straight out in front of your body. As you bring your right leg in, squeeze the abs tightly and take your Sit-Up, bringing your chest to meet your right knee.

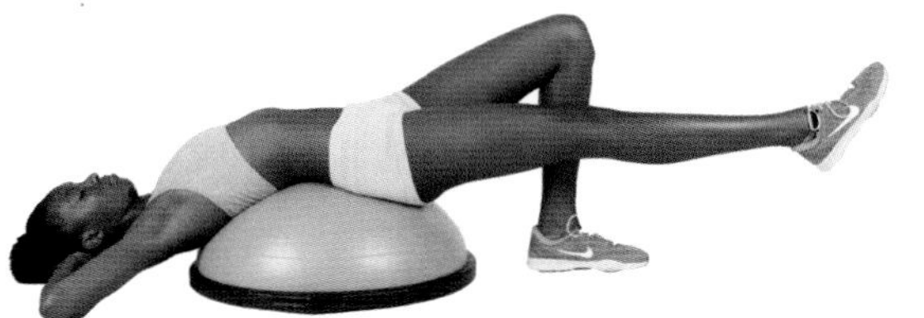

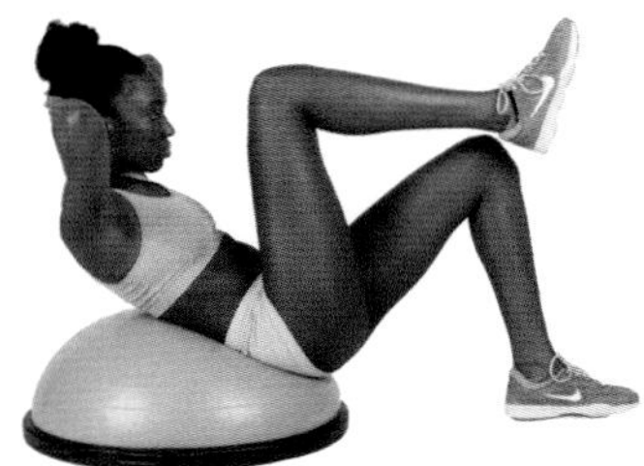

190 **Balance Ball Ab Roll-Backs**

Begin by sitting up on the balance ball. Ground your tailbone, down into the middle of the balance ball, for balance. Slowly lower your body back as far as you can manage with your feet still planted, then sit back up again.

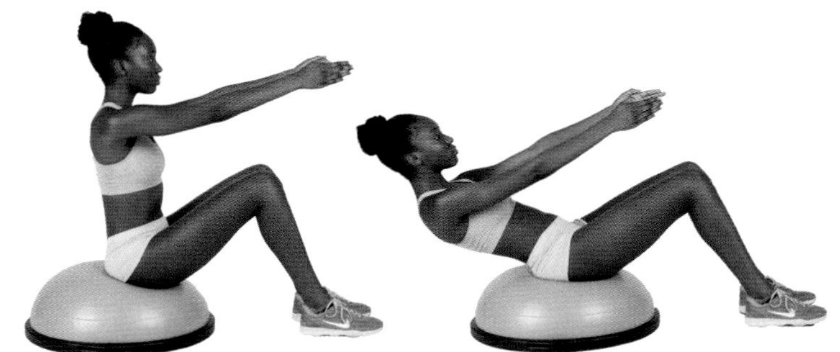

191 **Balance Ball Ab Twist**

Take a seat, balancing on the balance ball, and come up into your Crunch with your arms long out in front of you. Twisting side to side, let the knees be still each time you alternate your direction. Keep your torso on an angle, challenging the core.

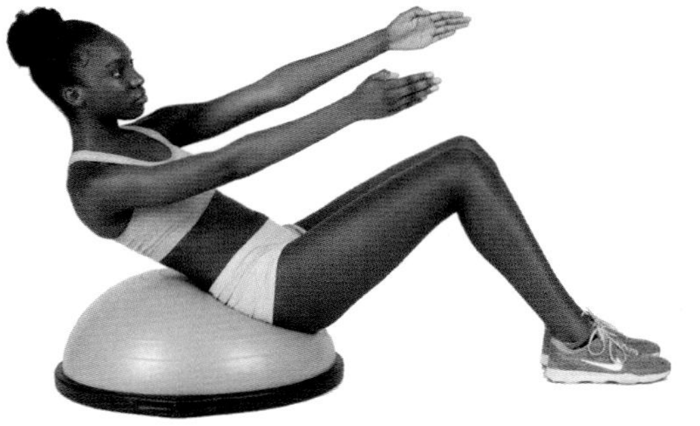

192 **Foam-Roller Diagonal Crunch**

Lie with your head and spine supported on the roller. With long legs, pull the abs in and sit up. Simultaneously, lift the right leg, and bring the left arm up overhead. Diagonally cross your left arm to meet your right foot.

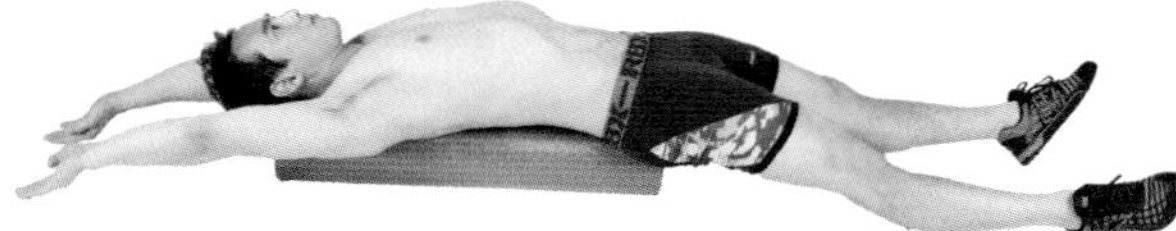

193 **Decline Oblique Crunch**

Hook your feet securely around the base of an incline bench facing downward. Lie back and engage your abdominals. Put your hands behind your head, and come into a Sit-Up, then twist the body to the right, once at the top of your movement. Alternate sides, and repeat.

194 **Crunch with Weighted Ball Hold**

From a lying position, take a weighted ball and hold it with both hands. Flex your feet and bring them up to the ceiling at a 90-degree angle from your hips. Keep your legs there, tuck in your chin, squeeze your abs, and come into a Sit-Up, reaching the ball up along your shins toward your feet.

195 **Diagonal Sit-Up**

Begin by sitting up with a strong core. Open your legs so that they are wider than shoulder-width apart. With a weighted ball, roll your body down to lying flat on the floor, stretching the arms diagonally to the left. In one move, lift the ball overhead and come into a dynamic Sit-Up. Repeat to the other side.

196 **Balance-Beam Crunch with Leg Lifts**

Lie down, balanced on the beam, with your legs bent. Grasp the beam with both hands overhead and scoop the lower abdominals. Bring your hands behind your head and prepare for your Crunch. Extend the right leg while squeezing the inner thighs together; go for your Crunch here. Switch legs, and repeat.

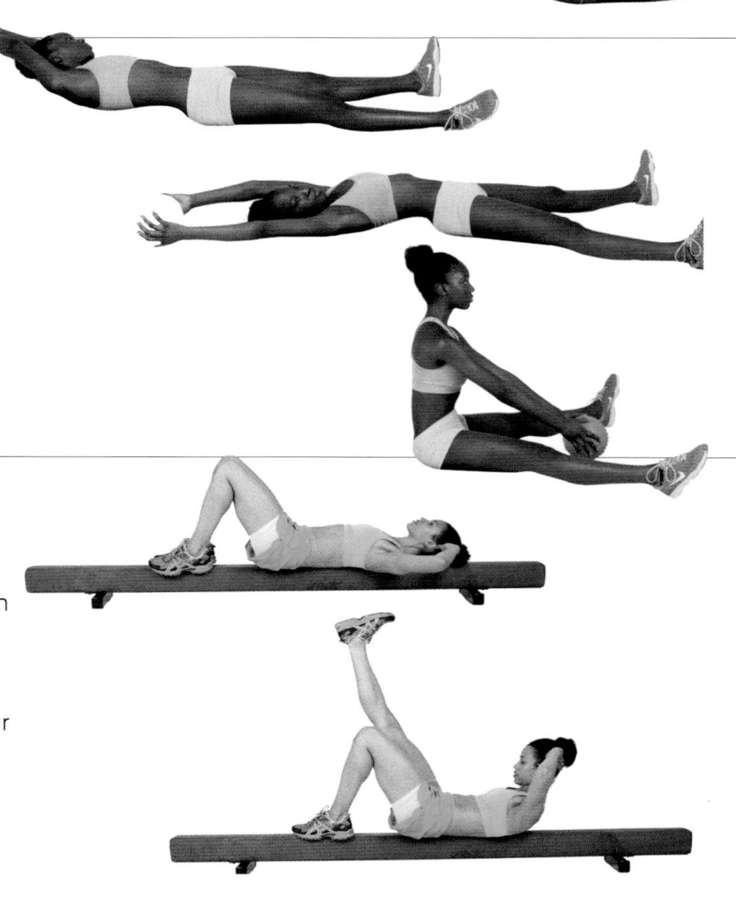

197 Rebounder Alternating Diagonal Ab Crunch

Lie back on a rebounder, with your feet on the floor and your hands behind your head. Begin by crunching and rotating your torso. As you twist and lift your trunk, bring your opposing knee toward your chest. Touch the opposite elbow to the knee, alternating from side to side. Perform each repetition on a quick but controlled tempo.

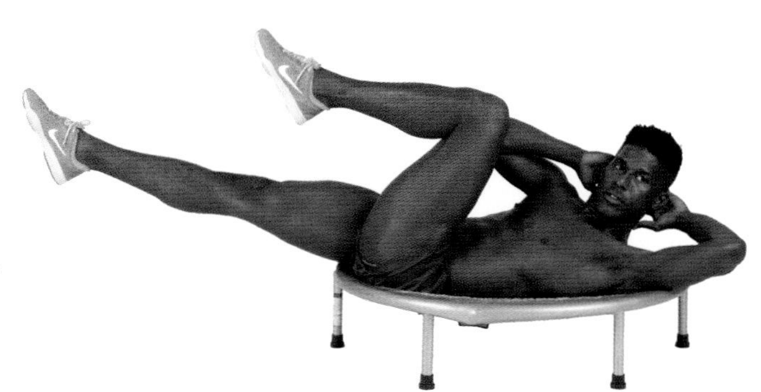

198 Suitcase Crunch

This Crunch variation targets the transverse abs, obliques, and the many layers of abdominals that run along the upper body. The aim is to bring the legs (alternated) and upper body together, closing them like a suitcase at the top of your movement. The weighted ball adds an extra degree of difficulty.

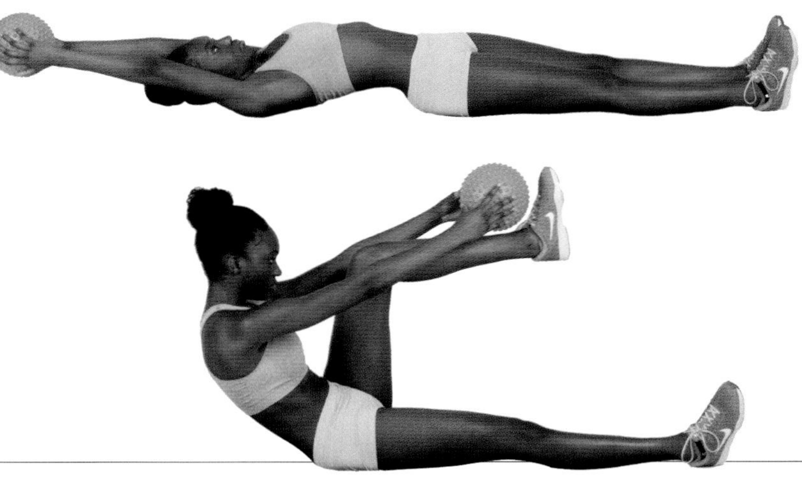

199 Toe Touch

Lie your body long on the floor. Take a Medicine ball and hold it with both hands. Flex your feet and bring them up to the ceiling at a 90-degree angle from your hips. Keep your legs there, tuck in your chin, squeeze your abs, and come into a Crunch, reaching the ball to your toes.

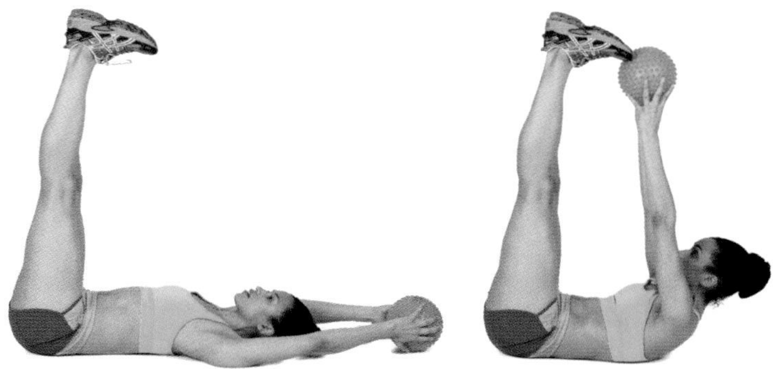

200 Oblique Roll-Down

Start by sitting up with your knees slightly bent and open. Bring the soles of your feet to the floor. Open your arms wide so that your body is facing the front. Rotate from your obliques to the left, keep the arms open, and roll your body down to the floor.

201

Sit-Up

The Sit-Up is a classic move that you are sure to find in just about all workout routines. Athletes and performers alike utilize Sit-Ups for their ability to stabilize and strengthen the upper body. The Sit-Up is a movement that works every inch of the core, from our multilayered abdominals through to our back bodies. Stabilizing the muscle groups that support our spine betters the total movement of our entire body, both upper and lower.

Correct form

When moving into your Sit-Up, curl through each part of your spine. This will ensure that you are really engaging each part of your abdominals.

Avoid

Don not pull on the neck with the hands to get your body off the floor. All of the work should be directly from the core.

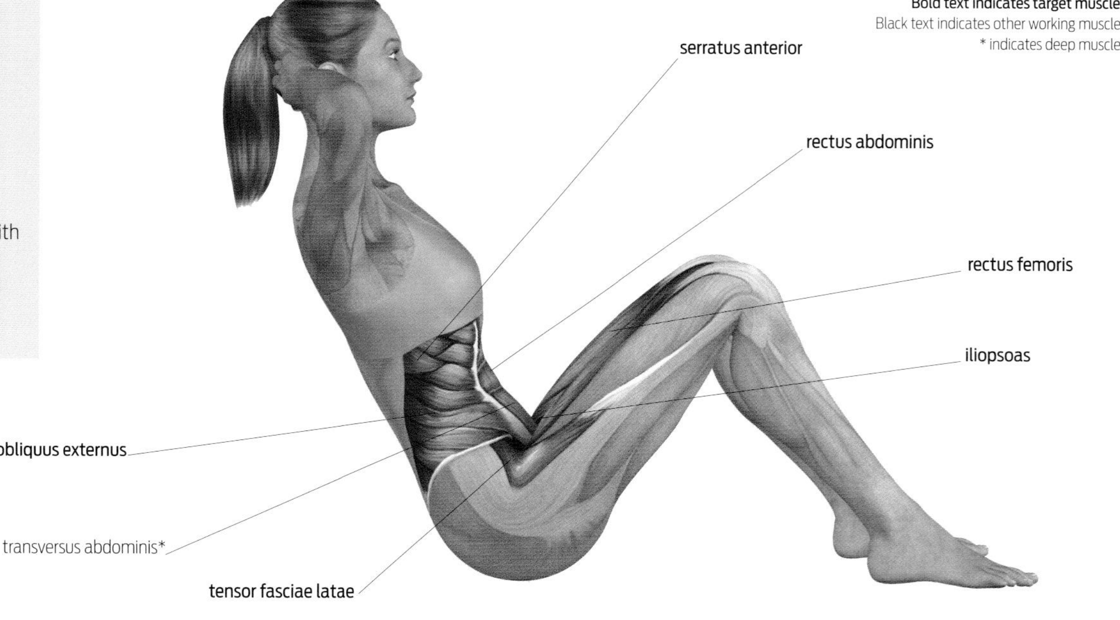

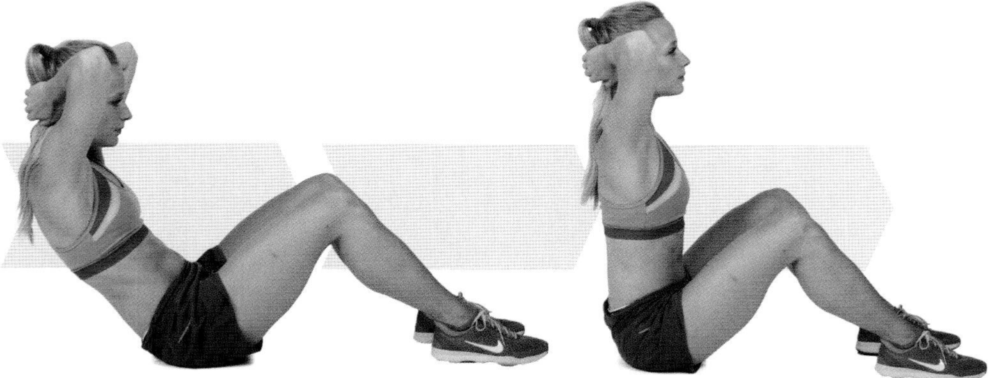

- Lie down on your back and bring your feet in, along the floor, toward your hips about 2 feet (60 centimeters).
- Stack your hands behind the lower part of your head.
- Engage your abs, tuck your chin into your chest, and curl your body up until your torso comes off the floor and is at a right angle to the floor.

202 Weighted Ball Sit-Up with Chest Press

Lie flat on your back with your legs bent. Hold a weighted ball in the center of your chest to begin. Squeeze your abs in and bring your torso all the way up into a Sit-Up. At the top of your Sit-Up, press the ball out in front of your chest on the diagonal.

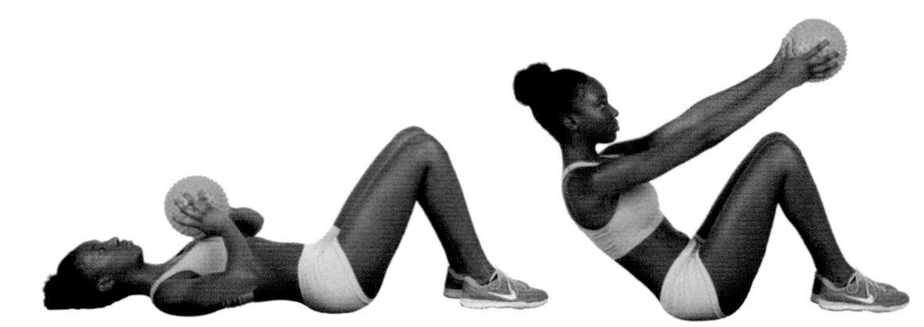

203 Alternating-Side Sit-Up

Lie supine with your legs slightly bent and your hands clasped behind your head. Push through your heels for support and raise your trunk off the floor, contracting your abs and rotating to the right so that your elbow touches your opposite knee. Lower and repeat, alternating to the other side.

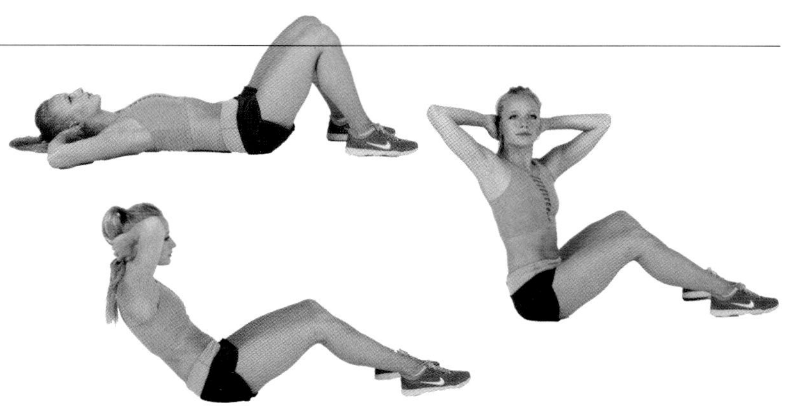

204 Roll-Up

Begin by lying down in your standard Sit-Up position. Bring your legs together and your arms to your sides. Engage the core muscles and squeeze your lower abdominals into the back. Reach your arms forward and off the floor, coming into a seated position.

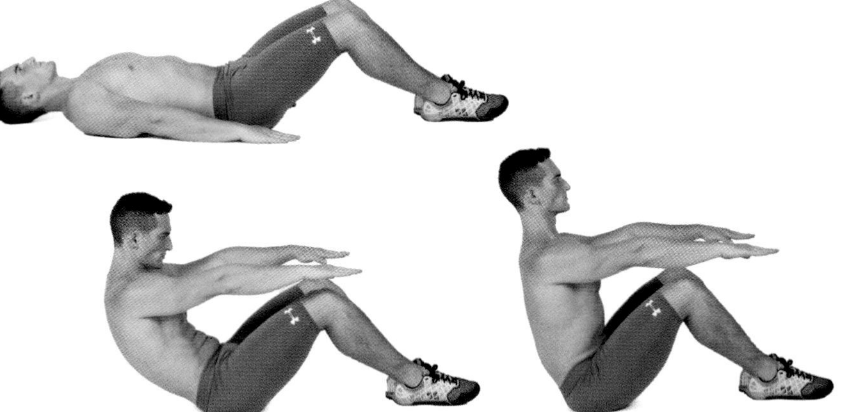

205 Weighted Ball Sit-Up

Lie flat on your back with your legs long and extended. Hold a weighted ball in the center of your chest to begin. Squeeze your abs in and bring your torso all the way up into a Sit-Up. Curl your body back down to lie flat, and repeat.

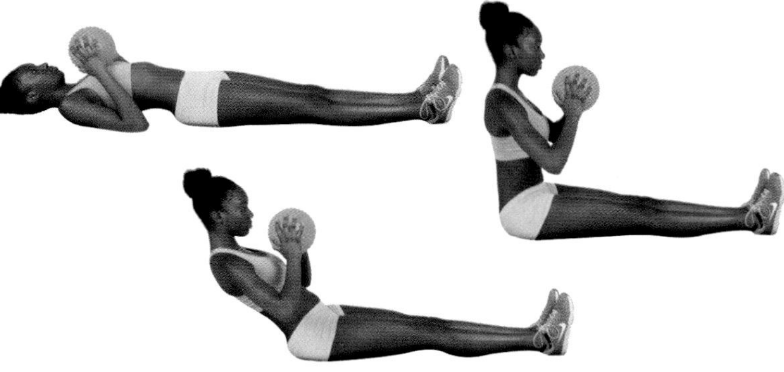

206 Straight-Leg Sit-Up

If you are looking to challenge the core a little deeper, and increase the stretch in your back and legs while performing your Sit-Up, try this straight-legged variation. This Sit-Up requires that you have a fair amount of flexibility in the hamstrings and hips.

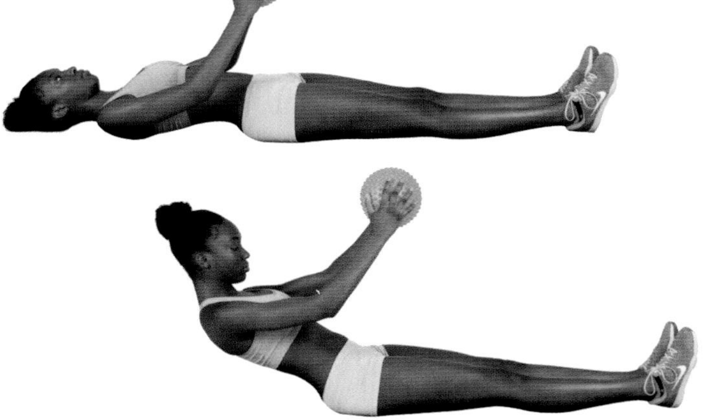

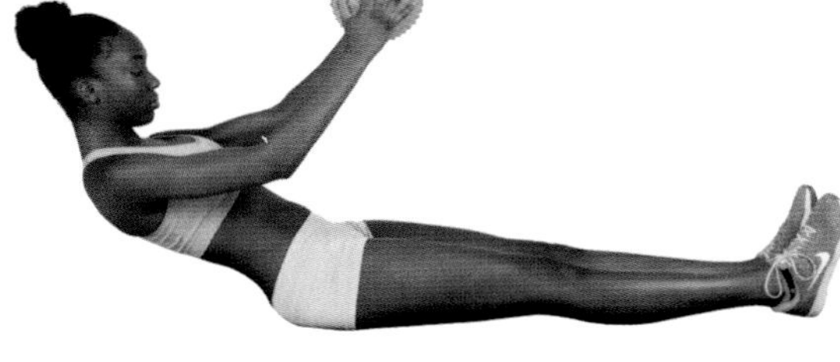

- Start by lying flat on your back with your legs long and extended.
- Hold a weighted ball over your head, along the floor, to begin.
- Squeeze your abs in and bring the ball over your chest, then reach it further forward until you have come all the way up into a sit up.
- Reach the ball directly up over your head, and curl your body back down to lie flat.

207 Balance Ball Sit-Up

Sit toward the edge of a balance ball with the flat side flush on the floor. The balance ball gives you an added element of balance and supports the lower back. Perform your Sit-Up here.

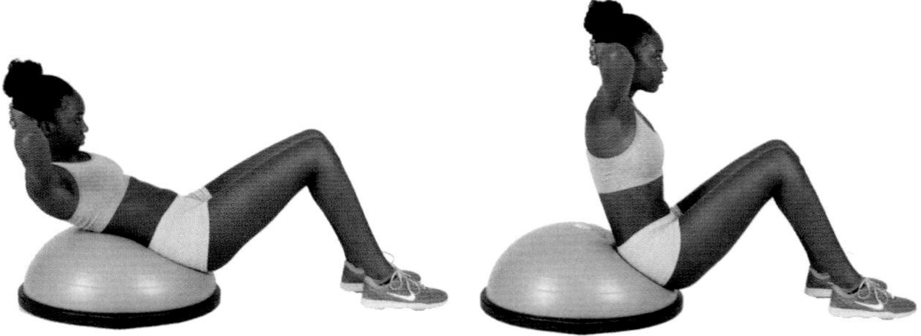

208 Foam-Roller Sit-Up and Reach

One of the most challenging ways to enhance your Sit-Up is by performing it on a foam roller. The cylinder shape of the roller asks you to find your balance while maintaining constant contact between the roller and your spine. Perform as you would a regular Sit-Up, but with your legs slightly more open to help you stay balanced.

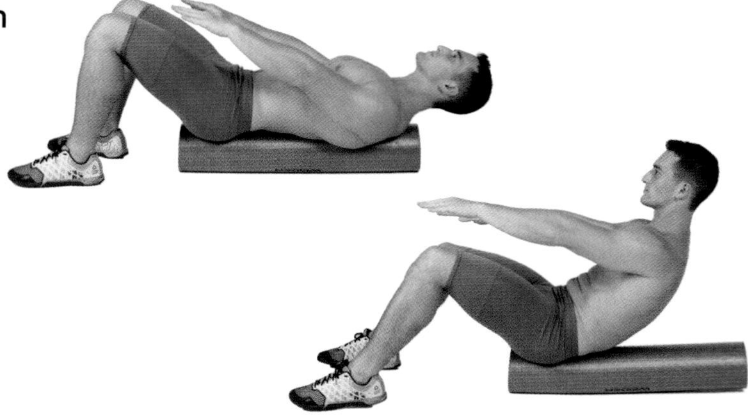

209 V-Up

Start by lying flat on your back with your legs long and extended. Hold a weighted ball over your head to begin. Squeeze your abs in and bring the ball over your chest. Simultaneously, pull your legs forward and up off the floor, and reach your arms toward your feet.

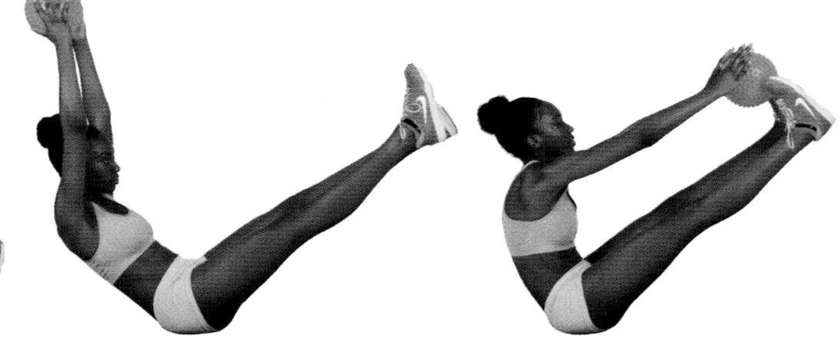

210 Sit-Up and Throw

Lie on your back with your legs bent. Hold a Medicine ball overhead, along the floor. Squeeze your abs in and bring your torso all the way up into a Sit-Up. At the top of your Sit-Up, launch the ball out in front of your chest on the diagonal.

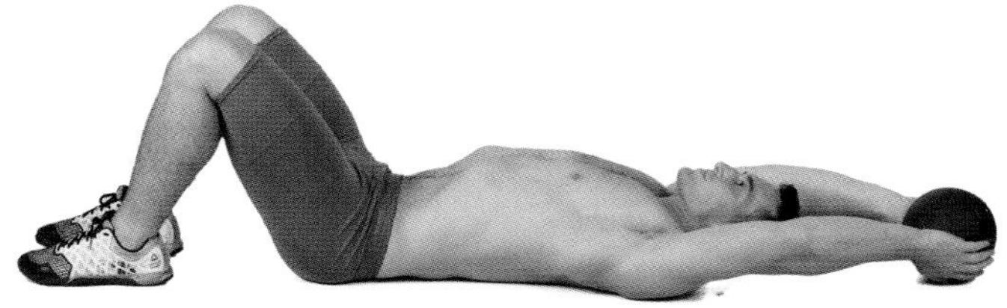

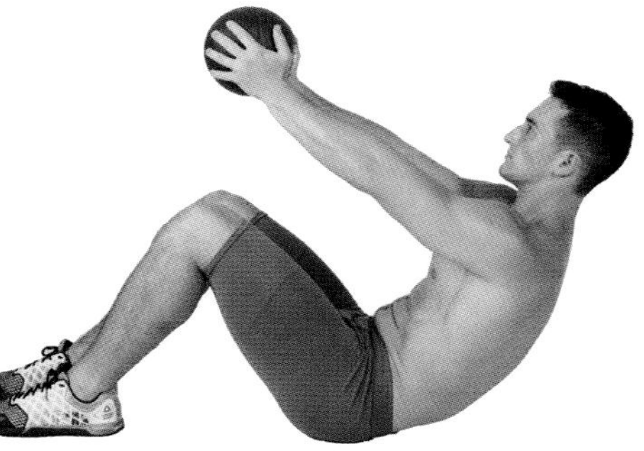

211 Side Lift Bend

Begin by lying on the left side of your body. Place your left hand behind your head and your right hand along your right side. Have the feet flexed and the body long and in one line. Squeeze in the abs, lift the legs, and crunch into the right side of your abdominals. Lower, and repeat.

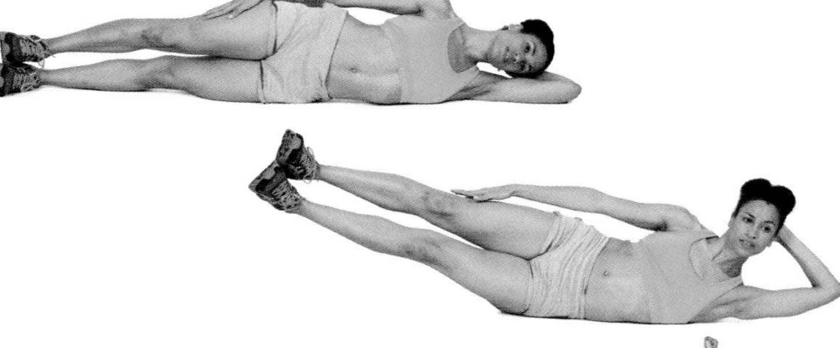

212 Turkish Get-Up

Lie straight along the floor and bend your right knee, bringing the right foot to the floor. Extend your right arm up, in line with your chest, and keep the left arm long along the floor. Slowly, keeping your right arm up, curl into a Sit-Up, bringing the left foot onto the ground, and then stand.

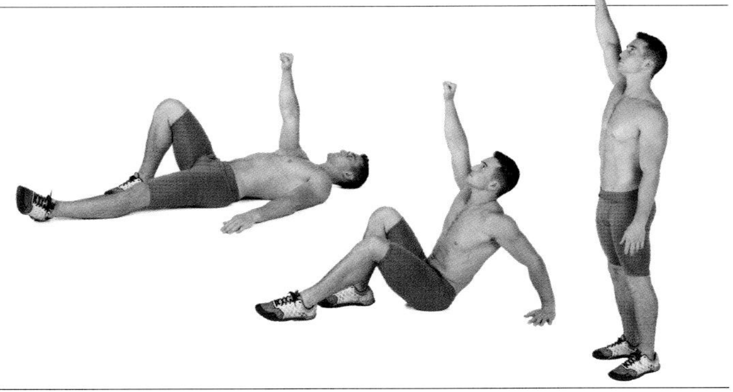

213

Plank

The Plank is a core exercise that can be found in almost all abdominal-focused workouts like yoga, Pilates, ballet barre, and calisthenics. Planking is all about keeping the core stabilized, suspended in the air, balancing on two arms and the balls of the feet. Not only does it strengthen the core muscle groups, it's also great for stabilizing the lower back and aiding with back pain.

serratus anterior

obliquus externus

obliquus internus*

rectus abdominis

transversus abdominis*

Annotation Key

Bold text indicates target muscles

Black text indicates other working muscles

* indicates deep muscles

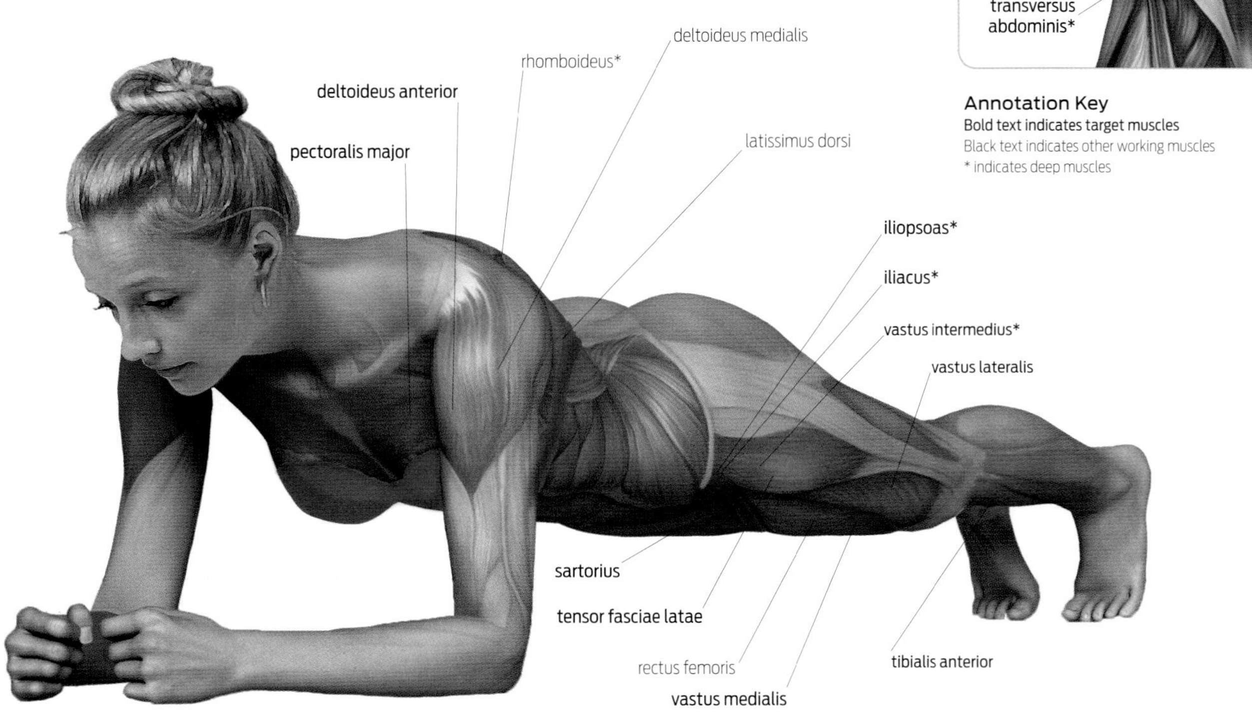

- Bring your body to balance on your forearms and the balls of your feet.
- Squeeze the abs in deeply, up and away from the floor underneath you.
- Lengthen the spine by reaching the top of your head away from your feet.

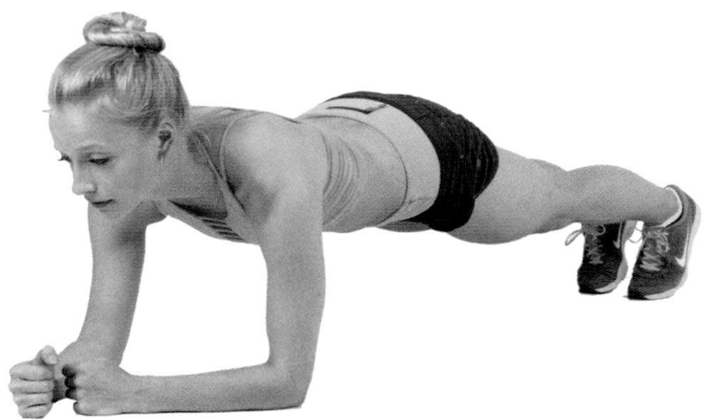

Correct Form

Keep proper alignment in your Plank by imagining that your body is reaching away from the core in both directions.

Avoid

Do not tense the neck or shoulders by trying to lift the focus of your eyes up further than you need to. Keep your gaze down and soft.

214 **Simple Plank**

Bring your body to balance on your forearms and knees. Squeeze the abs in deeply, up and away from the floor underneath you. Lengthen the spine by reaching the top of your head away from your knees, and bring your thighs down toward the floor.

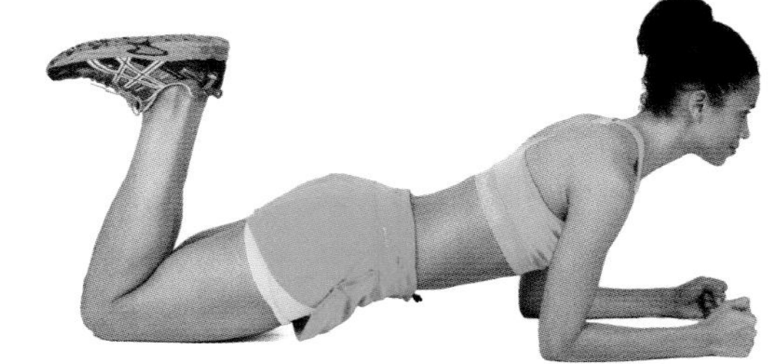

215 **High Plank**

Assume your Plank position with your hands shoulder-width apart on the floor. Engaging the abs up into the lower back, bring the knees down together to touch the floor briefly, then straighten them again.

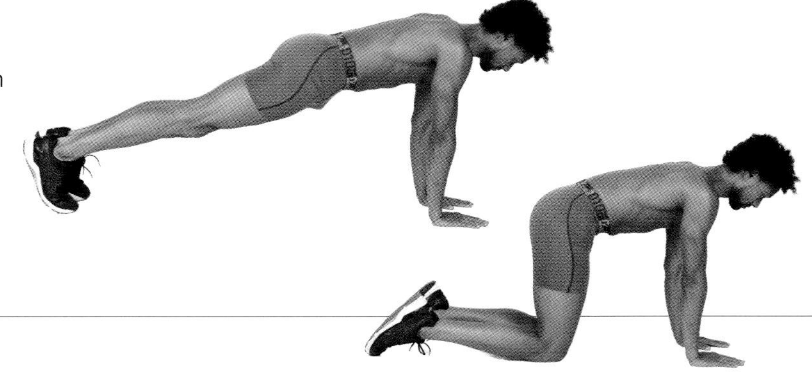

216 **Forearm Plank**

Bring your body to balance on your forearms and the balls of your feet in an upward Plank. Squeeze the abs in deeply, up and away from the floor underneath you. Lengthen the spine by reaching the top of your head away from your feet.

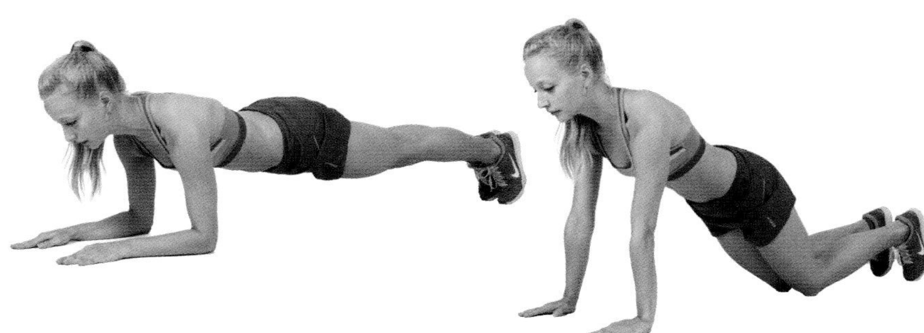

217 **Side Bend Plank**

Begin by sitting on the left hip. Reach your left hand out from your body and push your hips up, coming into a Side Plank. Let your right arm rest on the right thigh. Take turns sitting and pushing up into your Side Plank.

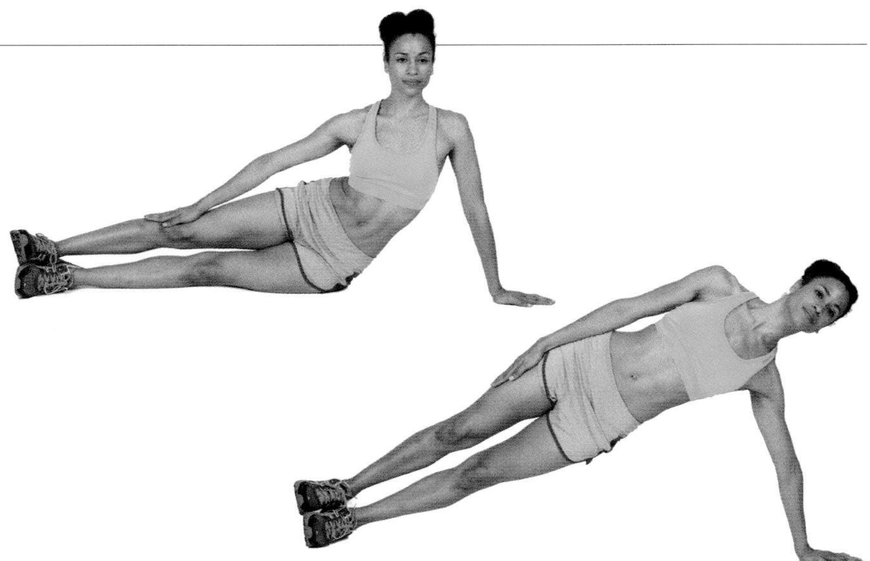

218 T-Stabilization

Start in your standard Plank with both palms flush with the floor beneath you. Shift the weight of your feet onto the side of one foot, stacking your feet on top of each other. Spin your upper body open and balance on one hand, stabilizing your side body and core.

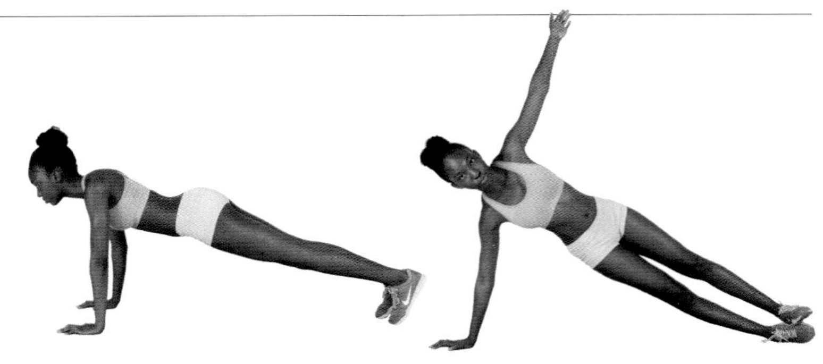

219 Twist

Start in your T-Stabilization with the right palm flush with the floor beneath you, your feet stacked on top of each other, and your left arm extended open. Inhale, exhale, squeeze the sides of your body into your center, and spin your upper body, reaching the left arm under your right side.

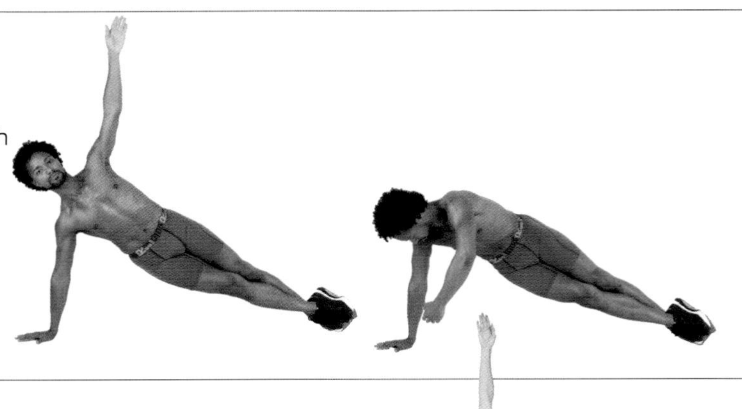

220 Balance-Beam T-Stabilization

Start in your standard Plank with both palms flush with the beam under you. Open your body to the right and stack your feet on top of each other. Extend your upper body open and balance on the left hand, engaging your side body and core.

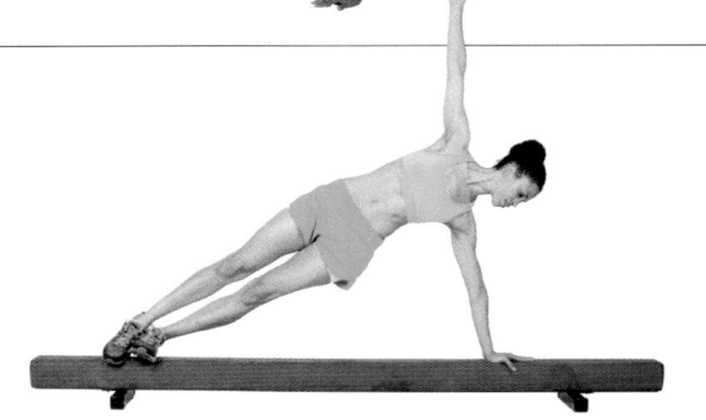

221 Plank Roll-Down

Begin with a long spine, standing tall. Lengthen your abs and pull in your core muscles. Bend at the hips, bringing your hands to the floor. Leave your feet planted where they are, and walk your hands out into a Plank position. Hold there, and then walk back in to stand.

Strengthen

Planks are one of the most simple moves to do. They are excellent for building up those deep inner core muscles that provide stability for your lower back. Planks are also excellent for improving posture, balance, and reducing back pain.

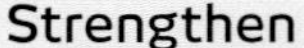

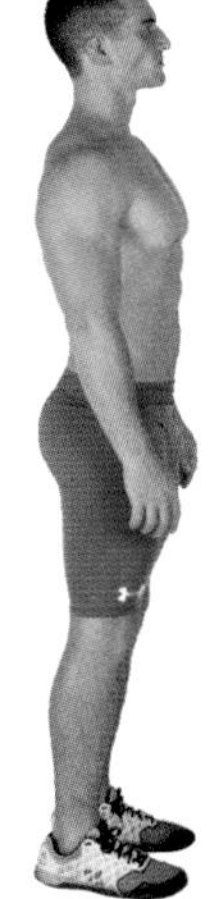

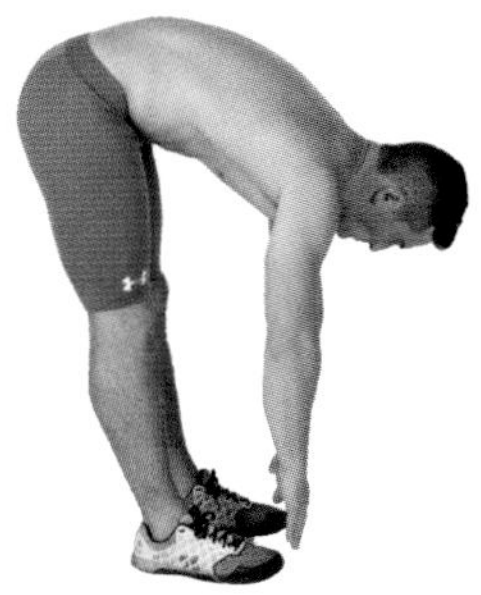

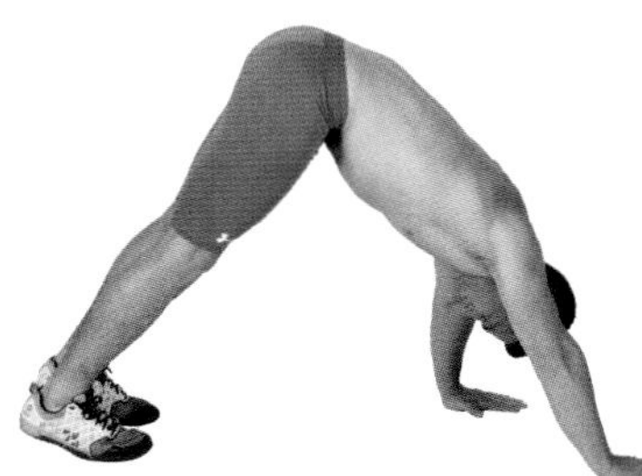

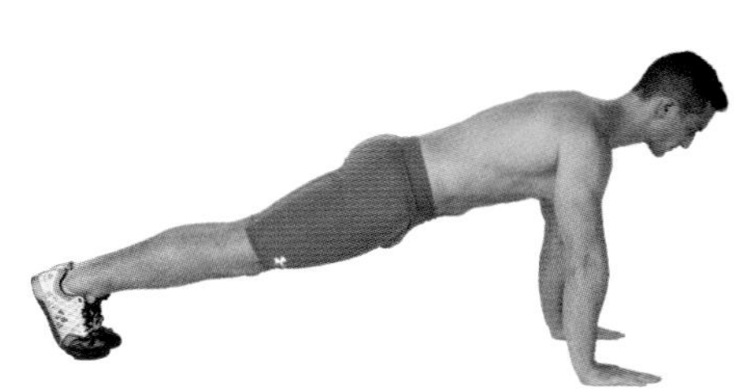

222 Hand Walk-Out

Start by standing with the legs in a shoulder-width position. Bend at the hips and reach your hands to the floor. Walk each palm out further forward and away from the feet. When you have reached a Plank position, hold there. Walk back in, and repeat.

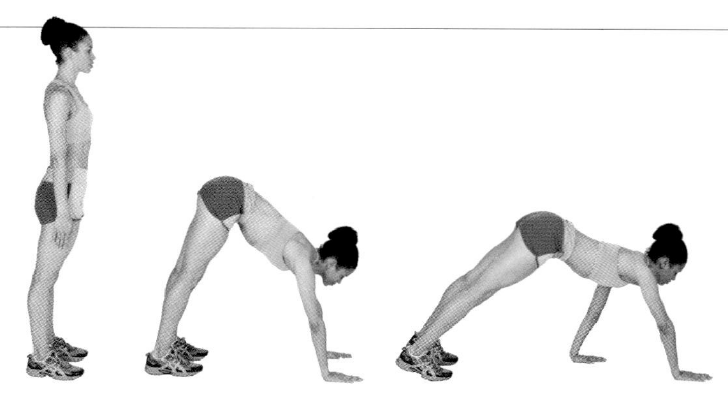

223 Pointer

Assume the drop position, and then extend your left arm straight forward while raising your left leg until your whole body forms a straight line from toe to shoulder. Pause at the top of the movement and lower back to the drop position. Repeat on the other side.

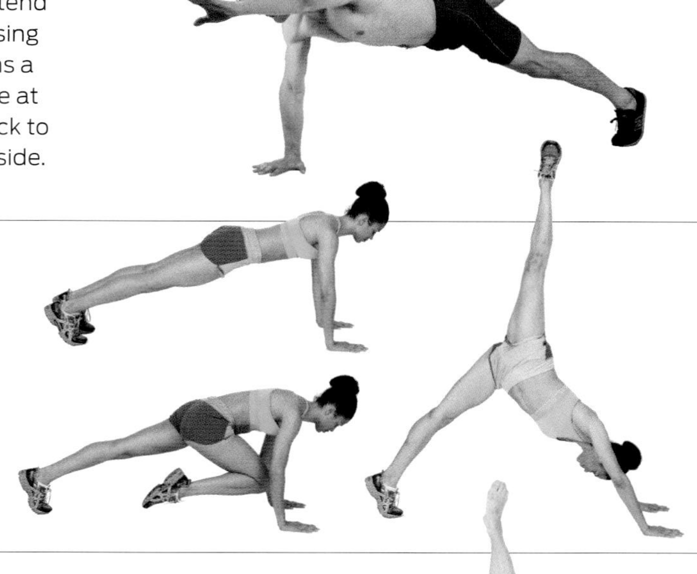

224 Knee-Pull Plank

Start in your Plank. Strongly pull your core up and bring your right knee close into your chest. Hold your Plank position and push your foot out and up to the ceiling, keeping your abs and core long and engaged.

225 High-Raise Plank

Balance in the standard High Plank with your palms down. Flex at the hips and bring your right leg up to the ceiling as you lower your torso so that it forms a straight line with the leg. Lower back into the Plank, and repeat on the other side.

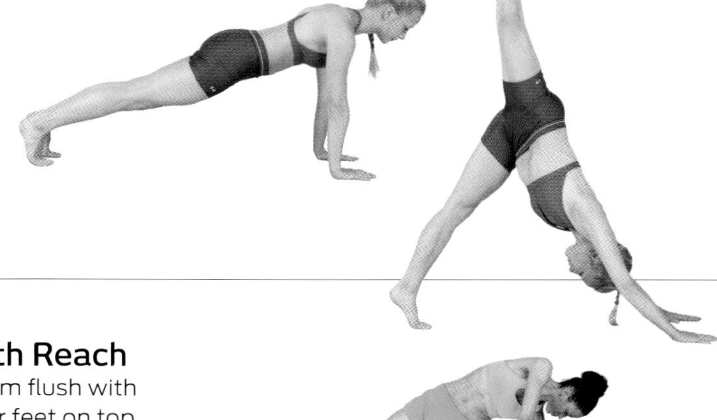

226 Balance-Beam Side Plank with Reach

Start in your Side Plank with the left palm flush with the balance beam under you. Stack your feet on top of each other and extend your right arm open. Inhale, exhale, squeeze the sides of your body into your center, and spin your upper body, reaching the right arm under your left side.

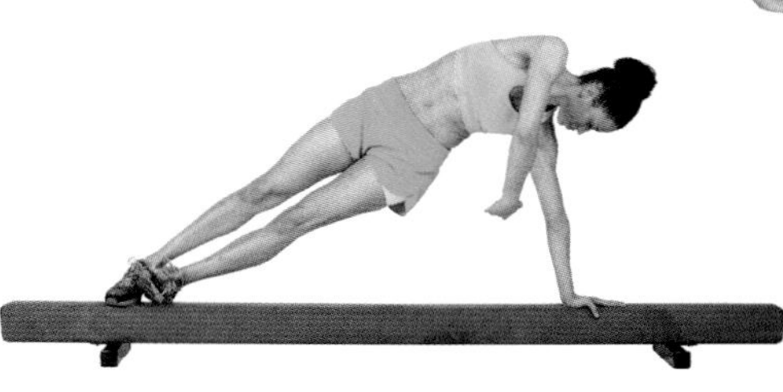

227 **High Plank with Jacks Variation**

Start in your Plank position with the legs and arms extended long. Put the weight in your hands, squeeze in the abs and jump your feet open wide. Jump the legs back together, and repeat.

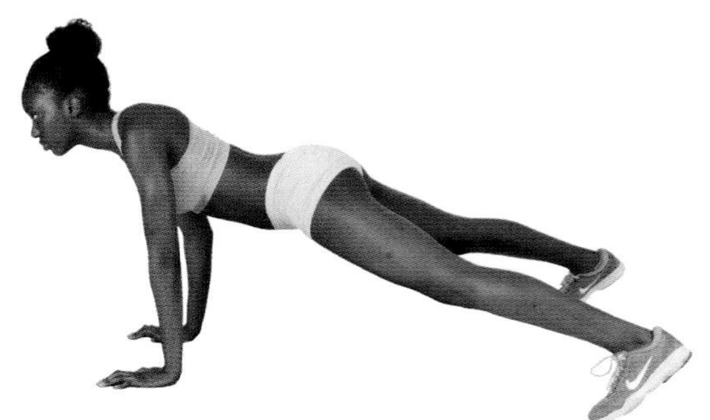

228 **Swiss Ball Transverse Abs**

Working the deepest layer of the core is this Plank variation. Bring the weight of your upper body into your forearms while balancing on the Swiss ball. Push your forearms into the ball and squeeze the abs very deeply.

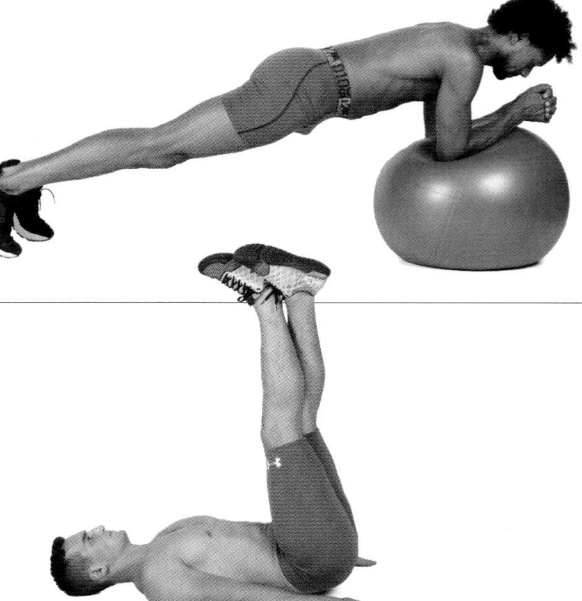

229 **Abdominal Hip Lift**

Lie on your back with your legs reaching long up into the air. Cross the ankles and bring your arms to the sides of your body, on the floor. Squeeze your lower abdominals into your back, engage the hips, and push your heels up to the ceiling.

230 **Balance-Beam Leg Lifts**

Lie down, balanced on the beam, with your legs extended out long from the hips. Grasp the beam with both hands overhead and scoop the lower abdominals. Raise your legs up into the air with your feet pointed. Keeping your back flat along the beam, pull the abs in again and lower the legs back down to the starting position.

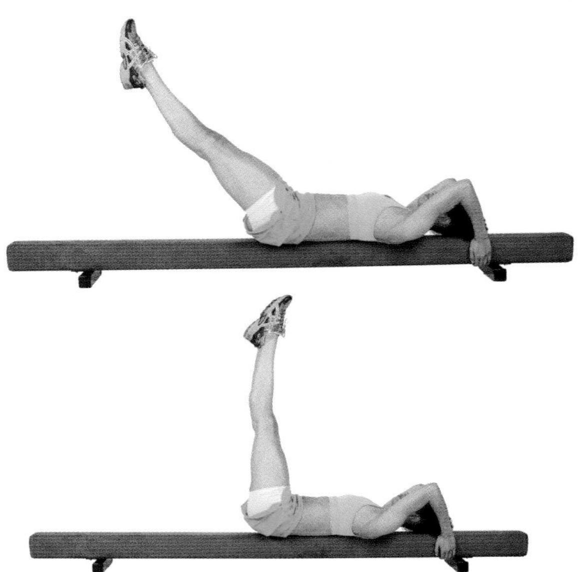

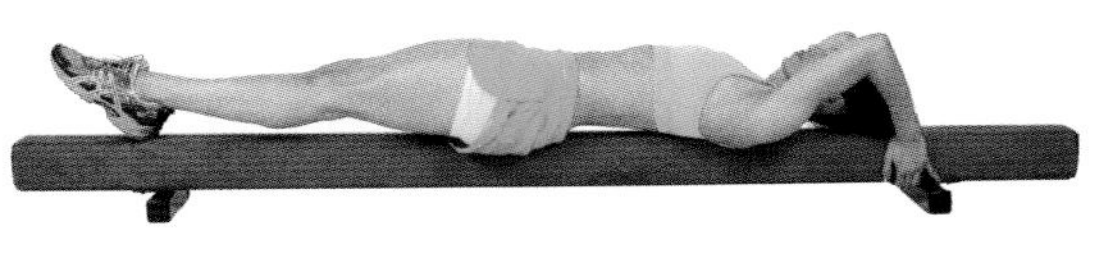

231 Hip Twist

This variation gives you the opportunity to work the deep inner core muscles, which can be hard to reach sometimes. By keepng the legs elevated in the air and stabilizing from deep inside your core, you will strengthen both internal and external abdominal groups.

- Sit down with your legs extended long in front of you.
- Lean back, putting some weight into your arms and hands.
- Scoop the lower abdominals and lift the legs up into the air with your feet flexed.
- Keeping your chest open to the front, sway your legs from side to side.

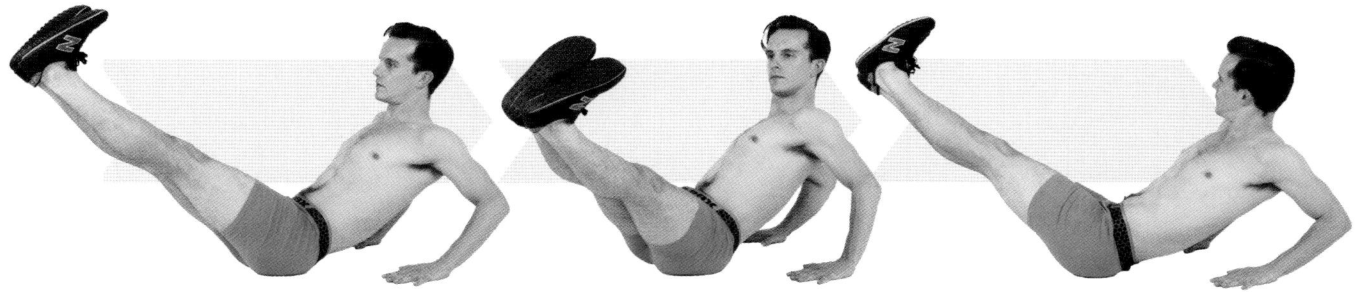

232 Front Plank with Leg Lifts

Front Planks are challenging because they require you to engage all muscle groups in the body in order to stay in perfect balance. They are great for stabilizing the shoulders and upper back, as well as the pelvis and hip rotators.

- Start by sitting on the floor with your legs extended out in front of you.
- Place your hands behind your hips and push into the floor.
- Elevate your hips up off the floor by squeezing your abs deeply.
- Lift your right leg and lower it, then the left. Take turns alternating legs.

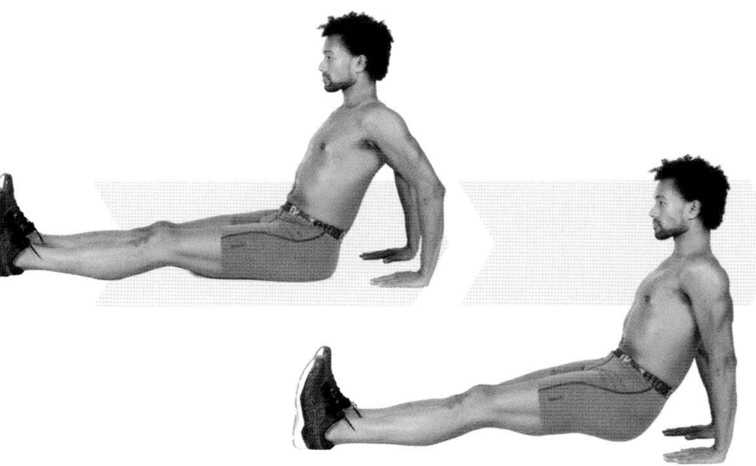

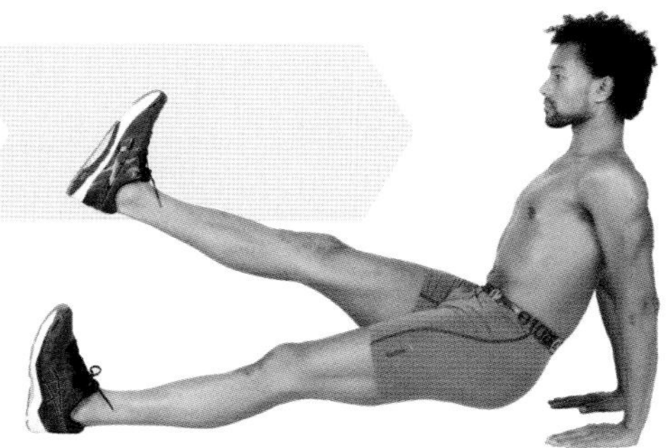

233 Reverse Plank with Leg Lifts

With your legs long out in front of you, place your hands down at your hips. Dig your heels into the ground and push your hips up into a Reverse Plank. Keeping the weight balanced between your hands and heels, take turns lifting each leg up to the sky.

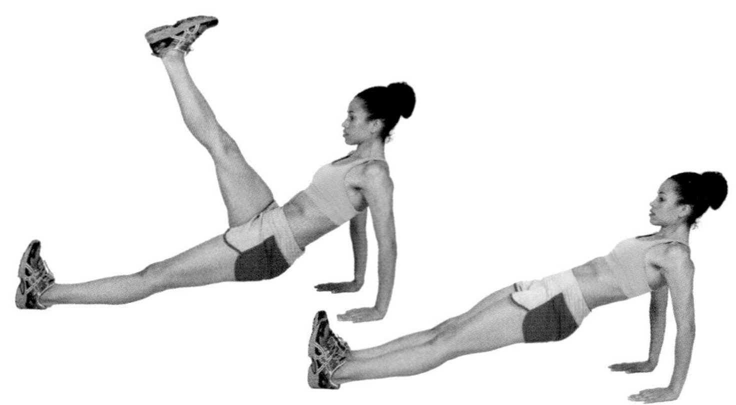

234 Swimming

Lie face down on the floor with your arms stretched overhead and the legs long. Pull the abs up into the back, lift the right leg off the floor and, simultaneously, reach the left arm forward. Alternate arms and legs as if you were swimming.

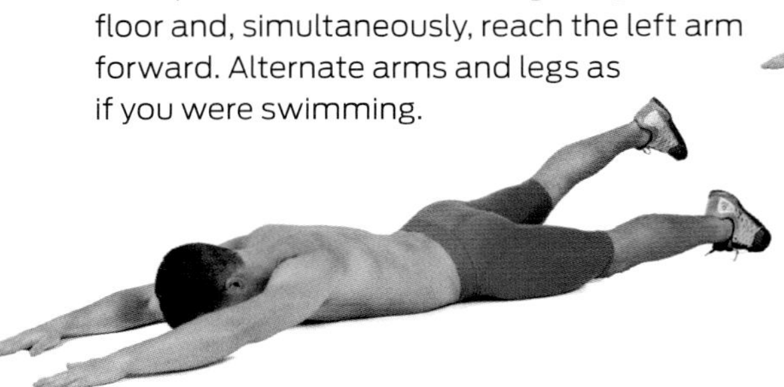

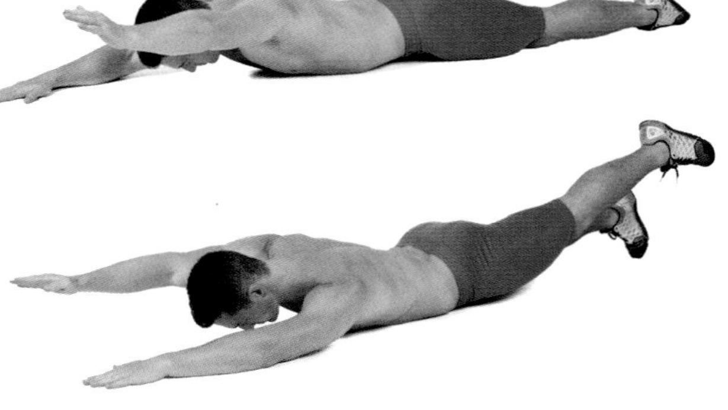

235 Superman

Extend your body long on top of a yoga mat. Bring your arms close together overhead and bring your legs to touch, squeezing the inner thighs tightly. Engage the abs strongly and, in one move, lift your arms and legs off the floor together.

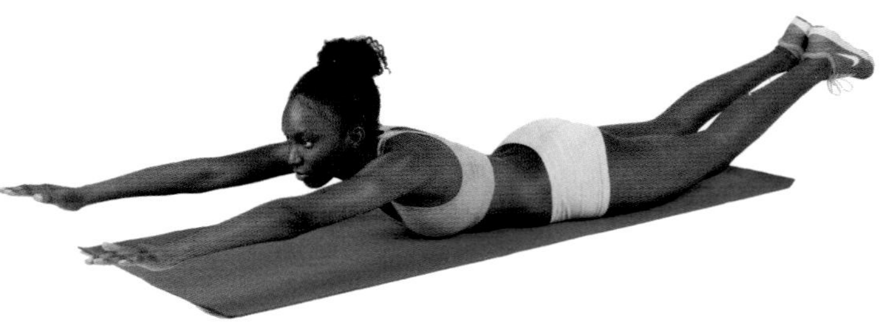

236 Advanced Superman

Lie face down along the floor. Bend your arms and bring your hands together at the base of your neck. Squeezing the inner thighs tightly, engage the abs strongly and, in one move, lift your torso and legs off the floor together.

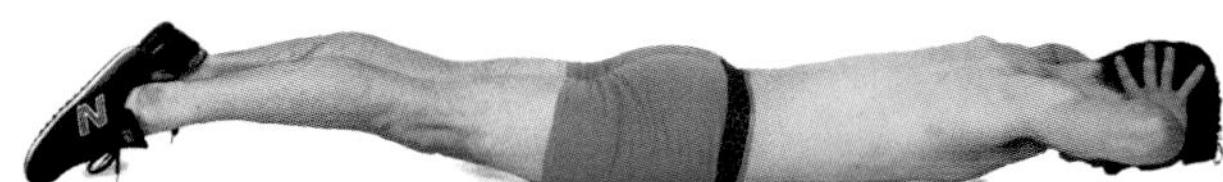

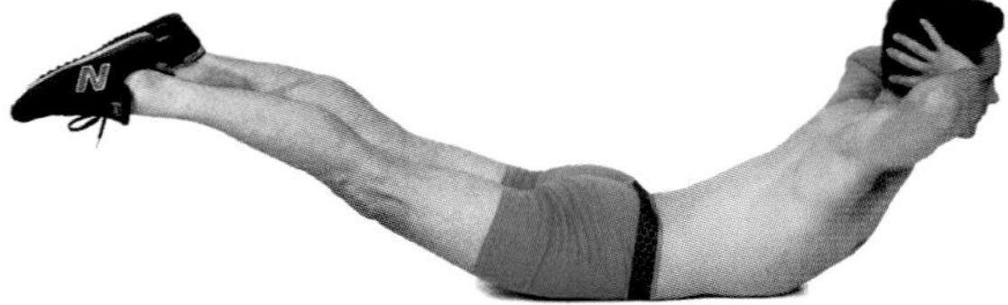

237 Weighted Superman

Perform your Advanced Superman holding a weighted ball. While lying long on the floor, take a weighted Medicine ball into your hands. Reach the arms forward and the legs back, bringing both ends of your body up off the floor.

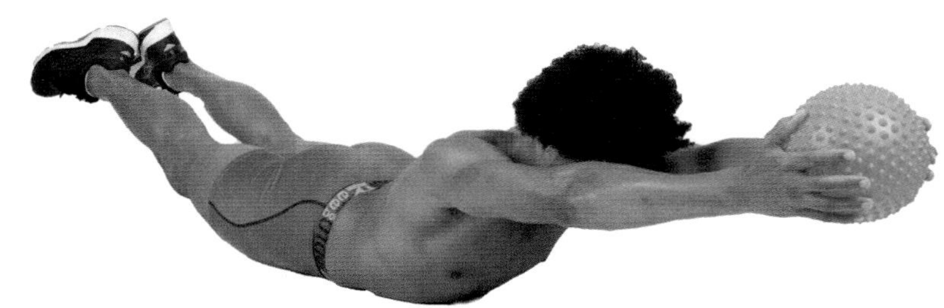

238 Balance Ball Superman

Lie face down with the balance ball underneath your abs. Bend your arms and bring your hands together at the base of your neck. Squeezing the inner thighs tightly, engage the abs strongly and, in one move, lift your torso and legs off the floor together.

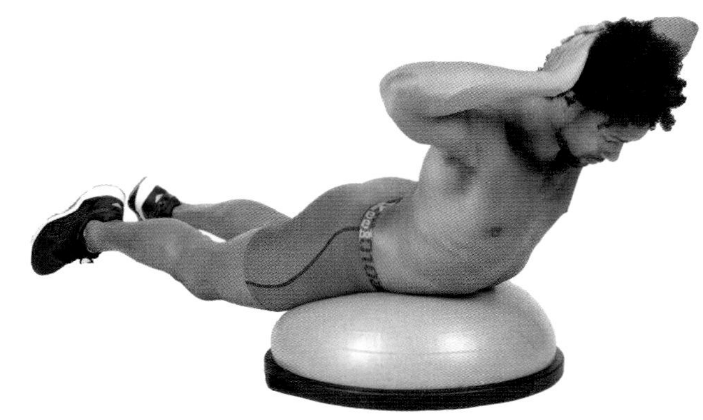

239 Foam Roll-Out

This is a Plank variation. It is challenging because it requires you to engage all muscle groups in the body in order to stay in perfect balance. Rollouts are great for stabilizing the shoulders and upper back, as well as the pelvis and hip rotators.

- Start by sitting on your foam roller with your legs extended out in front of you.
- Place your hands on the floor behind your hips and push into the floor.
- Pull your hips back and up behind you, curving the spine forward.

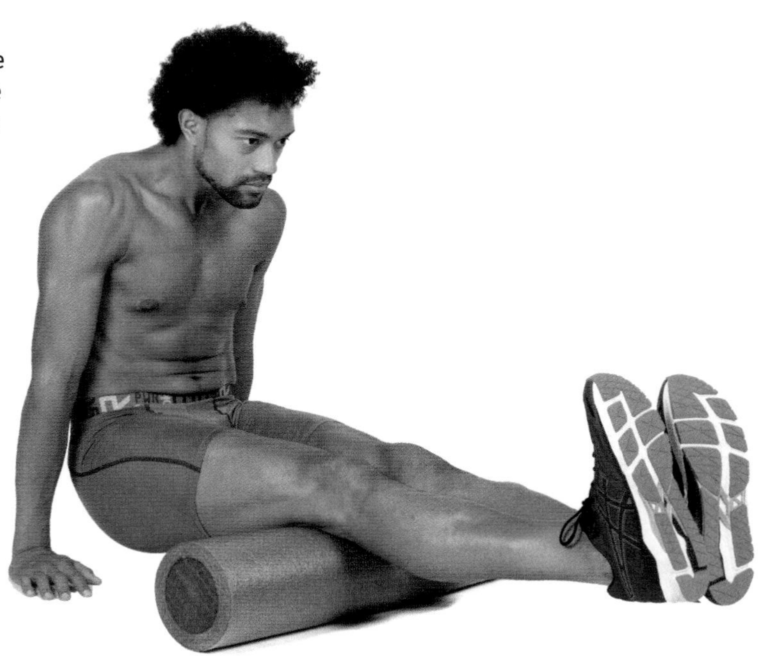

240 Foam-Roller Plank Alternative

Using your foam roller to balance on while in Plank is a good alternative to the balance ball, especially if you have weak wrists or elbows. The foam roller creates a more stable base, and is easier to balance on than the balance ball.

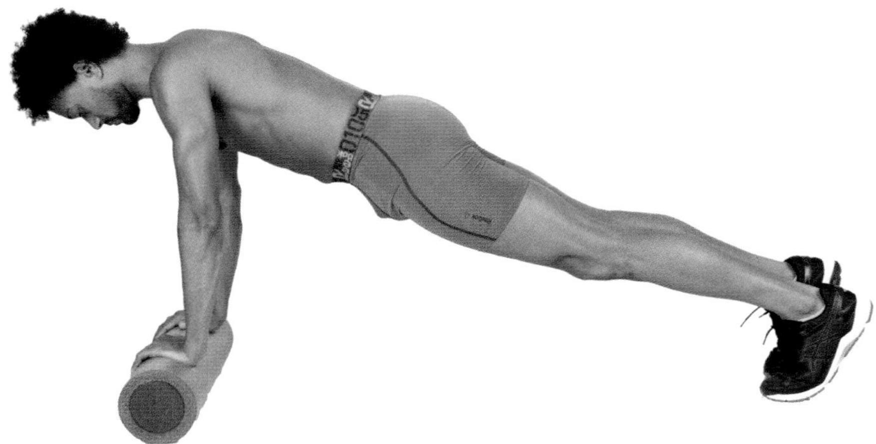

- Lay a foam roller perpendicular to your body.
- Stack your hands shoulder-width on the foam roller.
- Come up into your Plank, balancing with the weight equally divided between your feet and hands.

241 Foam-Roller Plank

Start with your lower legs propped up on a foam roller, knees on the ground. Place your forearms on the ground, shoulder-width apart, and come into your Plank by extending the legs long, and balancing the weight onto the fronts of your legs. Squeeze the abs in strongly.

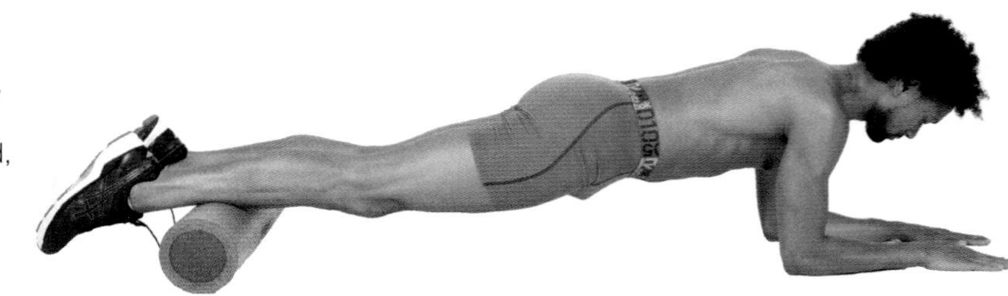

242 Rolling Foam-Roller Plank

Place a foam roller under your shins and come into a standard Plank. With your arms straight and hands flat on the floor, bring the weight of your body forward, suck your core in tight to your spine, bend your knees, and roll your legs up toward your chest.

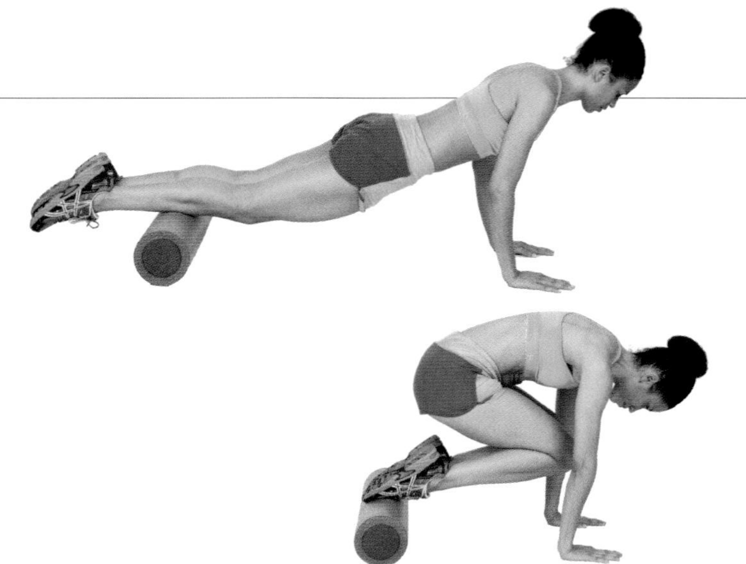

243 Balance Ball Plank to Tap Out

This variation is great for stabilizing the core and the lower back. If you have issues with lower-back pain, this is the exercise for you! By utilizing an unstable surface and your own body's weight in this Plank, you will create strong abs that support the whole core.

- Place the balance ball with the round side up.
- Come into a Forearm Plank position (#216) with the balls of your feet at the center of the balance ball.
- Keeping your body in one straight line, walk the right foot out to the side of the balance ball, then walk the left foot out.
- Step the right foot, then the left foot back up onto the balance ball. Repeat as much as you'd like.

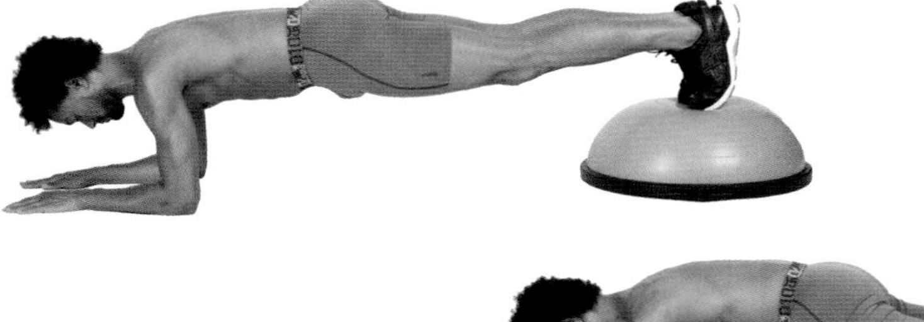

244 Side Plank and Hip Raise with Feet on the Balance Ball

Come into a Side Forearm Plank with your feet stacked at the center of your balance ball. Let your free hand rest on your hip. Slowly lower and lift the hips, down to and up off the floor. This is an awesome exercise for stabilizing the lower back and core.

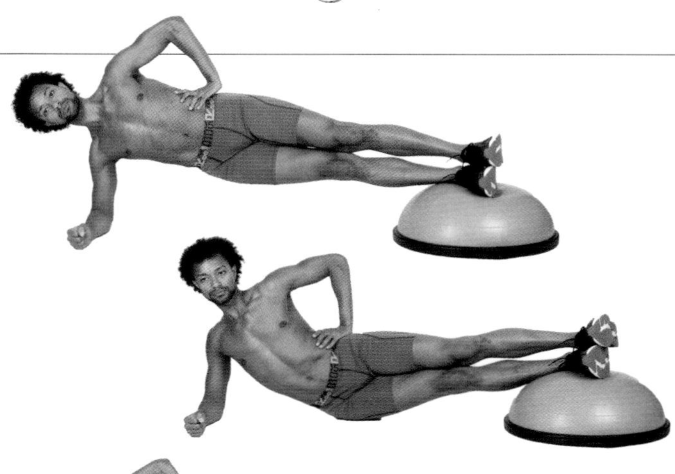

245 Side Plank with Hip and Leg Raise with Feet on the Balance Ball

Come into a Side Forearm Plank with your feet stacked at the center of your balance ball. Let your left hand rest on your hip. Lift your left leg up into the air while pressing your right leg down into the balance ball. Bring the legs back together, lower the hips to the ground. Repeat.

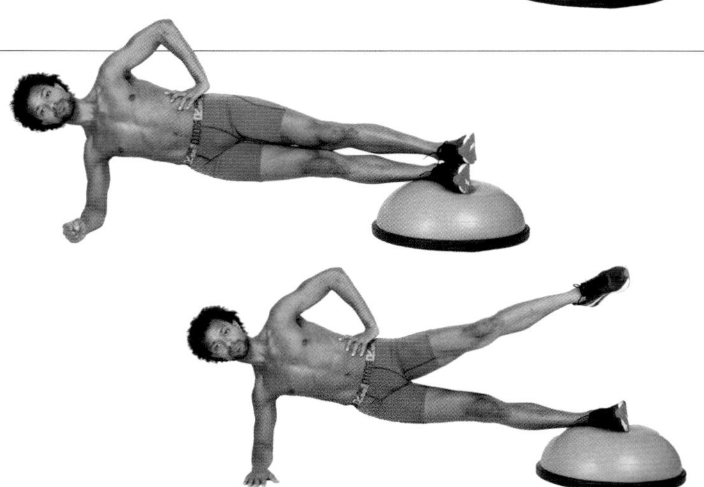

246 **Balance Ball Forearm Plank**

Start with your balance ball flat side down. Bring your forearms together with fingers clasped, on top and in the center of the balance ball. Come into your Plank by extending the legs long, putting the weight onto the balls of your feet. Squeeze the abs in strongly.

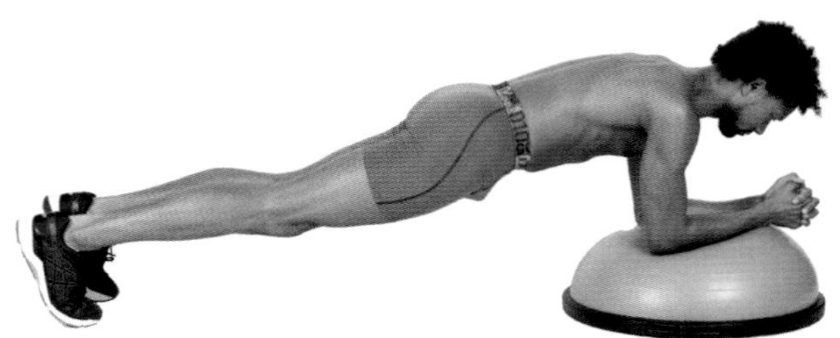

247 **Balance Ball Scissor Plank**

Start with your balance ball flat side down. Bring your forearms together with fingers clasped, on top and in the center of the balance ball. Come into your Plank by extending the legs long, putting the weight onto the balls of your feet. Slide your legs out wide and back, and repeat.

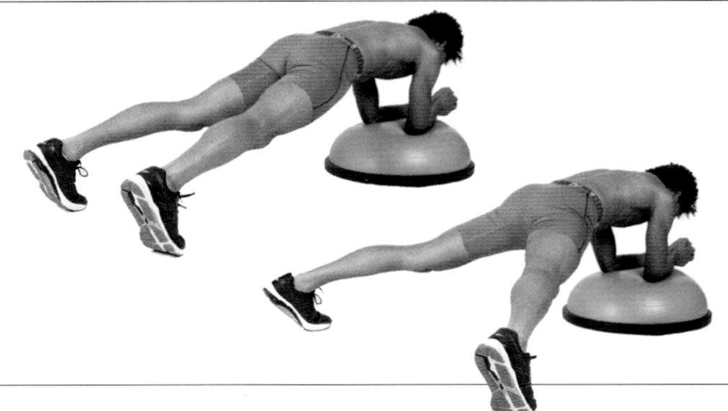

248 **Balance Ball Spiderman Plank**

Position your balance ball with the flat side down. Come into your Plank with your arms supported on the balance ball, fingers clasped together. Push down with your forearms into the balance ball and take turns bringing your left knee outside of your left elbow, then your right knee your right elbow.

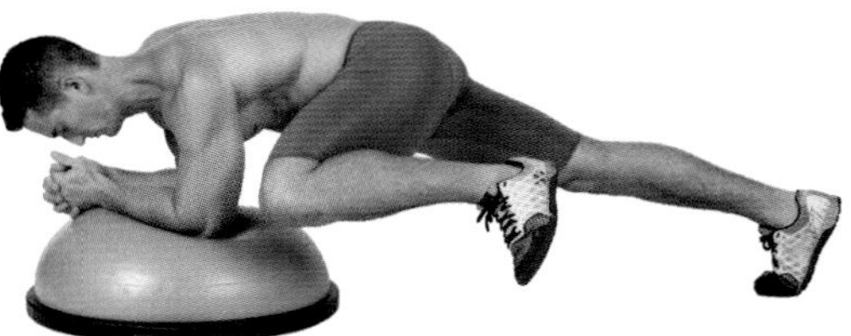

249 **Balance Ball Extended-Arm Plank**

Start with your balance ball flat side down. Bring your hands together with your arms extended, on top and in the center of the balance ball. Come into your Plank by extending the legs long, putting the weight onto the balls of your feet.

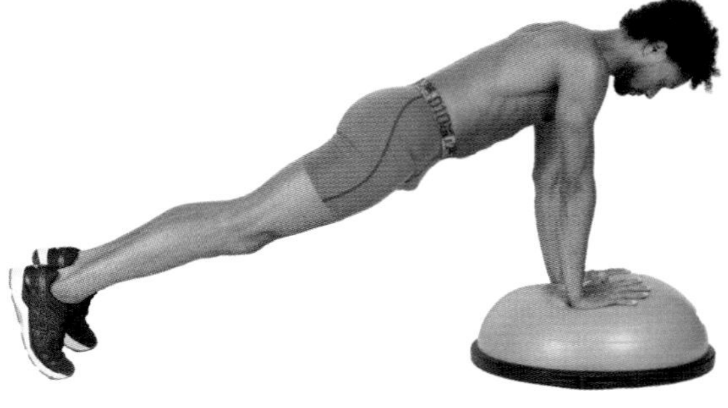

250 **Single-Leg Balance Ball Plank**

Start with your balance ball flat side down. Bring your hands together with your arms extended, on top and in the center of the balance ball. Come into a Plank. With the weight on the balls of your feet, lift the right leg up. Alternate legs, keeping the core engaged.

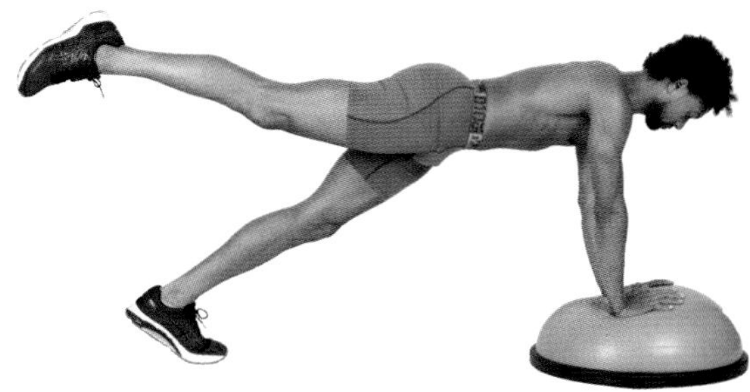

251 Side Plank and Hip Raise with Arm on the Balance Ball

Begin by sitting on the left hip, legs extended. Place your left forearm into the balance ball and push your hips up, coming into a Side Plank. Let your right hand rest on your right hip. Take turns sitting and pushing up into your Side Plank.

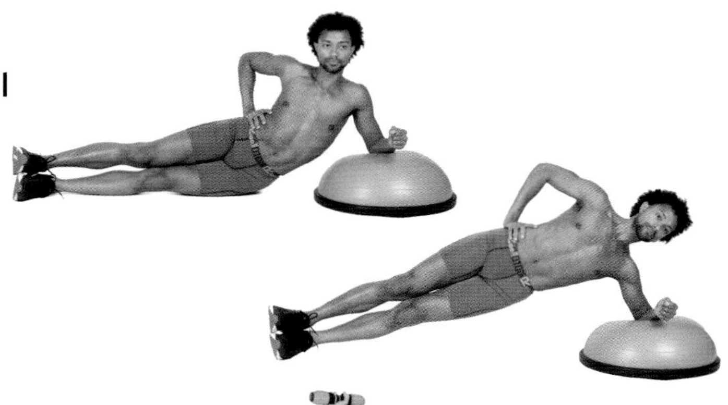

252 Balance Ball Side Plank with Lateral Shoulder Raise

Place your left forearm down and into the center of the balance ball. Push up into a Side Plank with your body supported by your left arm. Take a dumbbell in your right hand and open it up to your right side. Reach the dumbbell under your left ribs and, then, open back up.

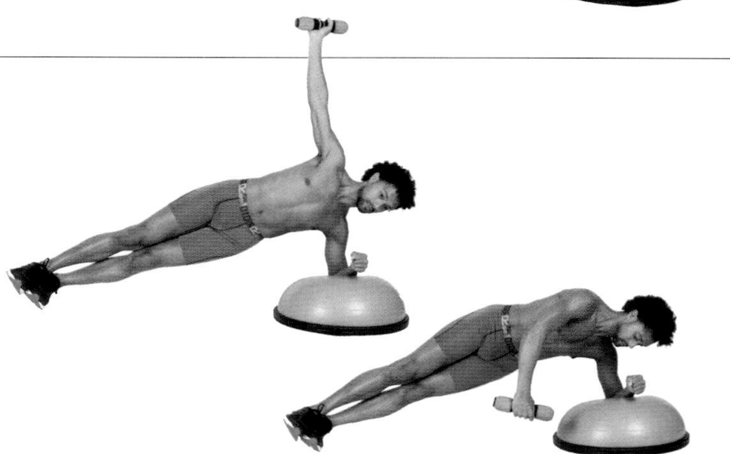

253 Balance Ball Side Plank with Leg Lift

Place your left forearm down into the center of the balance ball. Come into a Side Plank with your body long and in one straight line from head to toe. With your right hand on your hip, open your right leg up to the ceiling.

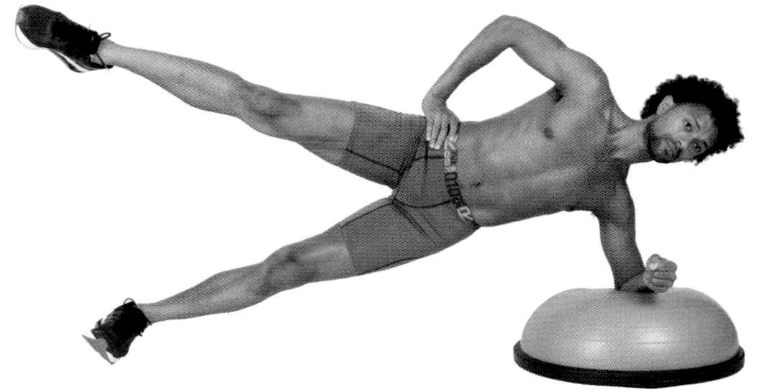

254 Balance Ball Upward Side Plank

Place your left hand at the center of a balance ball. Balance your body, and come into a Side Plank supported by the left arm. Place your right hand on your right hip. Hold in your Side Plank by engaging the core deeply.

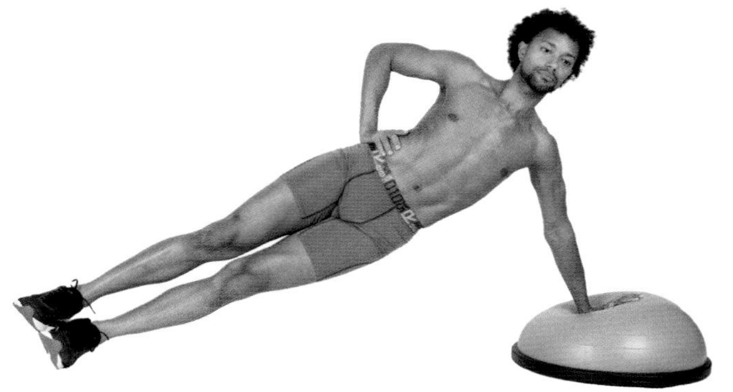

255

Lying Triceps Extension on Swiss Ball

The tricep is a muscle that runs from the elbow joint to the shoulder on the lower back arm. In this exercise, and the next few, we will focus on shaping and strengthening the tricep.

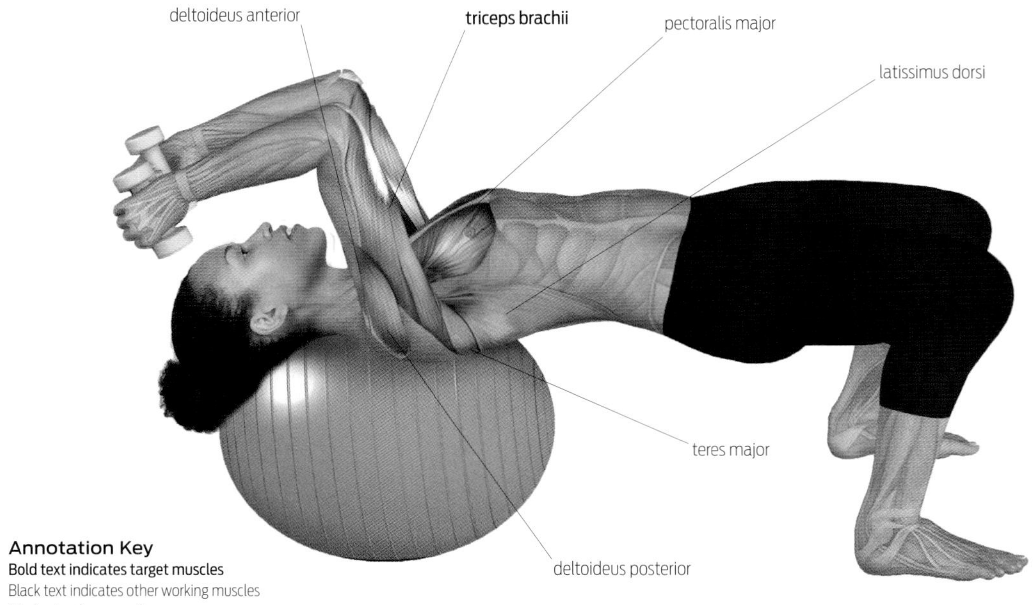

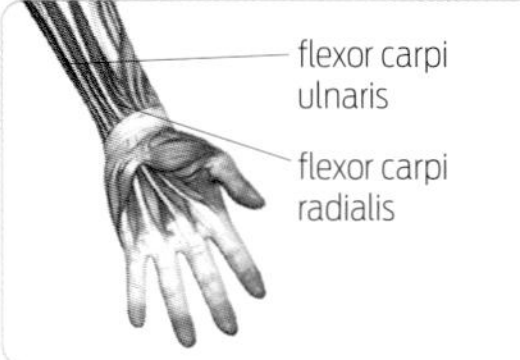

Annotation Key
Bold text indicates target muscles
Black text indicates other working muscles
* indicates deep muscles

Correct form

Be sure when working the triceps that the core muscles are all activated and helping to stabilize the arms so that they can work most efficiently.

Avoid

Avoid moving your arms too much in this exercise. Keep the movement isolated in the elbows.

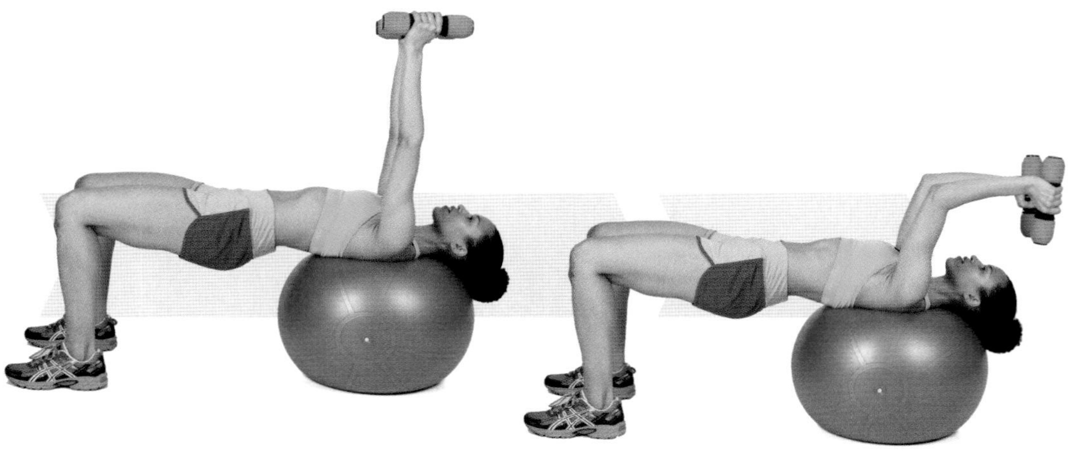

- Place a Swiss ball in between your shoulders so that it is supporting the weight of your torso.
- Take your dumbbells in your hands and bring them straight up above your chest.
- Isolate your elbows and bend your arms into right angles. Straighten the arms, and repeat.

256 EZ Bar Lying Triceps Extension

Incorporating the EZ bar into this variation works the triceps, the pectorals, and the upper middle back. The EZ bar is a heavier weight than dumbbells and challenges the work of the torso a little more. A standard grip with the palms facing away from the body is required.

- Start with the bar above your chest and your arms outstretched.
- Bend at the elbows and slowly lower the bar toward your head, and then raise it back up.

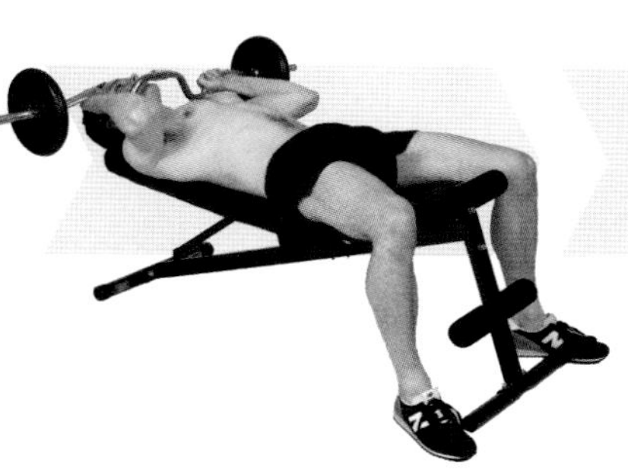

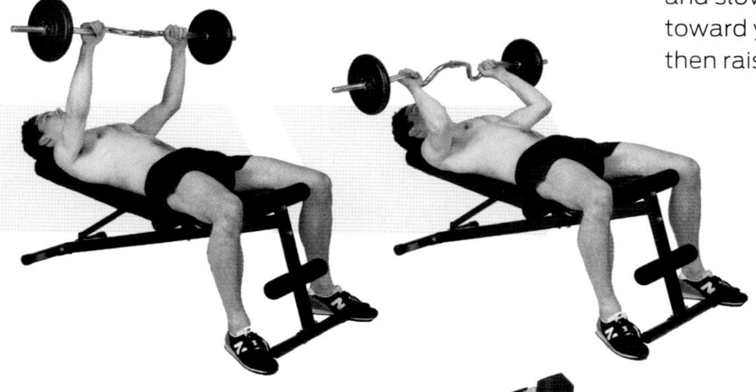

257 Single-Arm Lying Triceps Extension

Begin by lying flat on your bench with your legs apart. Take your dumbbell into your right hand and extend it directly out from the shoulder, in line with your chest. Use your left arm to hold your right tricep so that you can more easily feel the muscle activate. Bend your elbow to lower the dumbbell behind your head, then, with control, raise your arm back to the starting position.

258 Bottoms Up Kettlebell Clean

This exercises your whole arm, not just the tricep. Stand tall with your core engaged and your shoulders pressing down into your middle back. Allow the kettlebells to hang loosely at your sides. Begin by thrusting the right bell up into a 90-degree angle from the chest. Alternate, and repeat.

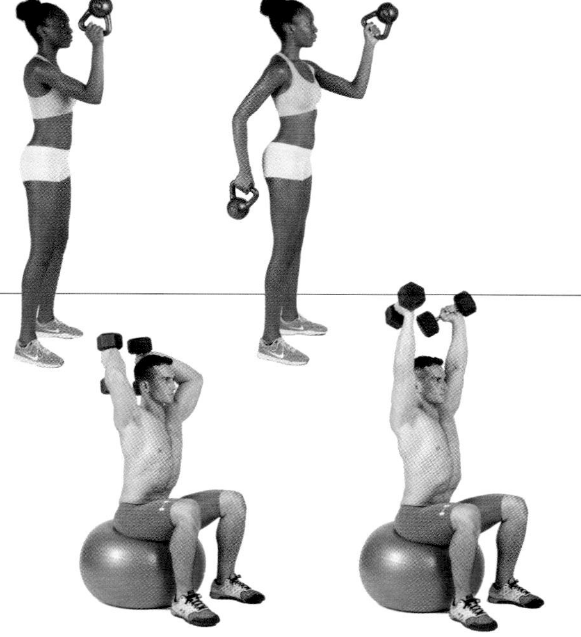

259 Swiss Ball Overhead Dumbbell Extensions

Sit on a Swiss ball with the back of the spine long and supported by your abdominals. Take your dumbbells into your hands and reach them long overhead in line with your ears. Isolate the elbows and bend the weights to touch your shoulders.

260 **Overhead Band Extension**
Secure your band under the middle of your feet. Stand tall with the abdominals in and the weight toward the balls of your feet. Pull the bands from behind your shoulders to straight overhead.

261 **Lying Triceps Press**
Lie down on a bench with your dumbbells in each hand along the sides of your chest. Engage your triceps and shoulders and push the weights up in line with your chest, straightening the arms. Lower back down, with control.

262 **Roll-Up Triceps Lift**
Lie on the floor with your spine in a neutral position. Hold a body bar or barbell bar with both hands straight up above your head. Engage your abs and smoothly roll your torso up, keeping your arms straight and the bar higher than your head. Slowly roll back to the starting position.

263 **Close-Grip Dumbbell Extension**
Lengthen your body along the bench with your legs slightly apart. Take a dumbbell into both hands, holding it directly overhead. Bend the elbows deeply, straighten the arms up over the chest, and then bend again.

264 **Rope Push-Down**
Begin by standing in front of a cable. Grasp the rope handles, pull in your abs, and push down on the handles. Each end of the rope handles should frame either side of your pelvis. With control, raise your ropes up again.

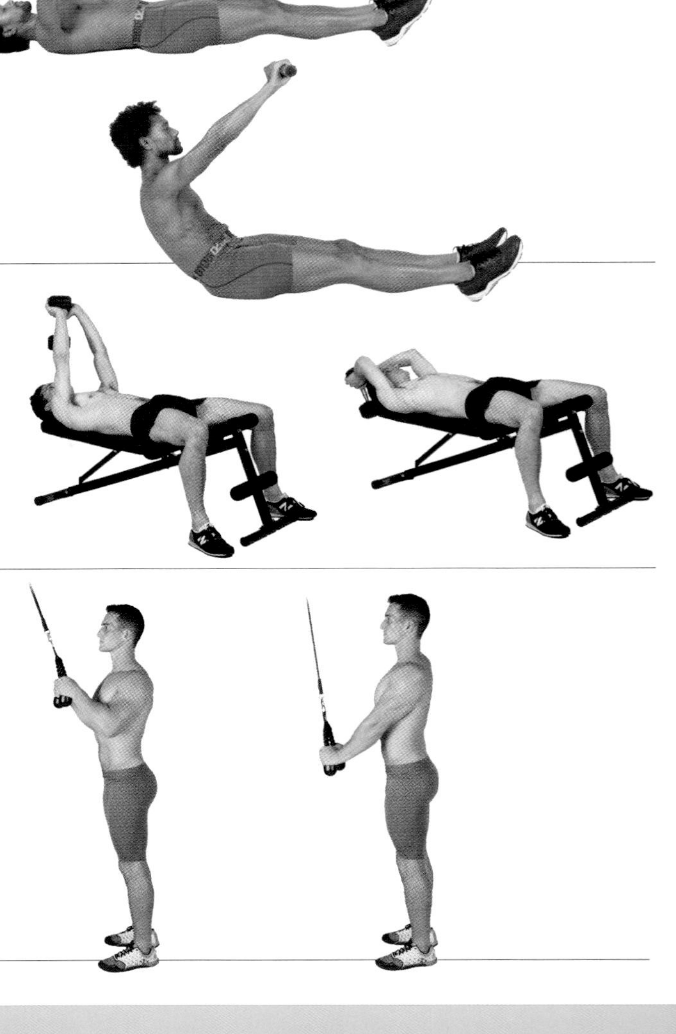

265

Swiss Ball Single-Arm Triceps Kick-Back

Kneel on the ground and rest your left forearm on a Swiss ball in front of you, while holding a dumbbell in front of your thigh with the other hand. Straighten your right arm, and slowly extend it behind you. Hold for 2 seconds, contracting the triceps muscles. Slowly return to the starting position, and repeat on the other side.

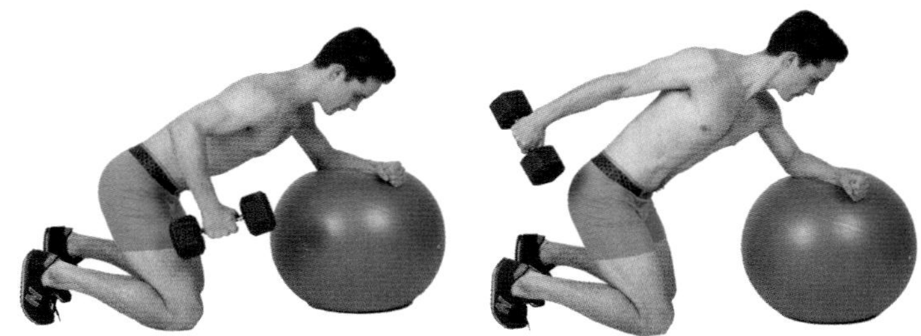

266

Band Kick-Backs

Secure a band under the middle of your feet. Bend at the hips with the abdominals in and put the weight toward the balls of your feet. Pull the band up into your chest and then straighten the arms back, in line with the hips.

267

Single-Arm Overhead Band Extension

Secure a band under the middle of your right foot. Stand tall with the abdominals in and the weight toward the balls of your feet. With the right hand, pull the cable from behind your shoulder to straight overhead. Switch sides, and repeat.

268

One-Arm Band Push-Down

Secure a band under the middle of your left foot. Allow the cable to reach over the back of the right shoulder. With your right hand, pull the cable from behind your shoulder straight down to the floor. Switch sides, and repeat.

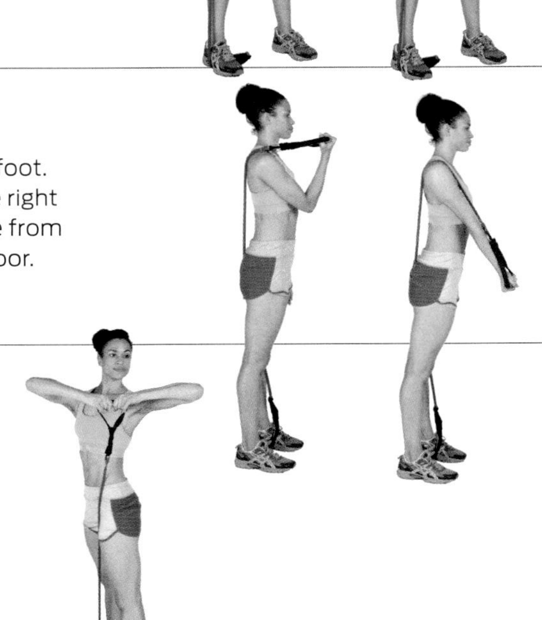

269

Twisting Lift with Band

Secure a resistance band under your right foot, while standing with your feet shoulder-width apart. Take the band into both hands, facing the front, and twist to your right side, pulling up on the band and opening the elbows out to the sides.

270

Swiss Ball Jackknife

The Swiss Ball Jackknife is a great combination of planking and isometric abdominal work. Utilizing the Swiss ball as a moving prop for the lower body to manipulate, you will strengthen your abdominal wall and stabilize the pelvis.

Correct form

Be sure to keep your Plank supported and balanced by engaging the abs deeply.

Avoid

Do not let the hips or back arch. Keep the body in one straight line from head to toe.

Annotation Key
Bold text indicates target muscles
Black text indicates other working muscles
* indicates deep muscles

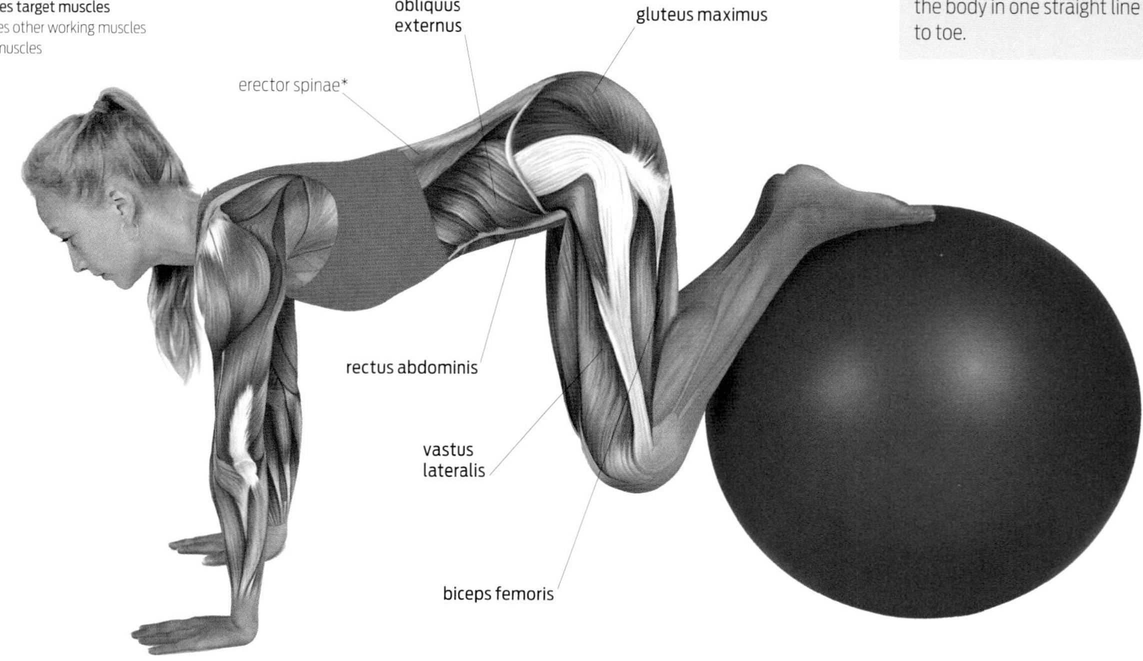

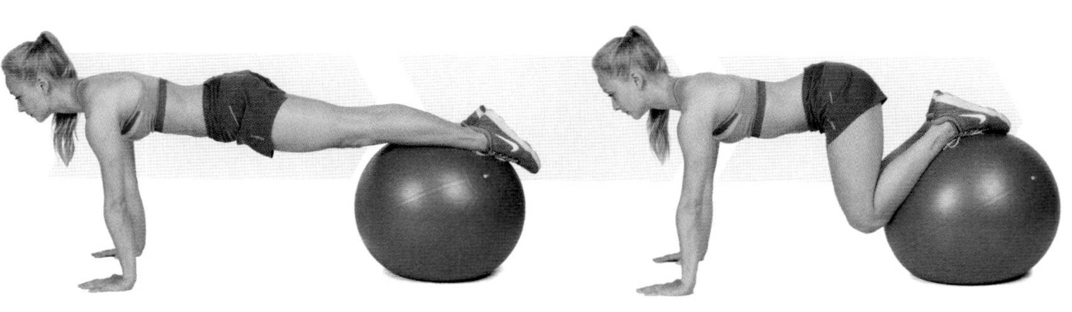

- Begin in your Plank position (#213) with the arms fully extended. Walk your feet up onto the Swiss ball.
- Squeeze the abs up and in a lot and pull your knees toward your chest, bringing the ball with you with your feet.

271 Swiss Ball Forward Roll/Roll-Out

Bring the weight of your upper body into your forearms while balancing on the Swiss ball. Lower the knees down in an extended kneeling position. Push the forearms into a ball and squeeze the abs very deeply, rolling the ball out away from you.

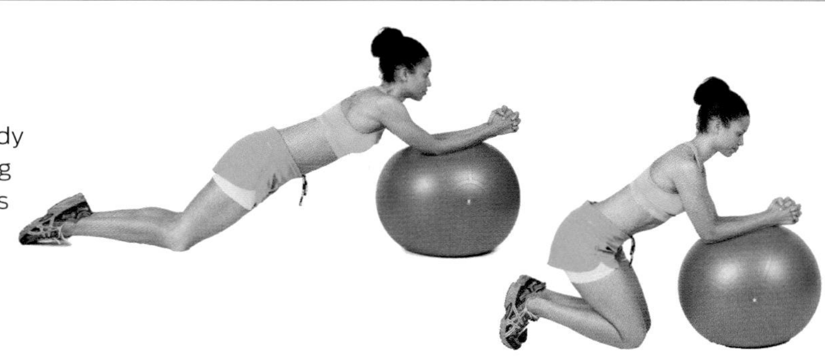

272 Swiss Ball Pike

Start in a solid Plank position with your feet supported at the center of a Swiss ball. Engage the lower abs and the lower back and bend at the hips. Allow the Swiss ball to roll in toward the body, and pike the hips up high.

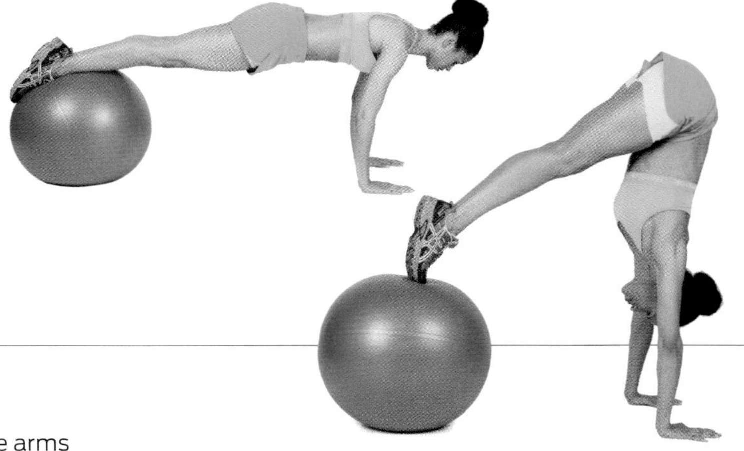

273 Swiss Ball Walk-Around

Come into your Plank position with the arms fully extended. Bend at the hips and pike the lower body up high. Hold in your pike position, pull in the abs strongly, and move the hands—toward the right then toward the left—then lower down.

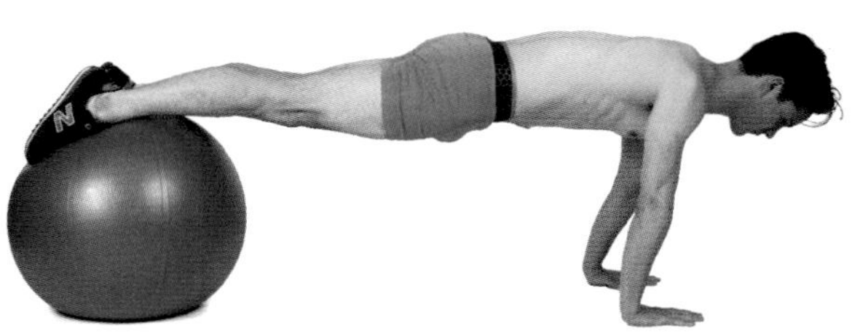

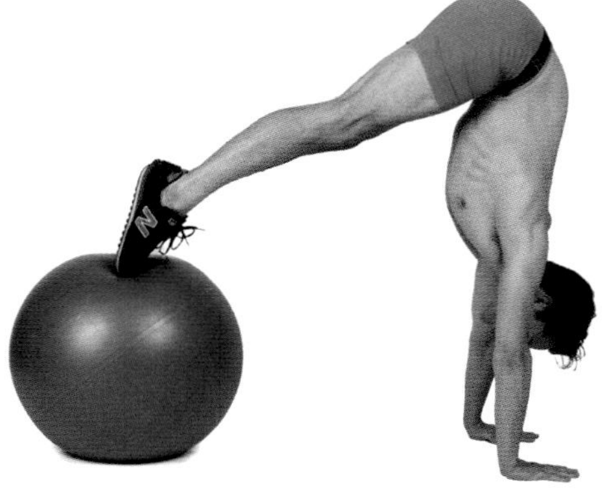

274 Medicine Ball Pike

Start in a solid Plank position with your feet supported on a Medicine ball. Engage the lower abs and the lower back and bend at the hips. Allow the ball to roll in toward the body and pike the hips up high.

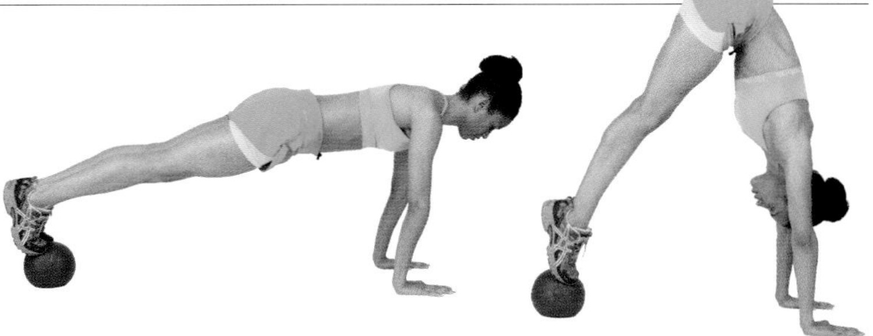

275

Foam-Roller Abdominal Roll-In

The foam roller is an unstable prop, meaning it moves. Using your foam roller to assist in your core workout is a great way to confuse the muscle groups, enabling the development of all the muscles, simultaneously, in new dynamic ways.

Correct form

From head to hips, keep the body in one even line. This will ensure that the work is focused in the core only.

Avoid

Do not let the weight of your body rest heavily on the foam roller. You want to be able to roll in and out with ease.

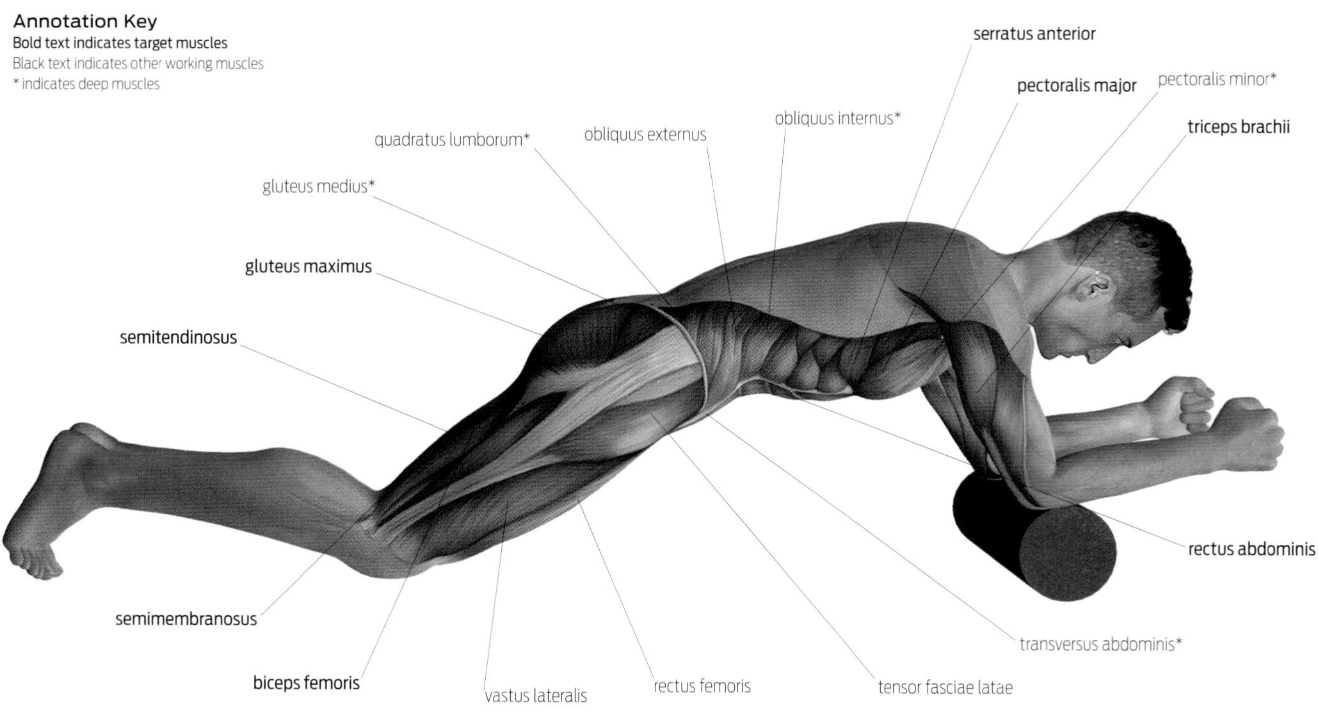

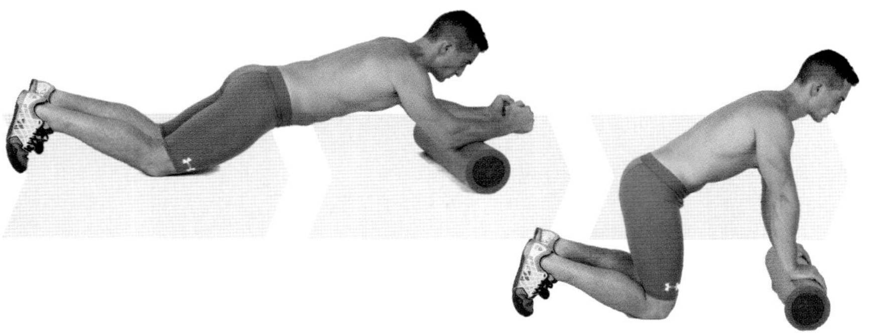

- Come into a Forearm Plank, with your lower arms resting on the foam roller.
- Bring your knees to the floor and pull in the foam roller with the abs, rolling the prop from your lower arms to the palms.

276 Triceps Roll-Out

In this variation, you will use your foam roller to activate the backs of the arms. Moving through your standard Plank position while focusing the weight into the triceps will create stabilization in the shoulders and strength in the chest and core.

- Start in a kneeling position, hands on top of the foam roller, arms straight, and abs braced.
- Using your abs, roll the foam roller straight out in front of you, bringing your lower arms to touch the roller.

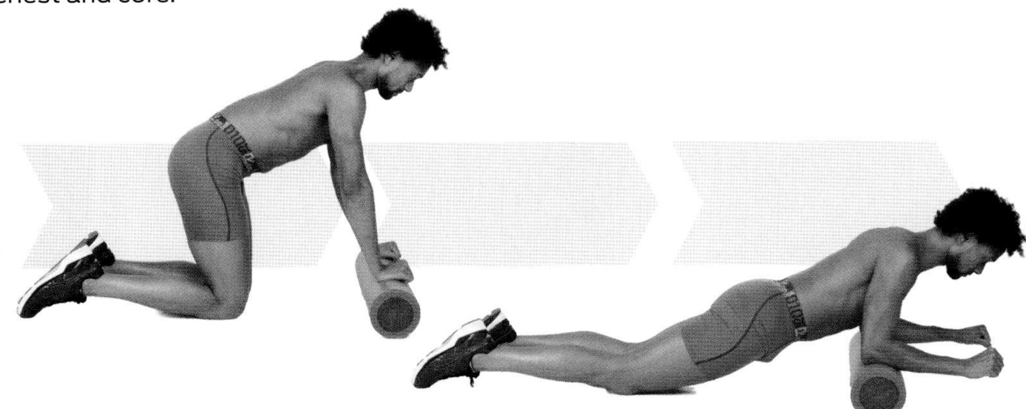

277 Ab-Wheel Roll-Out

Come to a kneel, holding the wheel between your hands. With the knees slightly apart, pull the abs and core in tightly and allow the weight of your body to roll out with the wheel. Pause when fully extended, and roll back in.

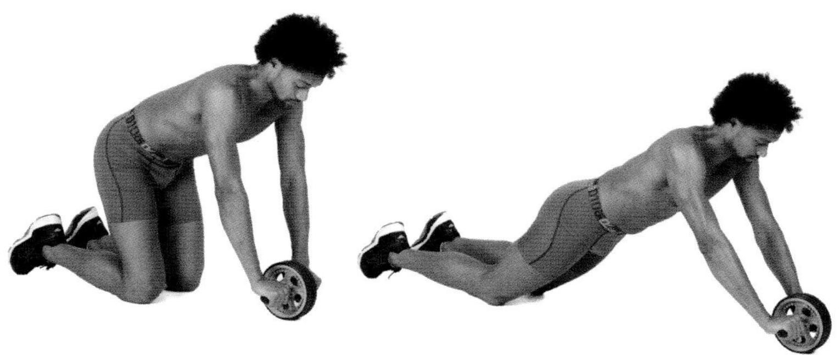

278 Oblique Ab-Wheel Roll-Out

Come to a kneel, holding the wheel between your hands. With the knees apart, pull the abs and core in tightly and allow the weight of your body to roll out with the wheel on a diagonal. Use the obliques on the side of your body to control the movement.

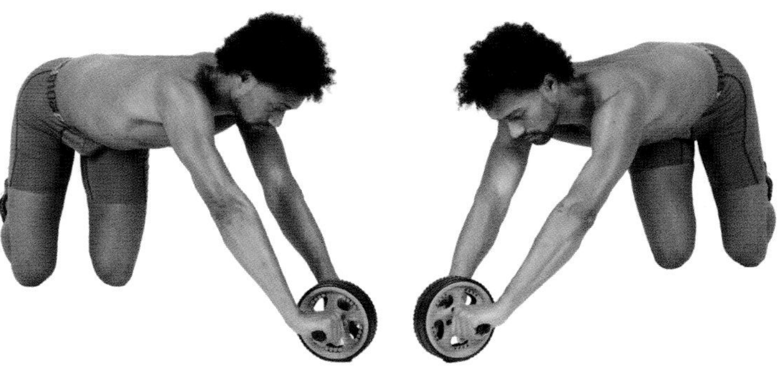

279

Hanging Leg Raise with Straps

Hanging suspended in the air, supported by straps, allows you to use the weight of your own body to enhance your strength. With your upper body stabilized and unmoving, the lower body can work freely, honing an intense core workout.

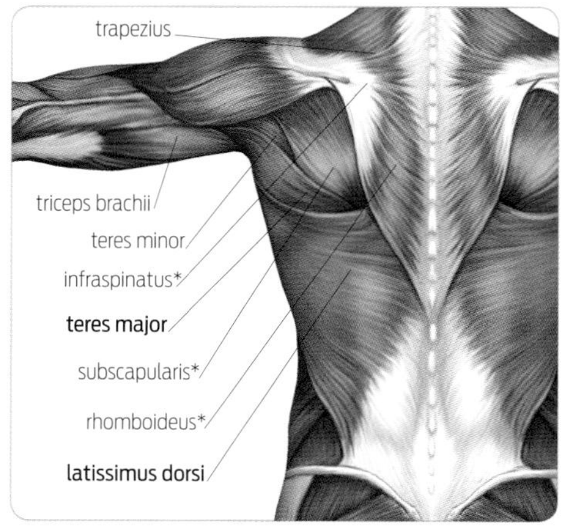

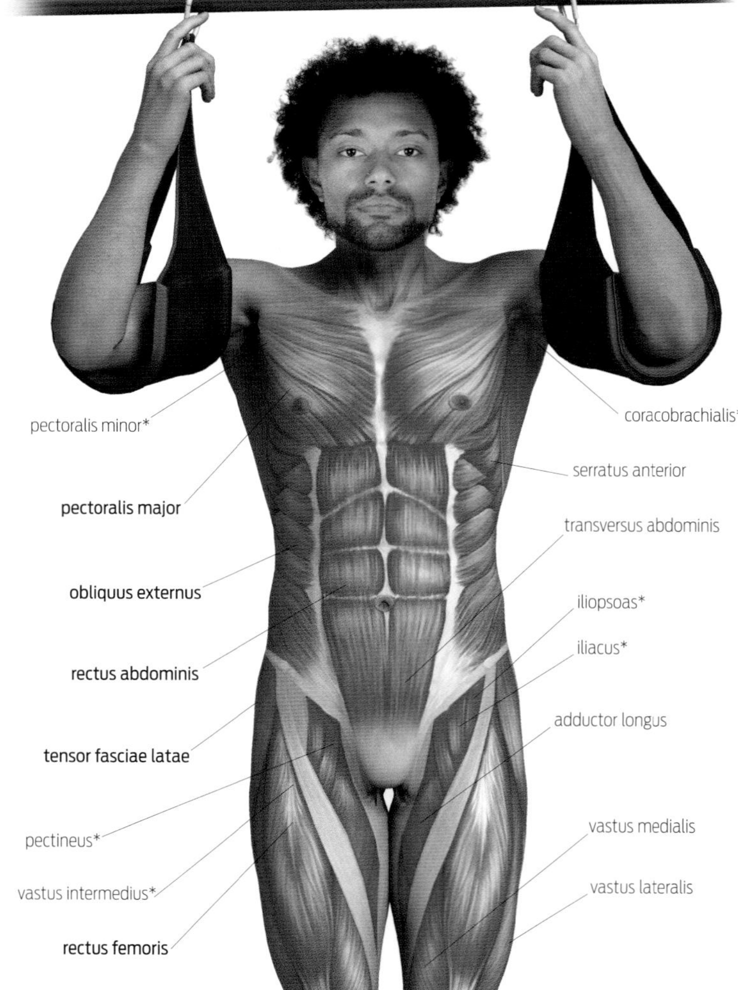

Annotation Key
Bold text indicates target muscles
Black text indicates other working muscles
* indicates deep muscles

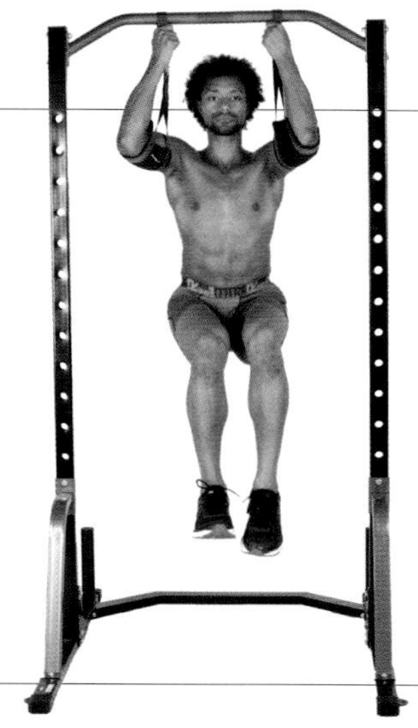

- Secure your upper arms by pressing your shoulders down into the straps. Hold the tops of the straps with both hands.
- With your legs hanging, activate your core by squeezing your lower abdominals into the back and pulling your knees up high into the core.

Correct form

Maintain alignment from shoulder to hip by engaging the core strongly up and in.

Avoid

Do not swing the legs with momentum. Instead, control the movement with the core muscles.

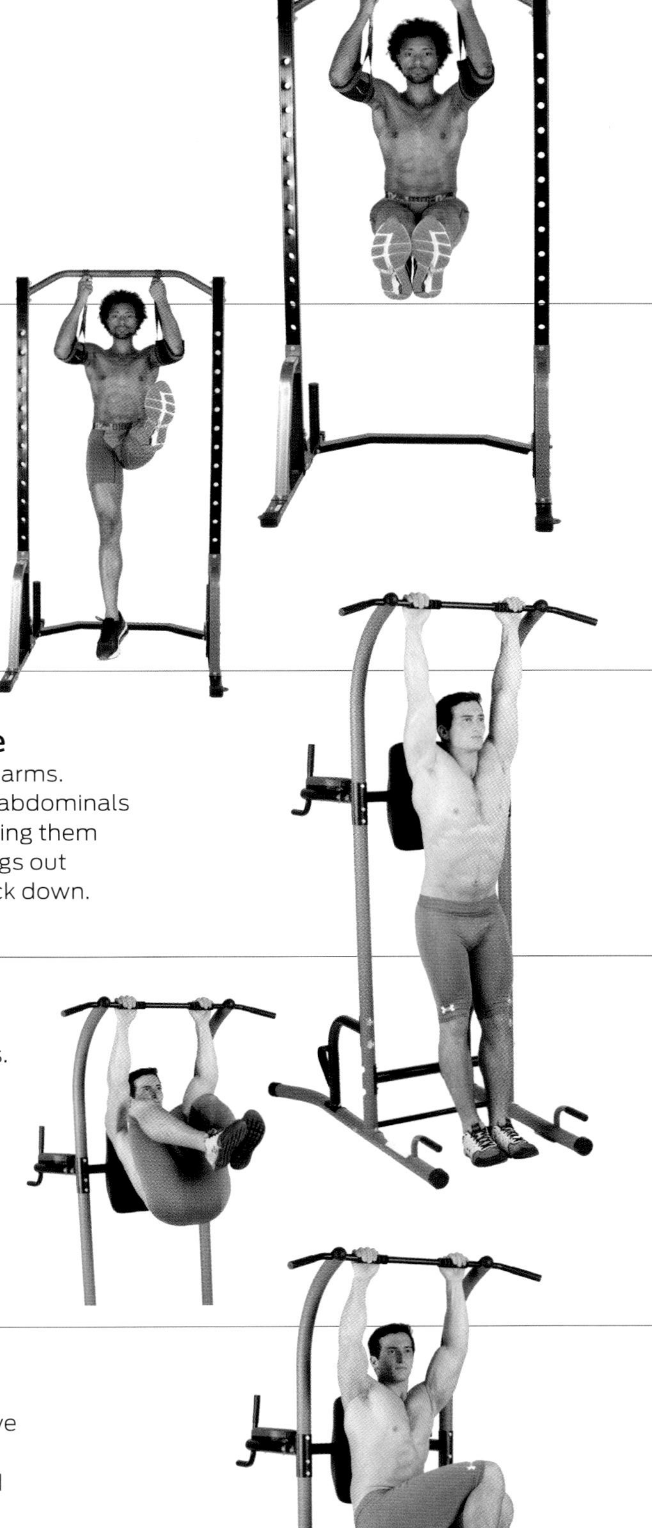

280

Hanging Straight-Leg Raises with Straps

Secure your upper arms into the straps. With your legs long, activate your core by squeezing your lower abdominals into the back. Lift the legs up high, bringing them straight out in front of your hips.

281

Hanging Single Straight-Leg Raises

Secure your upper arms into the straps. With your legs long, activate your core by squeezing your lower abdominals. Raise the left leg up, straight, and high to hip level. Hold there, flex the foot, and lower the leg back down. Switch legs, and keep alternating.

Straight-Arm Hanging Leg Raise

Hold the bar above you with extended long arms. Activate your core by squeezing your lower abdominals into the back, and lift the legs up high, bringing them straight out in front of your hips. Hold the legs out straight for a moment, then lower them back down.

283

Hanging Leg Raise Variation

Hold the bar above you with extended arms. With your legs long, activate your core by squeezing your lower abdominals, and pull your legs up high into your chest. Hold your legs there, then lower them back down.

Hanging Leg Raises with Twists

Start with a long spine, holding the bar above you with extended arms. Grip the bar firmly and pull the legs up and in, together, toward your left shoulder. Take turns alternating sides for the desired amount of repetitions.

285

Barbell Curl

The standard curl is featured in most upper-body workouts. Incorporating a barbell, weights, or resistance bands while performing curls will help chisel out beautiful arm muscles. Combining curls with exercises that focus on the core will help to strengthen muscles in the back, shoulders, and biceps.

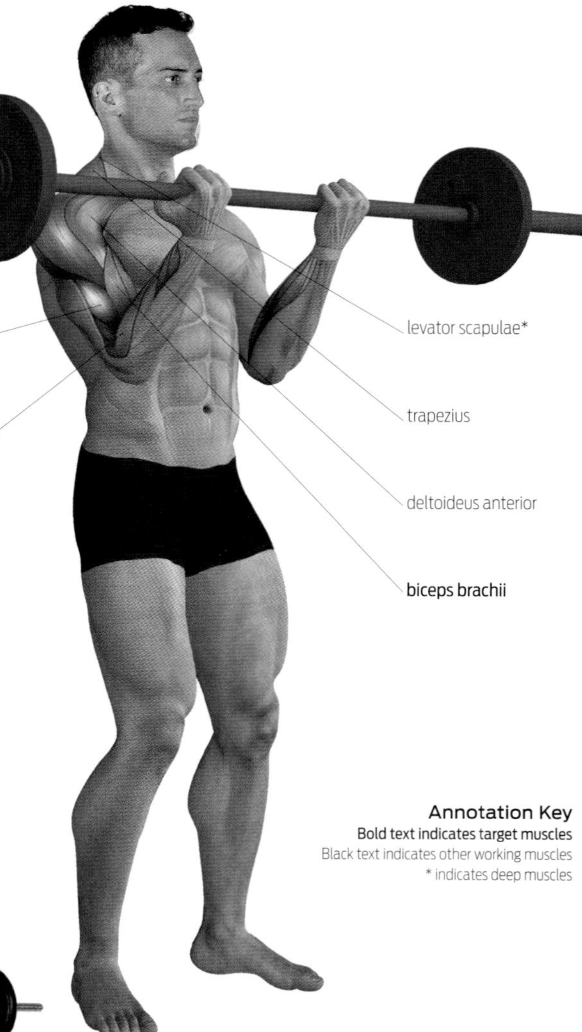

Annotation Key
Bold text indicates target muscles
Black text indicates other working muscles
* indicates deep muscles

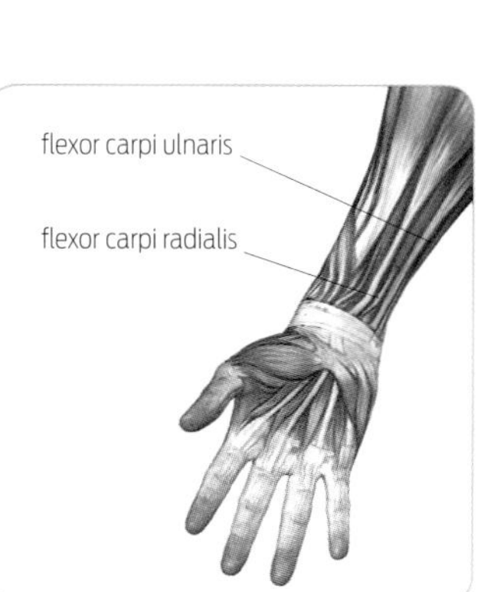

Correct form

Engage the shoulders down into the back, away from your ears. Imagine that the back of your neck is long and dropping down through your middle back.

Avoid

Avoid clenching your jaw or squeezing your neck in any way that may put unnecessary tension on your head. This includes lifting the chin too high.

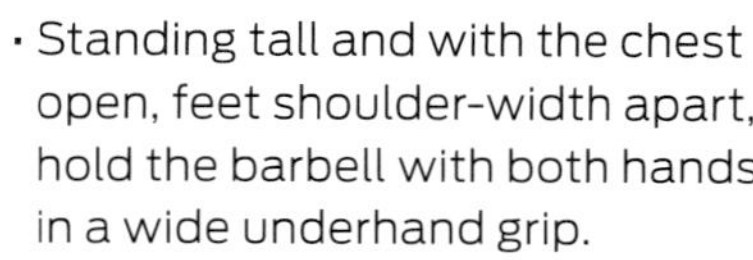

- Standing tall and with the chest open, feet shoulder-width apart, hold the barbell with both hands in a wide underhand grip.
- Pull the bar up along the front of your body, isolating the elbows at your sides.
- Once the bar has reached level with your shoulders, lower the bar, and repeat.

286 Alternating Hammer Curl

To perform these hammer curls you must keep an engaged core, while dynamically pulling and pushing your weights up and into the body. The benefits of this exercise include a strong set of abdominals, super developed triceps, biceps, core muscles, and sleek, shapely arms.

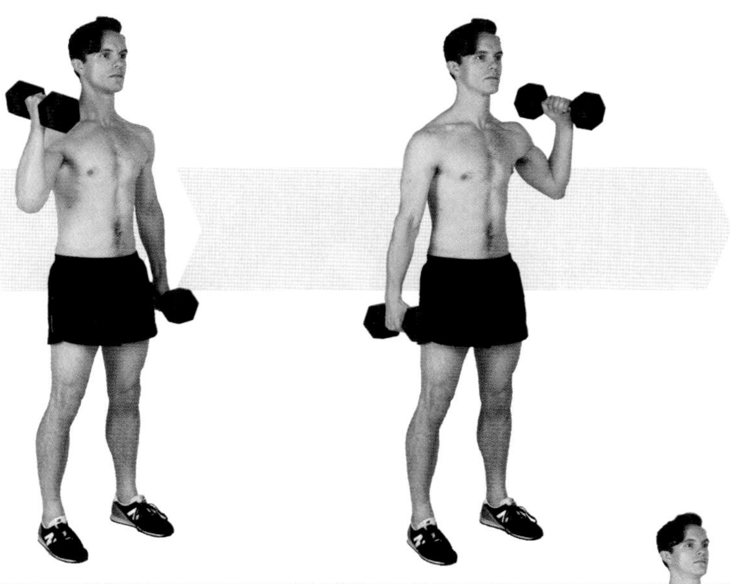

- With feet shoulder-width apart, suck the abs up and into the lower back, feeling the middle back long and strong.
- Holding a dumbbell in each hand, pull the right weight up and into the shoulder.
- Lower, and pull the left weight up into the shoulder.
- Keep alternating sides as you develop an even tempo.

287 Plate Curl

Open the legs to shoulder-width apart. Stand tall with a long spine, engaging the core and the arms. Holding a weighted plate in front of your hips, slowly squeeze the biceps and lift the plate up into the chest. Lower back down, and repeat.

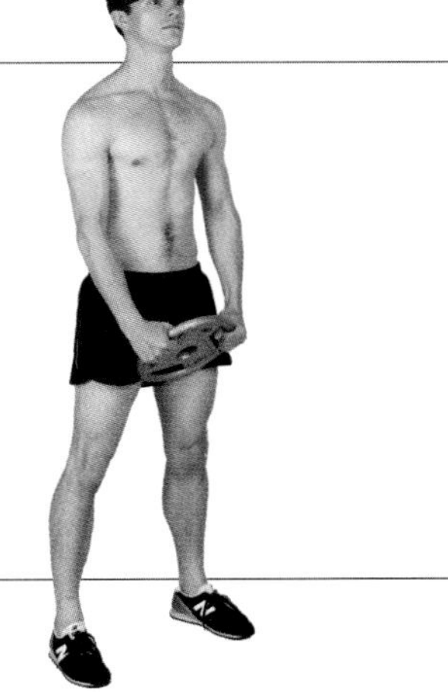

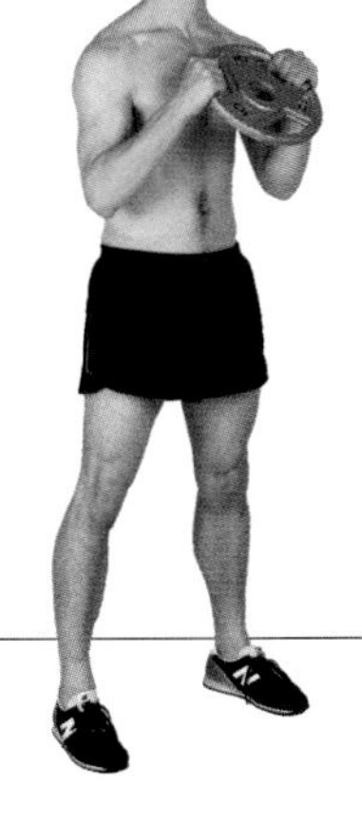

288 Single-Arm Concentration Curl

Sit up straight on an elevated surface. Bring the legs open wide and take a dumbbell into your right hand. Place your left hand on your left knee for balance. Slowly curl the weight up into your chest, bringing your bicep into full activation.

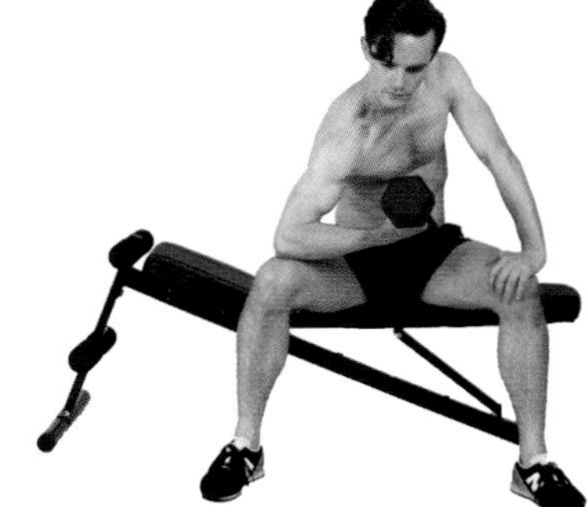

289 Incline-Bench Dumbbell Curl

Lie with your body extended long against an incline bench. With a dumbbell in each hand, loosely hanging on either side of the bench, isolate your biceps and pull the weights up into your shoulders.

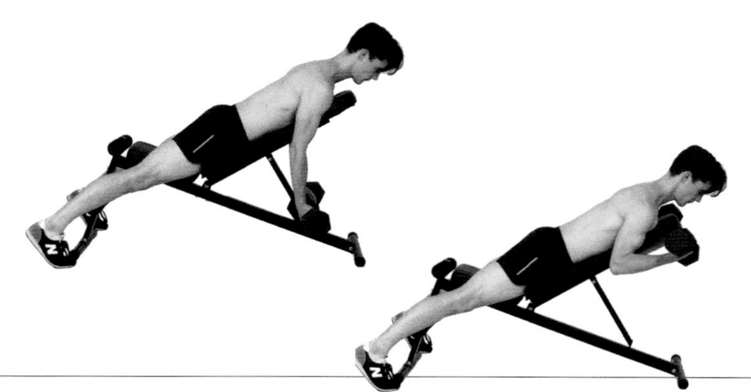

290 Incline-Bench Barbell Curl

Lie with your body extended long against an incline bench. Gripping a barbell with both hands, on the front side of the bench, pull your core into the lower back, isolate your elbows, and curl the bar into your shoulders.

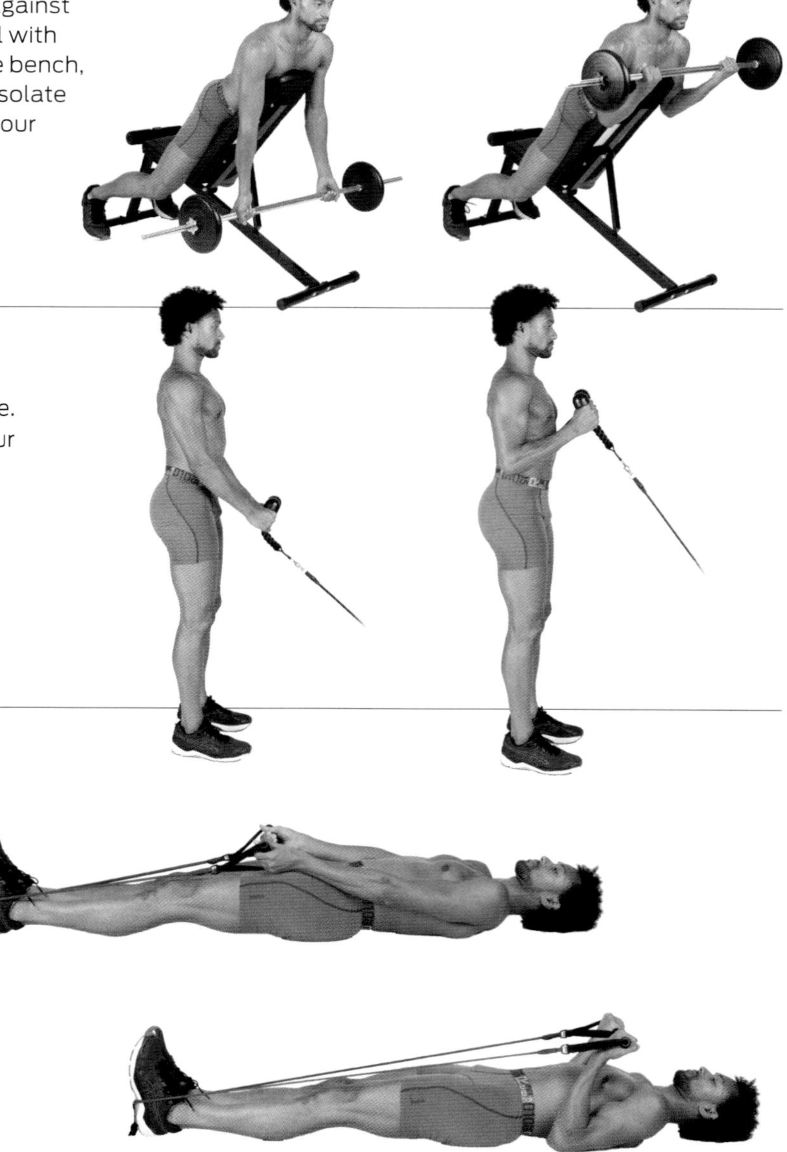

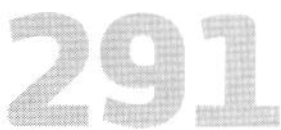

Rope Hammer Curl

Begin by standing in front of a cable. Grasp the cable handles, pull in your abs, and pull up on the handles. Each end of the handles should come to either side of your chest. Make sure your elbows stay glued into your sides.

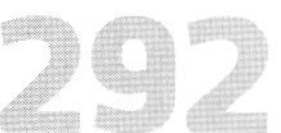

Reclining Band Curl

Lie down long and flat on the floor. Take a band and secure it around the center of your feet. Hold the ends of the band with the handles at each hip. Squeeze your core down into the ground, engage the biceps, and pull the handles into your chest.

293

Band Curls

Start by standing tall. Take a band and secure it under the center of your feet. Hold the ends of a band with the handles at each hip. Squeeze your core and stabilize the hips. Engage the biceps and pull the handles up into your chest.

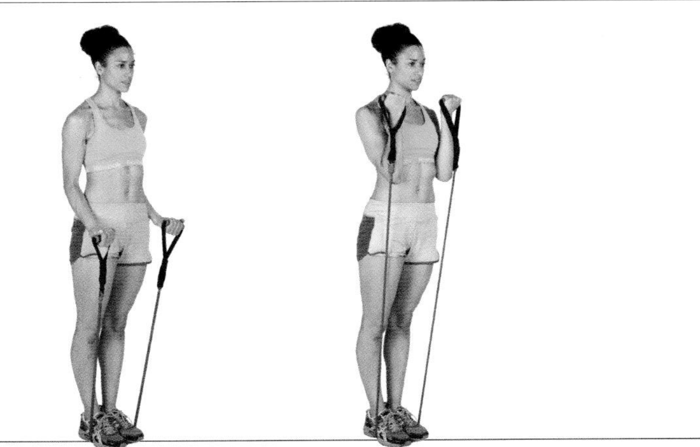

294

Swiss Ball Barbell Curls

Start by sitting on a Swiss ball, with your core engaged strongly into your back body. Take a barbell and hold it hanging out in front of your knees. Isolate the elbows, and bring the bar into your chest. Keep the elbows tight into your sides.

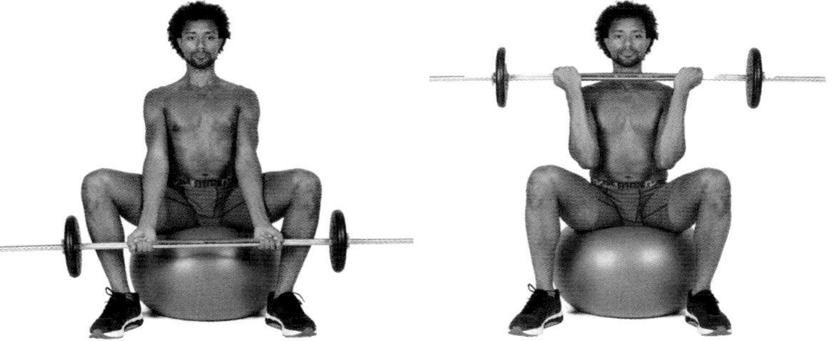

295

Swiss Ball Dumbbell Curls

Start by sitting on a Swiss ball, with your core engaged strongly into your back body. Take your dumbbells and hold them out in front of your knees. Isolate the elbows, and bring the weights into your chest. Keep the elbows tight into your sides.

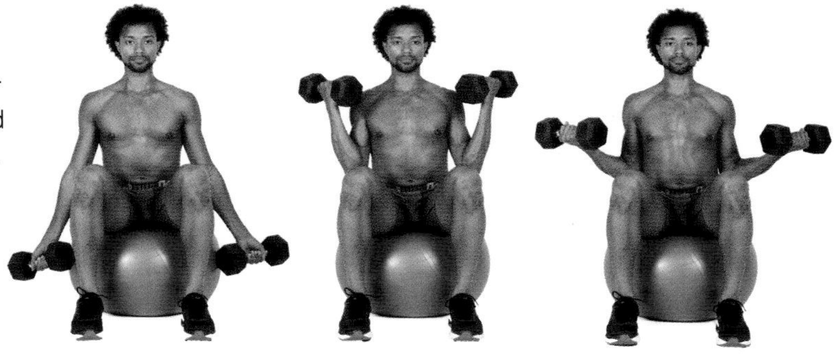

296

Alternating Incline Dumbbell Curls

Lying long on your bench, suck the abs up and into the lower back, feeling the middle back long and strong. Holding a dumbbell in each hand, alternate pulling them up and into the shoulders, making sure to keep the core tight. Lower, and repeat.

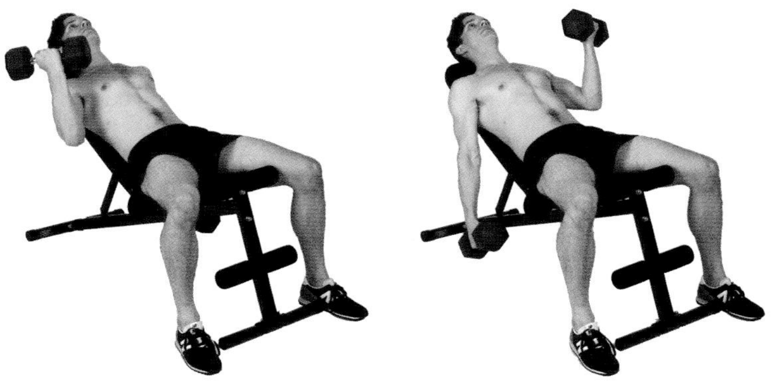

CHAPTER TWO

Lower Body

In this book, when we refer to the "lower body," we are describing the muscle groups and anatomy of all parts below the ribcage. The lower abdominals and spine, pelvis, thighs, glutes, knees, calves, ankles, and feet all encompass the glorious "lower body." Lower-body exercise routines and movements are varied and come in a myriad of styles. Some of the more well-known lower-body workouts combine isometric exercises, such as balances, planks, and bridges, with more dynamic, explosive plyometric movements like jumps, kicks, and thrusts. As you move through the lower-body exercises in these next few pages, you will discover that when you focus on developing lower-body strength, you simultaneously boost stability and power in every other section of the body—including your core and upper body.

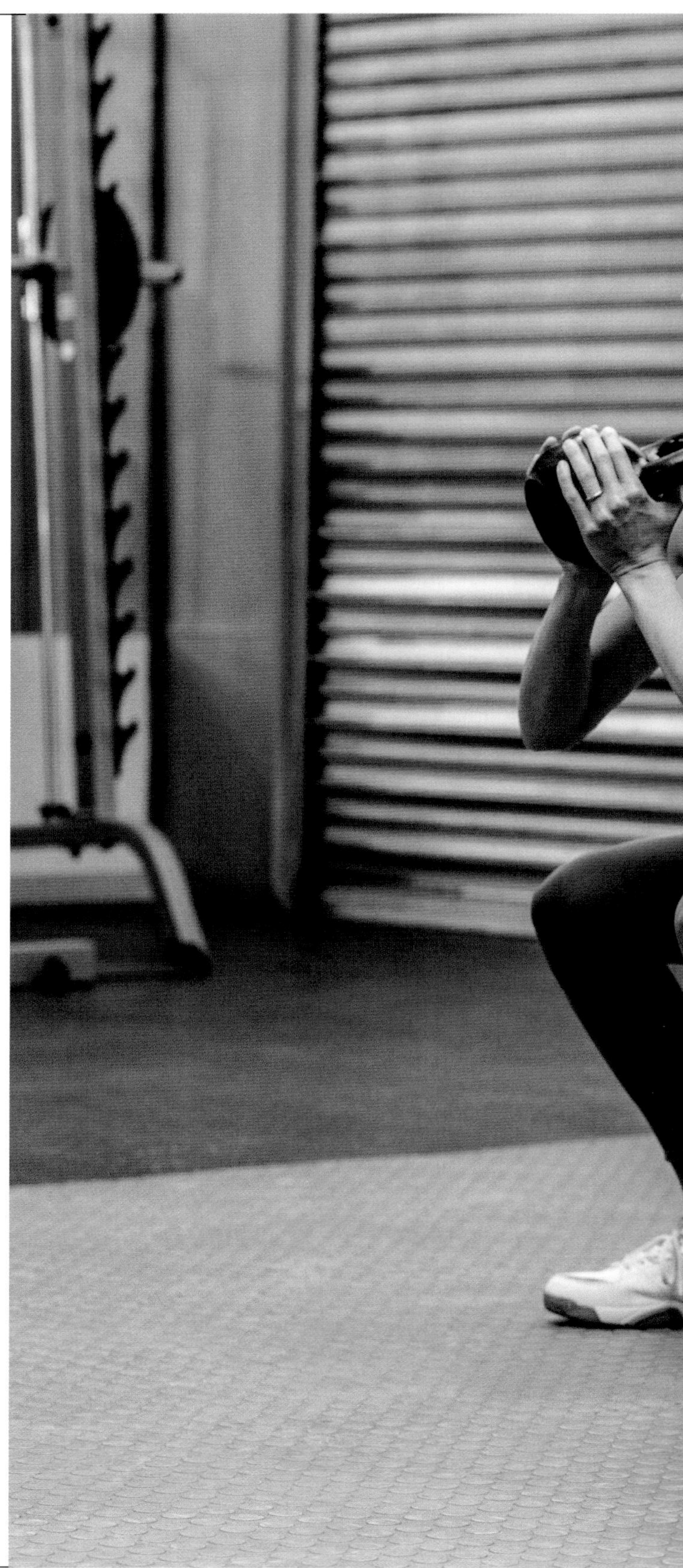

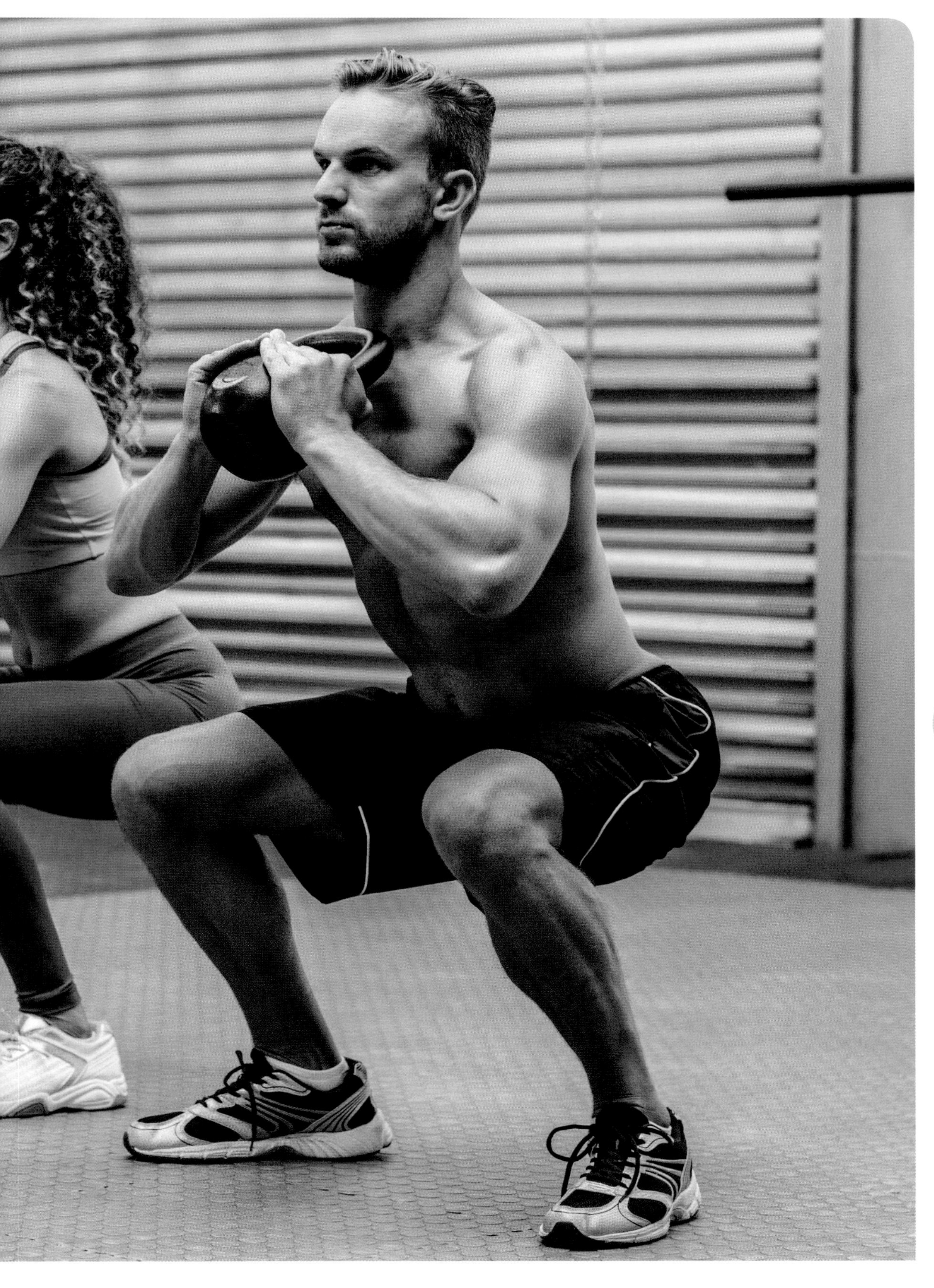

Lower Body

297

Basic Squat

The Squat is a basic movement that can powerfully strengthen and shape the abdominal core, lower back, and legs. It is a pretty straightforward move that relies on perfect square alignment from the top of the head to the base of the foot. The better your Squat form, the better your results will be!

Correct form

Aim for each joint to be stacked and supported on top of each other in a straight line during your Squat.

Avoid

Do not sit down too far in your Squat. Try to keep the back up very straight as you descend.

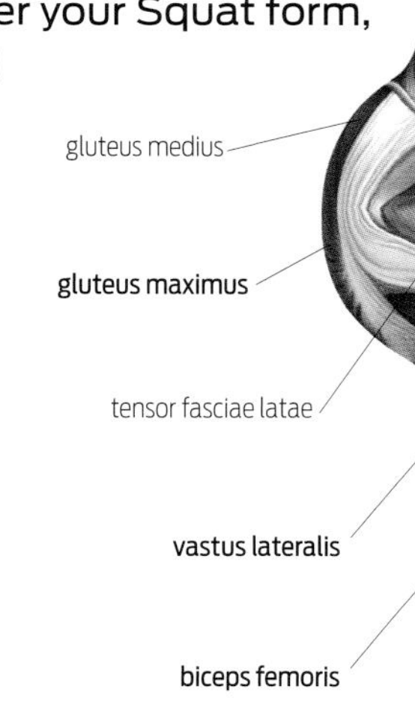

- Stand with your feet shoulder-width apart. Shift your weight so that it is poised over the balls of your feet, toward your toes.
- Lift your arms to a 90-degree angle out from your torso with your palms down.
- Bend your knees so that they track above your ankles, and keep your heels down. You should feel the work in the quads and hamstrings, with the core tight.
- Slowly lift back up to stand.

298 **Speed Squat**

A more difficult variation of the basic Squat, this exercise calls for the exact same movement, performed in a fast-but-smooth up and down movement that is repeated until you are unable to continue.

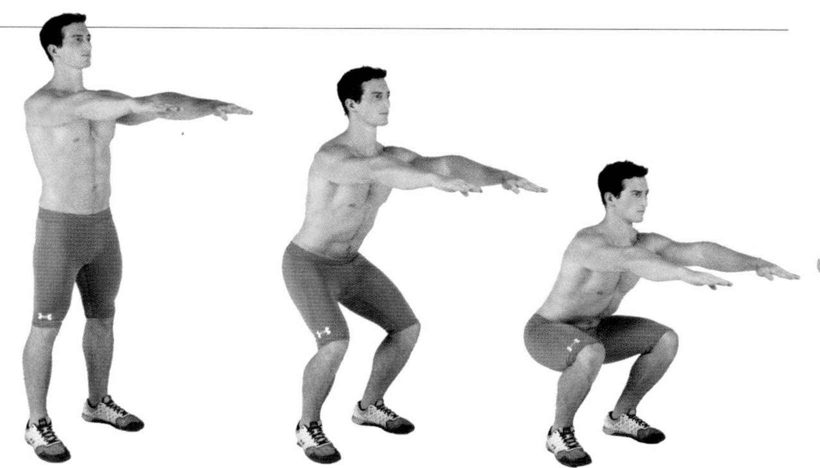

299 **Medicine Ball Squat**

Stabilize your two feet hip-width apart. Keep your abdominals and core engaged, squeeze your legs, reach your ball out in front of you, and come into your Squat stance. Hold at the bottom of your Squat and squeeze the ball between your palms.

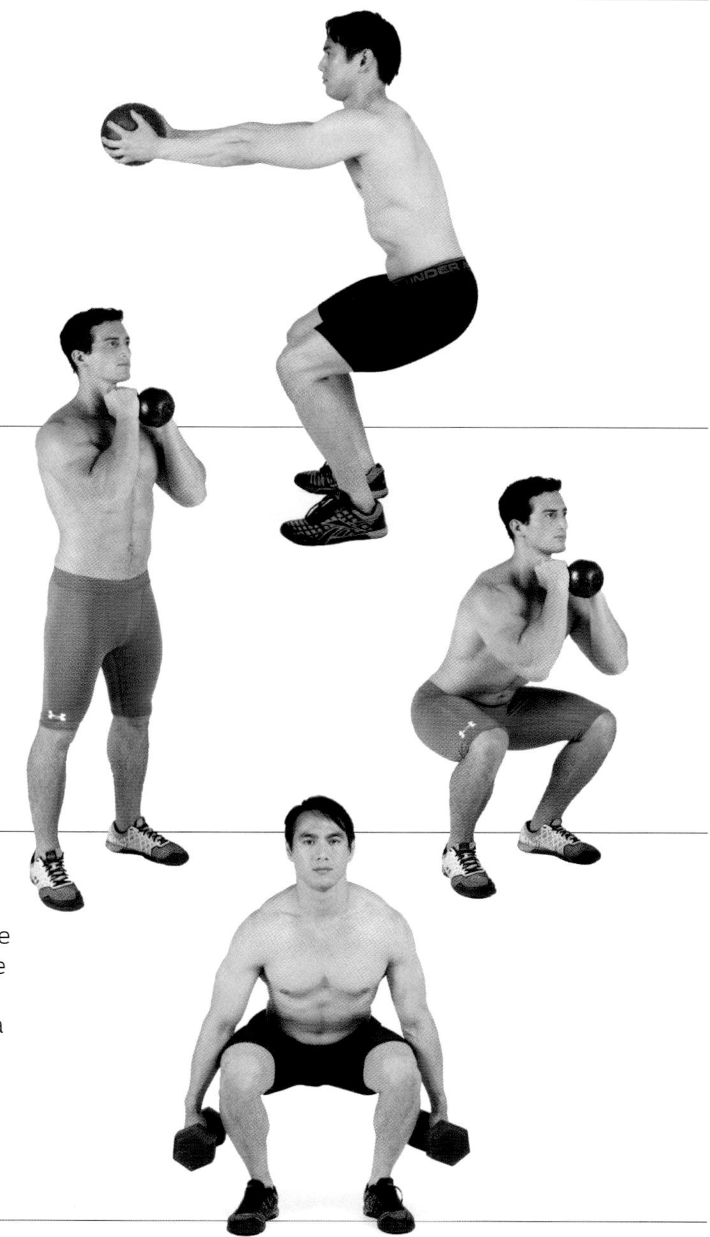

300 **Kettlebell Squat**

Stand with both feet hip-width apart. Hold a kettlebell in both hands, secured at the upper chest. Squeeze the core, glutes, and hamstrings tightly. Slowly, descend into your Squat, keeping a long spine and the kettlebell at your chest.

301 **Dumbbell Squat**

Stand with both feet hip-width apart while holding a dumbbell in each hand. Squeeze the core, glutes, and hamstrings tightly. Slowly descend into your Squat, keeping a long spine and the weights securely long and held at your sides.

302

Sandbag Squat

Stand up straight with a long spine. Open your legs wide and securely hold a sandbag on the tops of your biceps. Lengthen your spine, with abdominals pulled up, and bend deeply at the knees. Once your hips and knees reach 90-degree angles, return to standing.

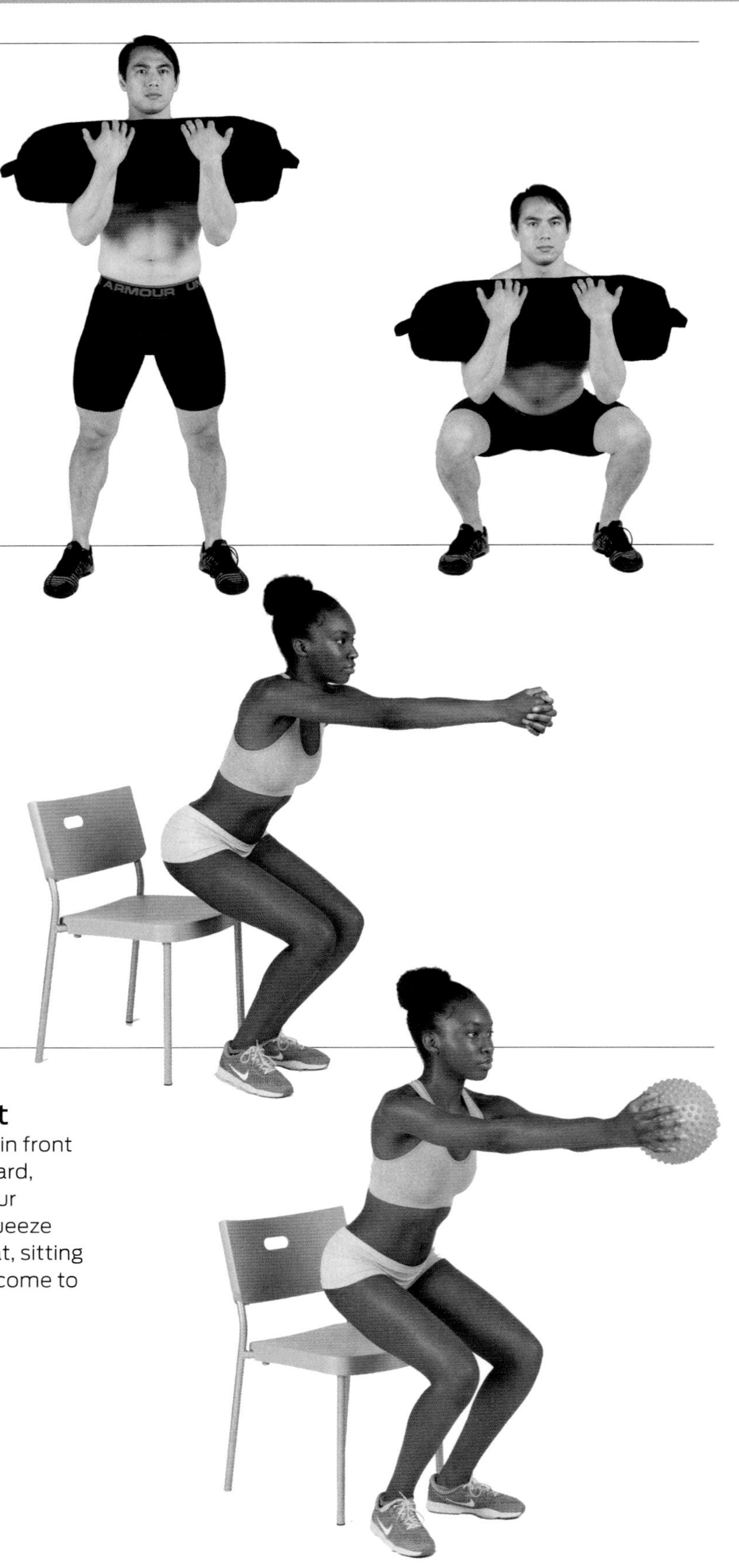

303

Chair Squat

Stabilize your feet hip-width apart in front of a chair and reach the arms forward. Keep your abdominals and core engaged, squeeze your legs, and come into your Squat, sitting onto the chair behind you. Quickly come to standing again, and repeat.

304

Weighted Ball Chair Squat

Stabilize your feet hip-width apart in front of a chair and reach the arms forward, holding the weighted ball. Keep your abdominals and core engaged, squeeze your legs, and come into your Squat, sitting onto the chair behind you. Quickly come to standing again, and repeat.

305 Balance Ball Squat

Stabilize both feet hip-width apart on a balance ball. Keep your abdominals and core engaged, squeeze your legs, and come into your Squat stance, reaching the arms forward. The balance ball is great for challenging the body's balance!

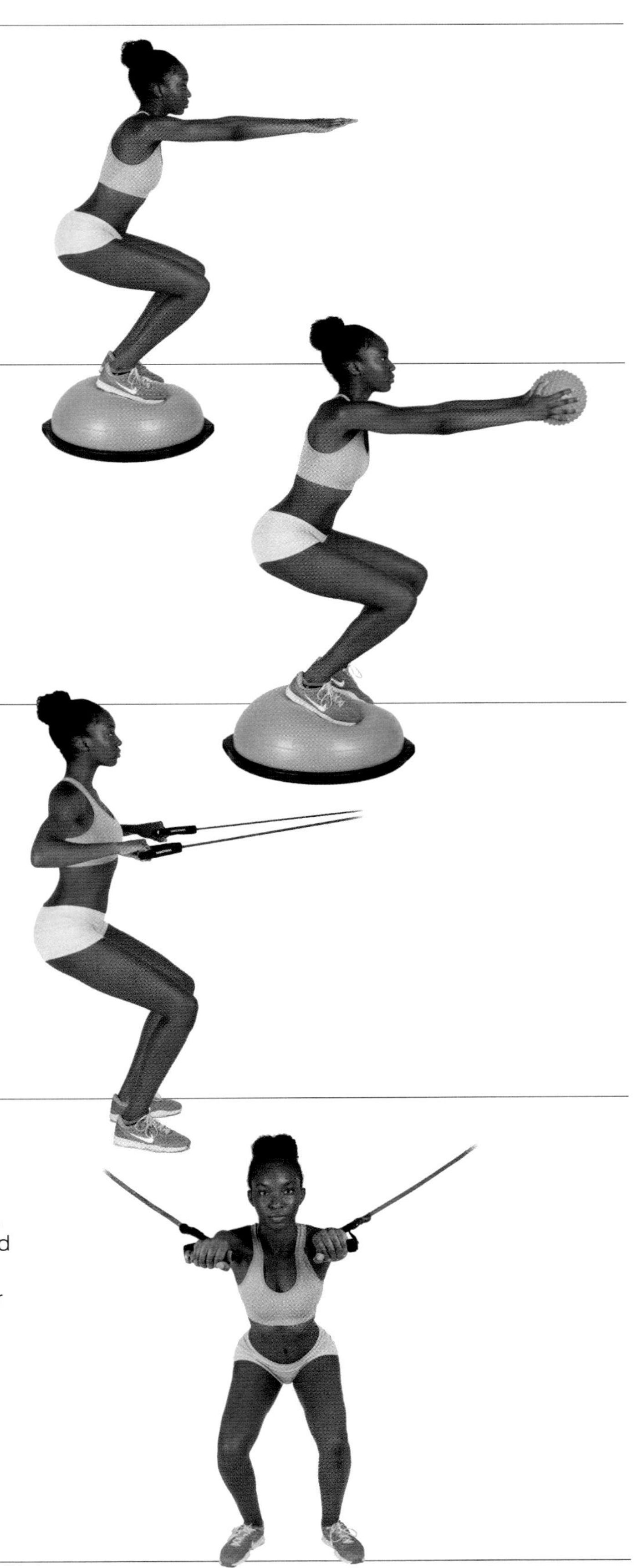

306 Weighted Ball Squat on Balance Ball

Stabilize your feet hip-width apart on a balance ball. Keep your abdominals and core engaged, squeeze your legs, reach your weighted ball out in front of you, and come into your Squat stance.

307 Band Squat and Row

Secure your resistance band around a fixed object at chest height. Balanced with slightly bent knees, with the band handles in each hand, take your Squat. Using your upper-back muscles, bend at the elbows and draw the band handles in toward your chest. Hold at the bottom, and repeat. Keep resistance in your legs and spine.

308 Press and Squat

Stand with your feet shoulder-width apart. Shift your weight over the balls of your feet, holding the cables in each hand from behind you. Push your arms straight out from your chest with your palms down and bend your knees into a Squat.

309 Cable Squat and Row

Balanced with slightly bent knees, with both hands wrapped around the cable handle, take your squat. Using your upper-back muscles, bend at the elbows and draw the cable handles in toward your waist, hugging the elbows into your sides. Hold at the bottom, and repeat. Keep resistance in your legs and spine.

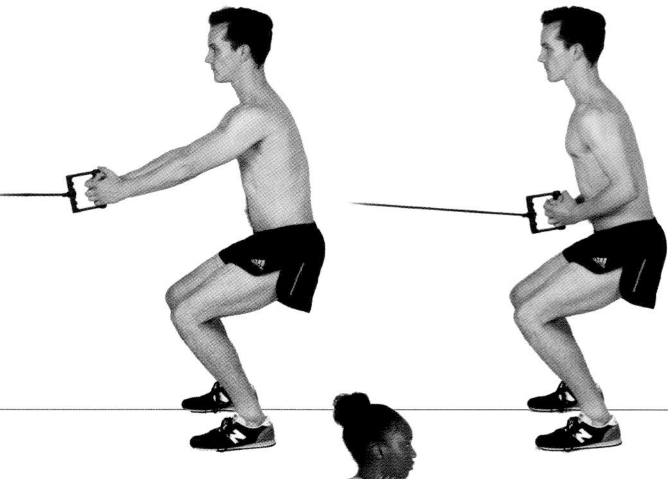

310 Resistance-Band Squat

Start upright with a long spine. Secure your band under the centers of both feet. Holding the handles in each hand, hug the elbows into your sides and keep them still while you squat. Hold at the bottom, and repeat.

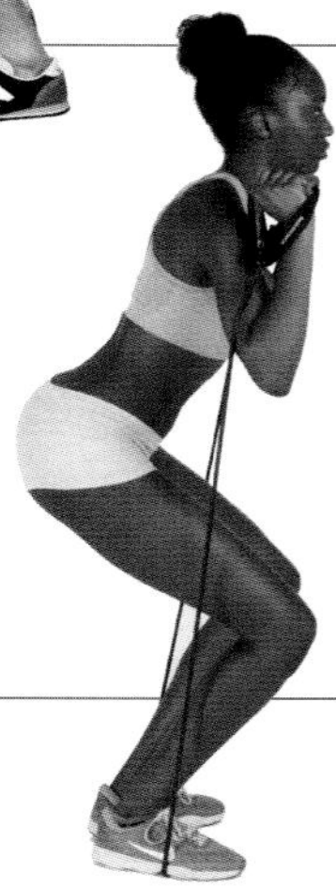

311 Jump Squat

Stand in a large, open-legged stance. Bend into a wide Squat and, with both legs bent, suck the abdominals in tightly, engage the hamstrings, and quickly jump up high. Land as you began, in your standard bent-leg-squat position. Use the arms as needed.

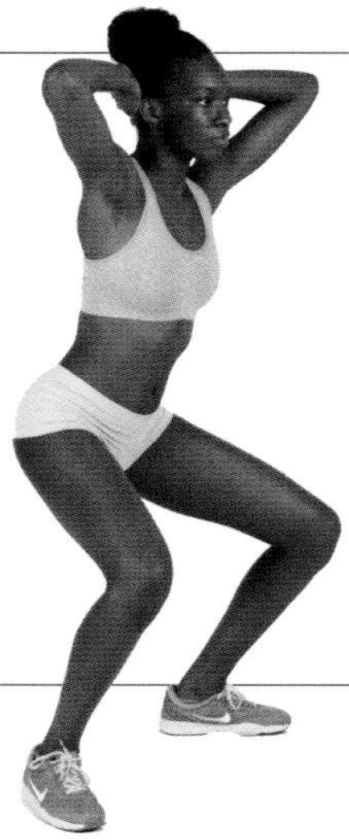

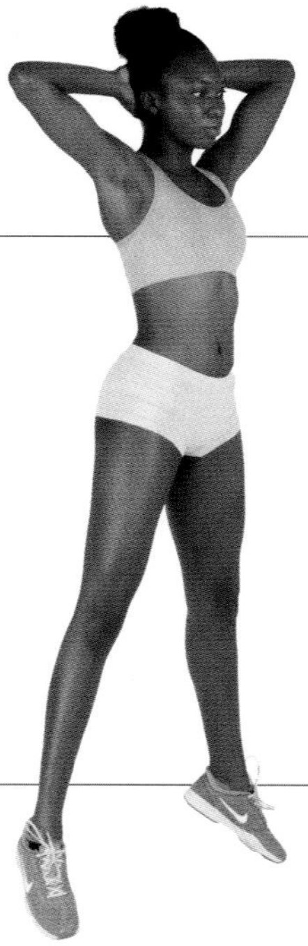

312 Resistance-Band Jump Squat

Start upright with a long spine. Secure your band under the centers of both feet. Holding the handles in each hand, hug the elbows into your sides and isolate the bend of your arm while you squat. Hold at the bottom and lightly hop once there, bending only at the ankles, holding your handles tightly. If performed correctly, the effort in your torso and legs in the exact same position, provides great benefits to both.

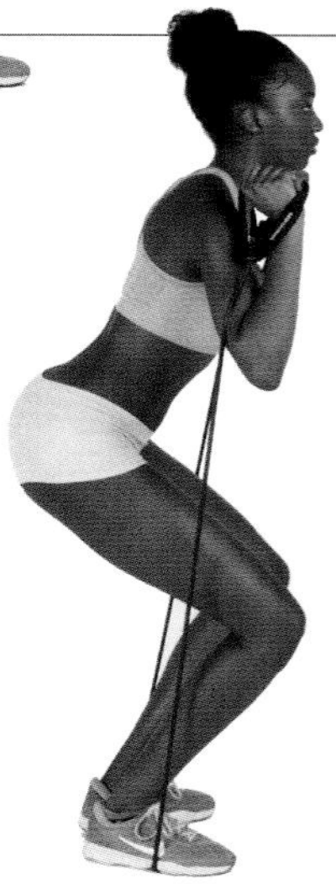

313 Suspended Squat

This variation of the Squat enhances the movement stretch by holding onto a strap. Hold the strap with both hands and descend into the Squat position. Use a strap for a deeper Squat stretch or simply to help assist your with you balance.

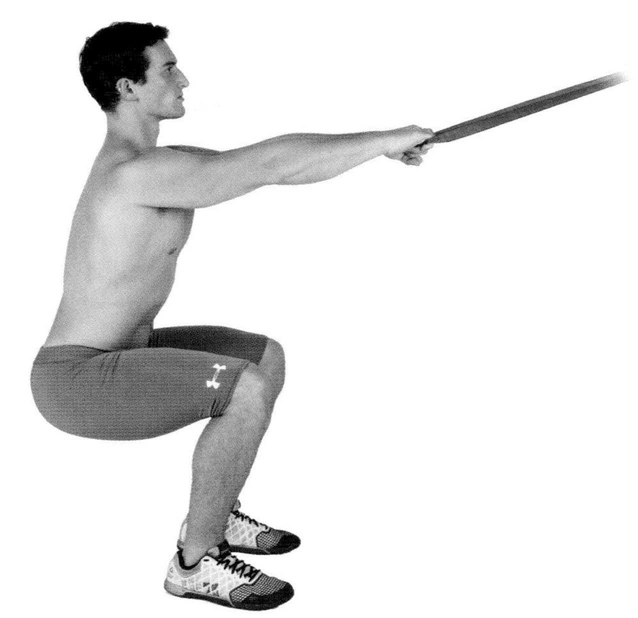

- Stand with an erect, long spine, bringing your feet shoulder-width apart.
- Take the secured strap and hold it tightly in both hands. Pull in the core tightly.
- Bend the knees and hinge at the hips, coming into your Squat position. Pull on the straps, and let your hips and body stretch back against the strap's resistance.

314 Suspended Single-Leg Squat

Stand with an erect, long spine, bringing your feet shoulder-width apart. Take the secured strap and hold it with both hands. Pull in the core tightly. Bend the knees and hinge at the hips, coming into your Squat position. Pull on the strap and lift the right leg, squeezing the inner thighs in toward each other. Return to the start position, and repeat.

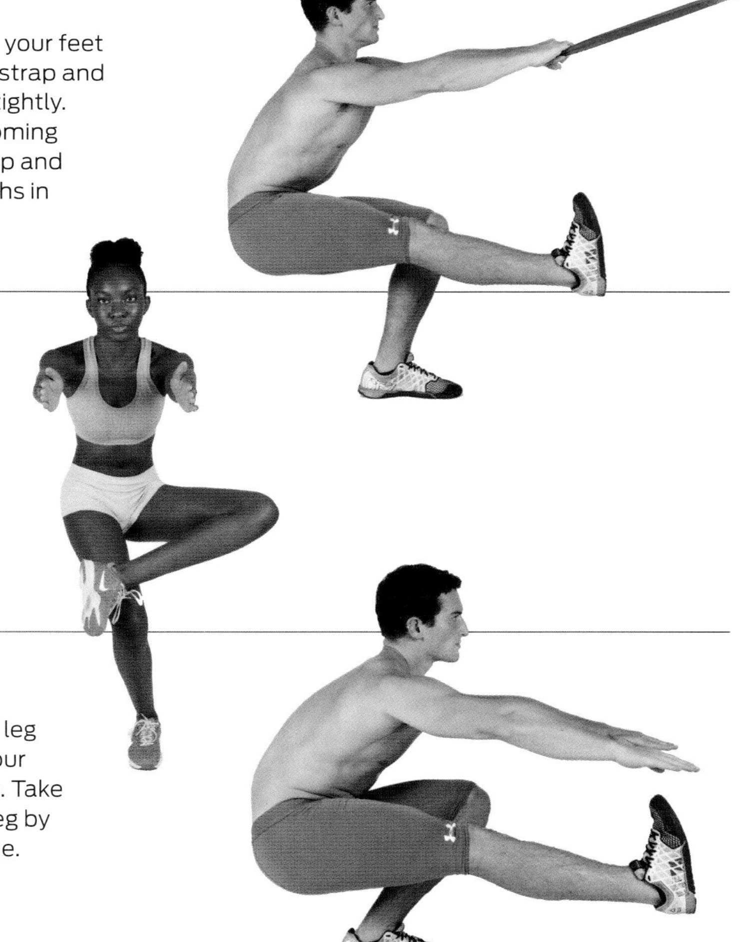

315 Single-Leg Squat

Reach your arms forward and place the left ankle on top of the right knee. Squeeze your glutes and squat, stretching your left knee open against the right leg. Let the hips push back while the arms reach forward in opposition.

316 Pistol Squat

Pull the core in strongly and lift the right leg off the ground. With the leg raised, tip your hips back, and lower slowly into a Squat. Take care to stabilize the working squatting leg by strongly engaging the abs the whole time.

317 **Sumo Squat**

Open your legs wide and turn your feet out with your hands on each thigh. Lengthen your spine, with the abdominals pulled up, and bend deeply at the knees. Once the thighs reach a 90-degree angle to the knee, return to standing.

318 **Sumo Squat with Toe-Touch and Reach**

Come into your Sumo Squat with your hands on your thighs. In one move, tip the hips back, bend forward, touching your toes with one hand, twisting your torso, and reaching your other arm straight up. Stand, and repeat on the other side.

319 **Side-Leaning Sumo Squat**

Take your Sumo Squat and hold deeply at the bottom of it, engaging your glutes, hamstrings, and abs. Place one hand on your thigh, extending the other arm up high and then over to your side. Stretch and hold here.

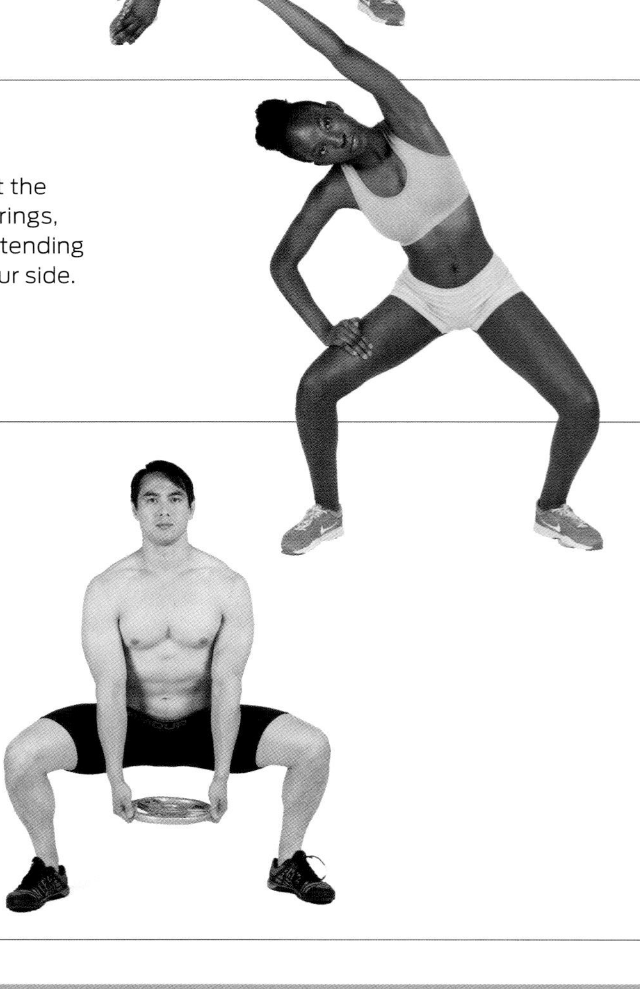

320 **Weighted Sumo Squat**

Open your legs wide and turn your feet out, with your hands gripping a weighted plate. Lengthen your spine, with the abdominals pulled up, and bend deeply at the knees. Once the thighs reach a 90-degree angle to the knee, return to standing.

321 Medicine Ball Sumo Squat with Overhead Lift

Come into your static Sumo Squat stance, with your hands holding the Medicine ball overhead. As you squat, isolate the arms to press the ball down below the pelvis, in between the thighs. Keep your spine straight and shoulders down.

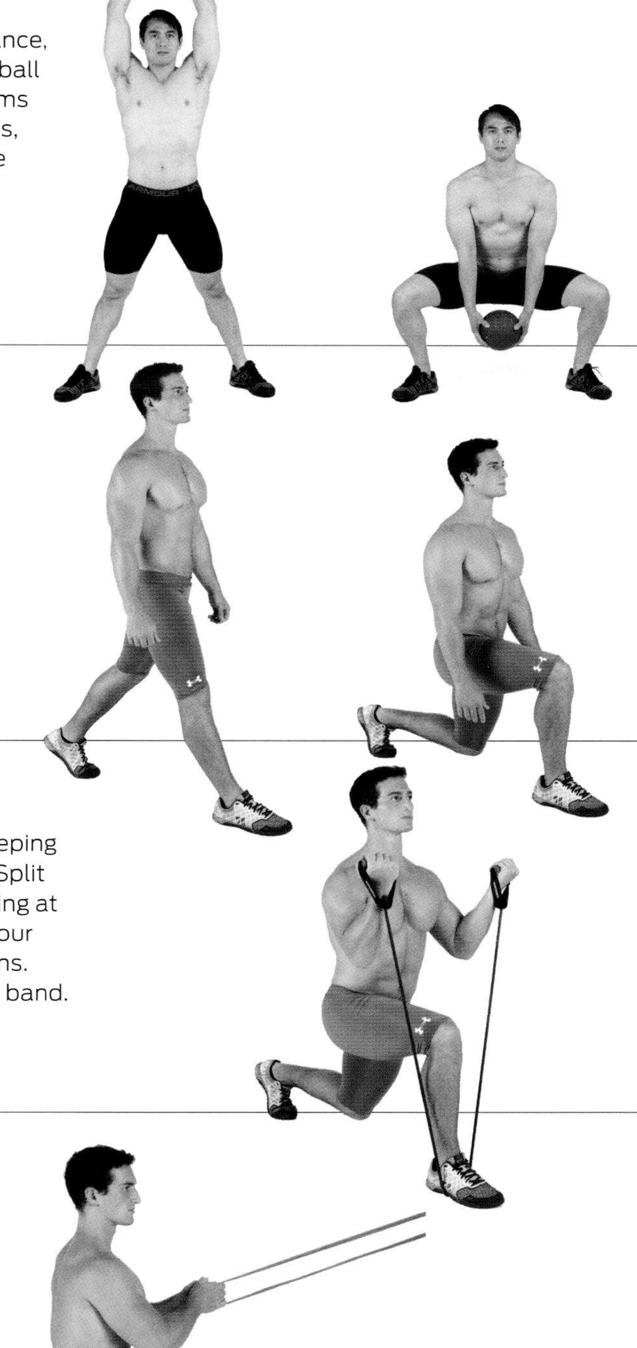

322 Split Squat

In a staggered stance, bend both knees into 90-degree shapes, parallel to the ground. Keep the abdominals tucked into the spine and the front knee over the ankle . Straighten the front leg, and come to stand back up. Switch legs. Feel the burn!

323 Split Squat with Band Curl

Place a band under your front foot, keeping a good grip on the band. Lower into a Split Squat, arms glued to your sides. Bending at the elbows, pull the band up toward your shoulders, working the front of the arms. Then stand, keeping resistance on the band.

324 Split Squat with Strap Row

Stand with an erect, long spine, and bring your feet shoulder-width apart. Take the secured strap and hold it tightly in both hands. Pull in the core tightly, stepping back into a Split Squat with the right leg. Pull the straps into your chest.

325 Dumbbell Split Squat

With a dumbbell in each hand, take a staggered stance. Descend into a Split Squat, lifting the dumbbells overhead, and quickly recover back to standing. Adding speed to the recovery with dumbbells will create quicker muscle response and better balance throughout the body.

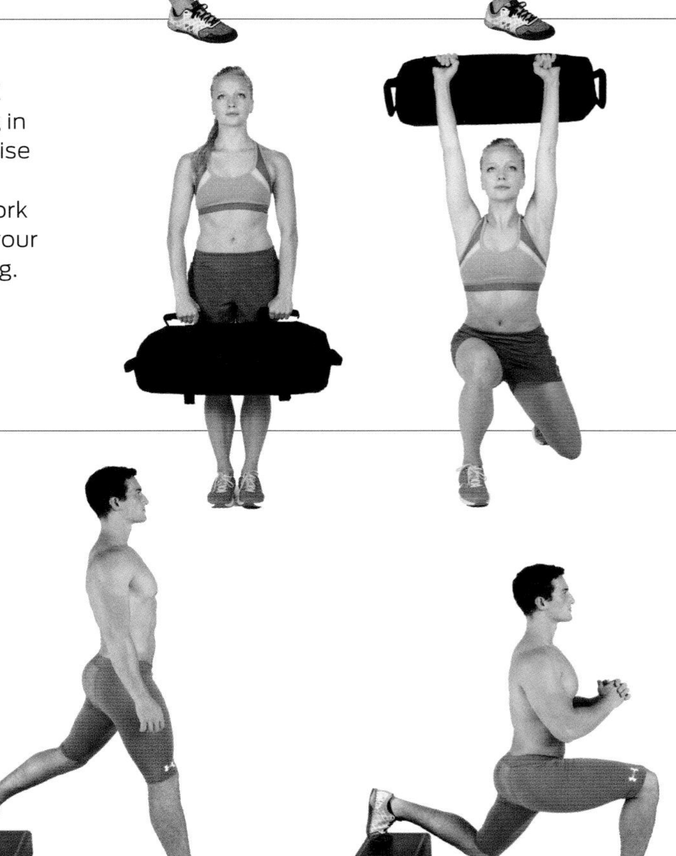

326 Medicine Ball Split Squat

In a Split Squat stance, hold the ball with both hands firmly against the chest. Now, lower into a deep Squat, holding the ball straight out in front, and pulling the core in tightly while engaging the backs of the arms. With control, return to standing.

327 Overhead Sandbag Split Squat

Standing with your feet together, sandbag in hands, make a deep forward lunge, and raise the sandbag straight up above your head. Challenge your core and leg muscles to work a little deeper, and hold at the bottom of your squat. Return to standing, lowering the bag.

328 Bulgarian (or Romanian) Split Squat

Start in a well-staggered position with your right leg in front of the left. Place the left, back leg on an elevated bench or step. Perform a Split Squat (#322). Lengthen the front of the back hip and stretch it forward. Switch legs, adding hand weights if you wish.

329 Bulgarian Split Squat and Overhead Press

Bulgarian Split Squats are famous for toning the rear leg muscle groups. They also provide you with a good, deep stretch in the front of the hip and down through the quad. Holding at the bottom of any Split Squat, for a moment, will also help create stability in the hip joint.

- With one foot elevated behind the other, find your Split Squat stance.
- As you bend into the Split Squat, raise your arms overhead and hold there.
- Your front thigh should be parallel to the floor. Squeeze your glutes here.

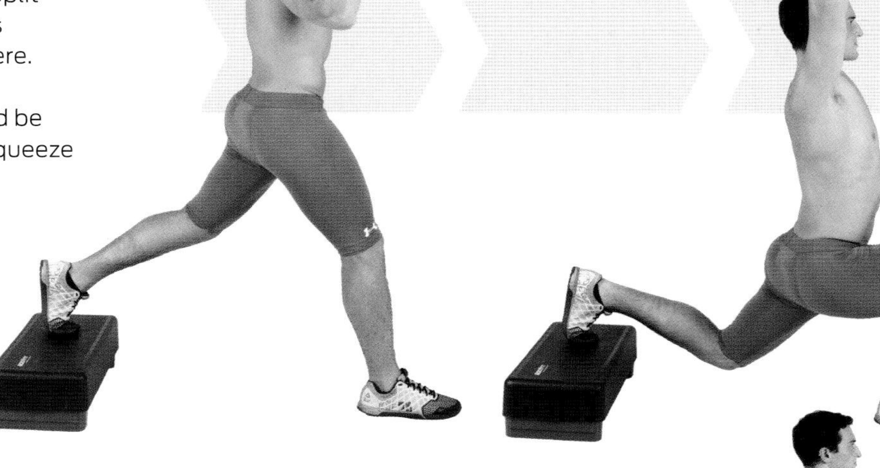

330 Bulgarian Split Squat on Swiss Ball

Put the top of your foot onto a Swiss ball and stabilize your standing leg by activating your core and hamstrings. Pull the core in tightly and bring your hands together in front of your chest. Lower into a Split Squat, bringing your knee and back leg into one long line.

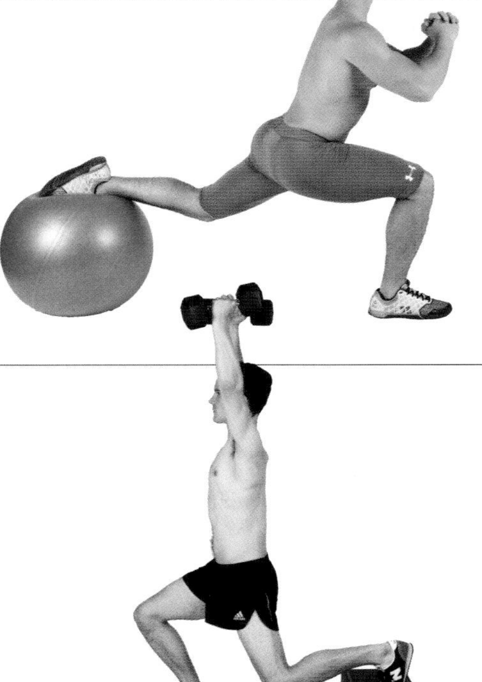

331 Bulgarian Split Squat and Dumbbell Overhead Press

Get into a Bulgarian Split Squat stance with your arms at your sides, dumbbells in hands. As you squat, isolate the elbows to bend and then press up overhead. Keep your spine straight and shoulders down.

332 Medicine Ball Power Squat

The Medicine Ball Power Squat is great for those looking to stabilize their core while, simultaneously, developing a wider range of flexible upper body movement. You can challenge your range by adding a weighted Medicine ball, kettlebell, dumbbell or disc. Move quickly for an added stability challenge.

- Stand on one leg with your back leg raised slightly off the floor. Balance your Medicine ball above your shoulder.
- In one move, bend forward and squat down, sweeping the ball across the body.
- Then stand, lifting the ball back up. Making this sequence quickly develops lateral core and glute power.

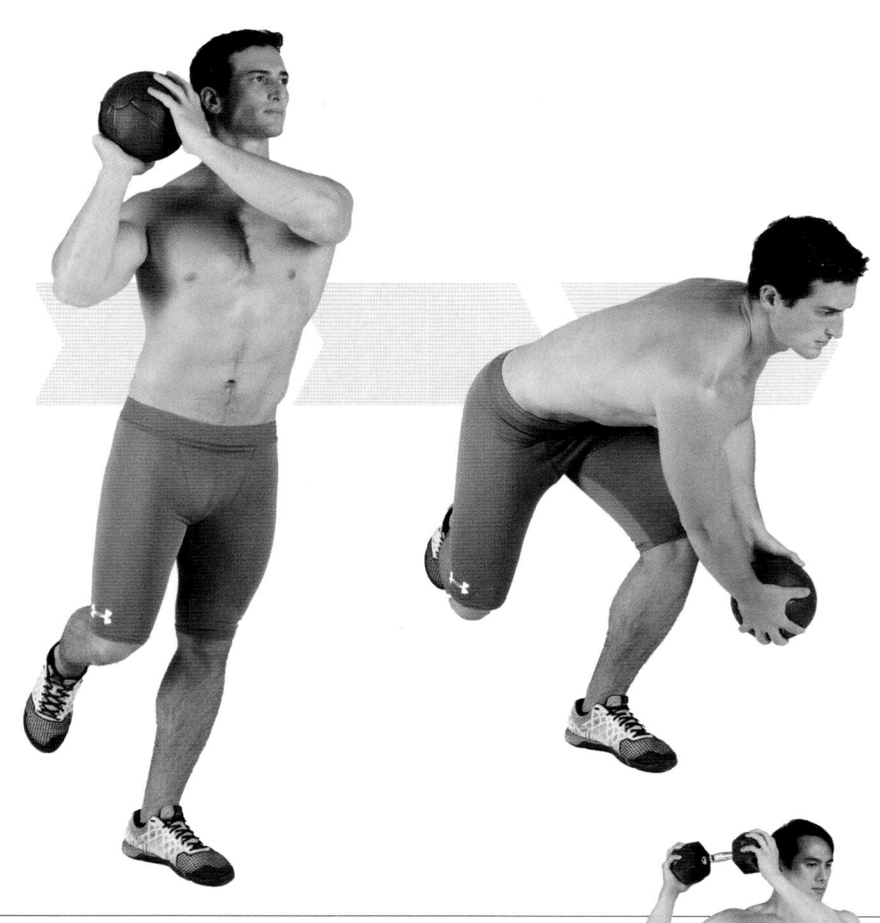

333 Dumbbell Power Squat

Stand on one leg, holding a dumbbell above your shoulder. In one move, squat down, sweeping the weight across the body, then stand, lifting it back up. Making this sequence quickly, develops lateral core and glute power.

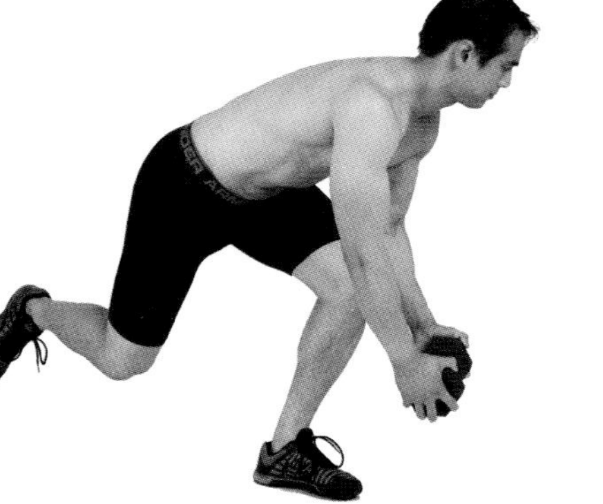

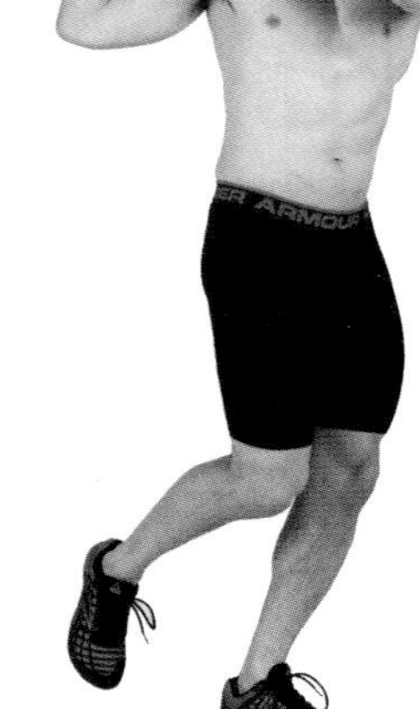

334 Weighted Ball Skater Squat

The advanced variation of the Medicine Ball Power Squat (#332) further engages the core, while adding a challenge to your balance with a deeper bend and high-raised back leg.

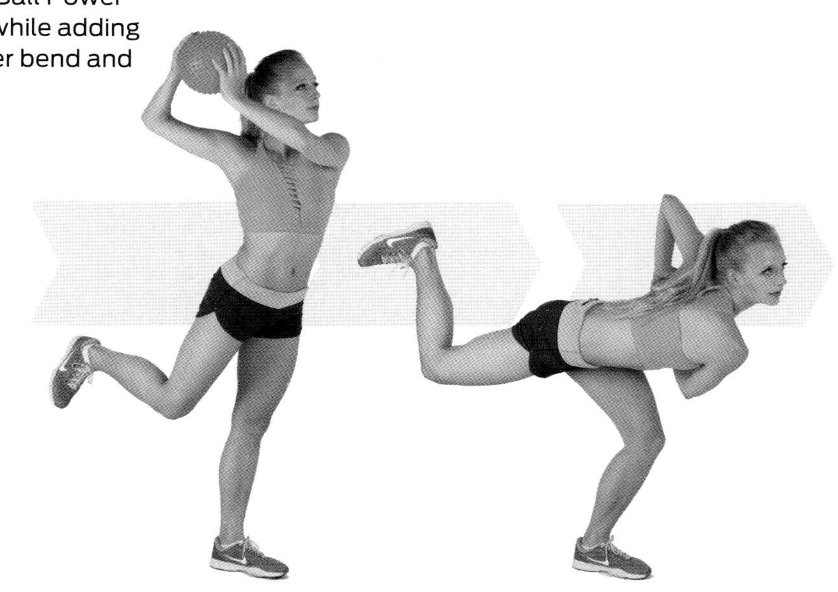

- Stand on one leg with your back leg raised slightly off the floor. Balance a weighted ball above your right shoulder.
- In one move, make a deep forward bend and squat down, sweeping the ball across the body, and raising your rear leg as high as you can.
- Then stand, lifting the ball back up. Making this sequence quickly, develops lateral core and glute power.

335 One-Arm Kettlebell Clean

In this variation you will use a kettlebell to enhance your body alignment and stabilization as you move through your basic Squat. Incorporating the kettlebell adds an element of pulling and pushing for the upper body.

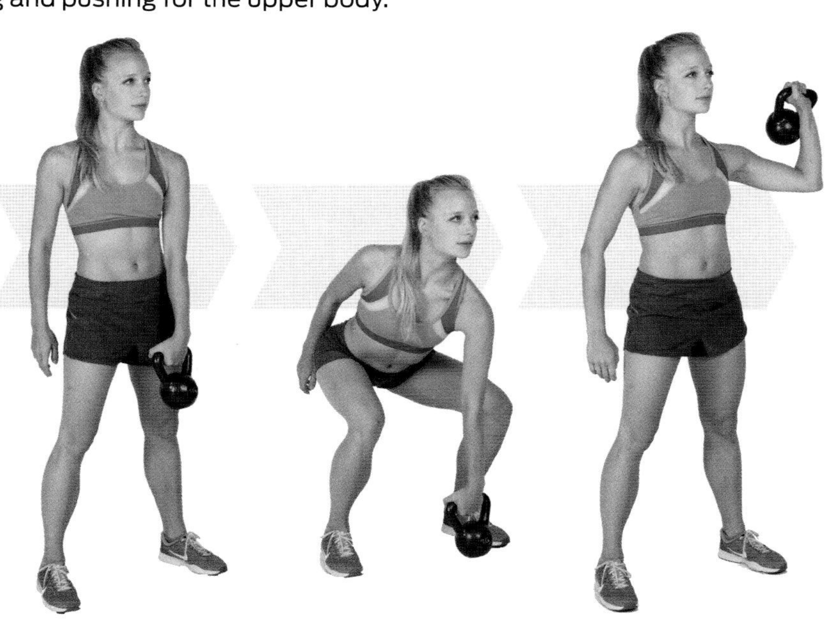

- Start by standing with your core pulled in tightly, grasping a kettlebell in your left hand.
- Deeply bend the knees and hinge the hips back into your standard Squat.
- Extend the legs and pull the kettlebell up alongside the front of the body in a quick, smooth movement, and open to the left shoulder.

336 Wall Squat and Hold

Incorporating a flat surface, such as a wall behind you, puts your upper body in perfect anatomical alignment. Executing your Squat position against a wall will yield optimal results, as you are activating deep into the squatting muscles.

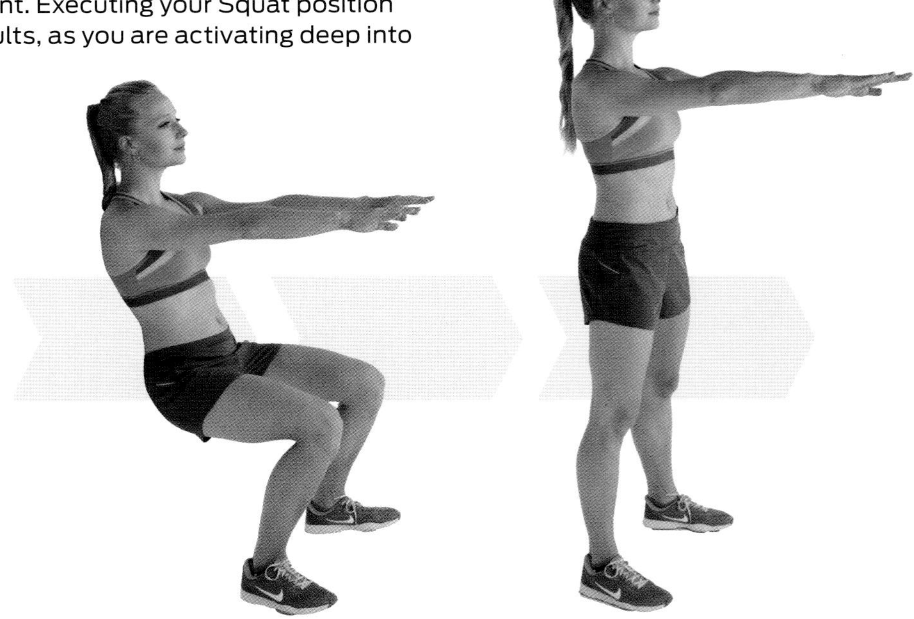

- Stand against a wall, with a long, supported upper spine. Walk your feet out away from the wall by about 2 feet (60 centimeters).
- With arms at shoulder level, and feet hip-width apart, squat down, keeping your back against the wall, until your knees reach a 90-degree angle. Hold there.

337 Swiss Ball Wall Squat

Engage your abs and balance standing against a Swiss ball, with your arms straight out in front of you. With a straight spine and the legs active, bend slowly into a Squat, keeping pressure on the ball. Pull the abs up and in to stand.

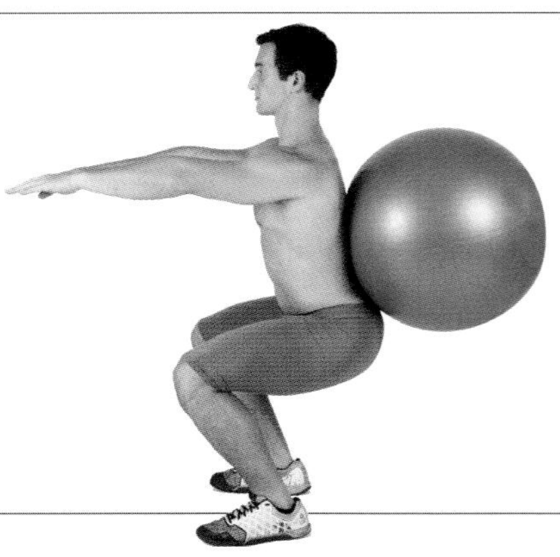

338 Swiss Ball Squat with Dumbbell Curls

Place a Swiss ball between your upper spine and the wall behind you. Come into a Squat, with dumbbells in each hand. Hug the elbows in and isolate the bend of your arm while you squat. Hold at the bottom, and repeat.

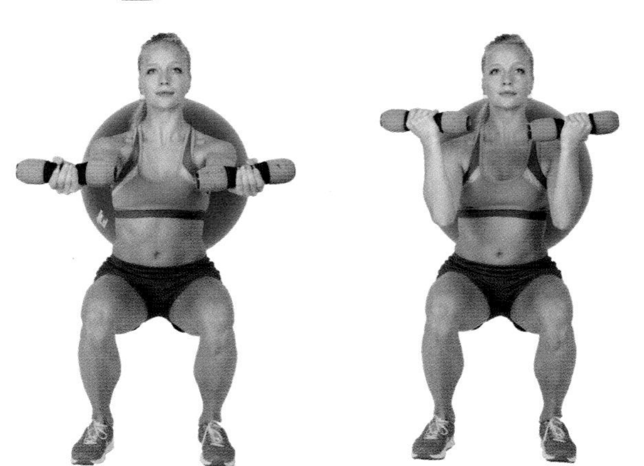

339 Single-Leg Swiss Ball Squat with Dumbbell Curls

Go for your Swiss Ball Squat with Dumbbell Curls, but with one leg off the ground. Your standing leg will need to work much harder to keep the knee aligned over the toe. Pull in those abs, and lower up and down with ease.

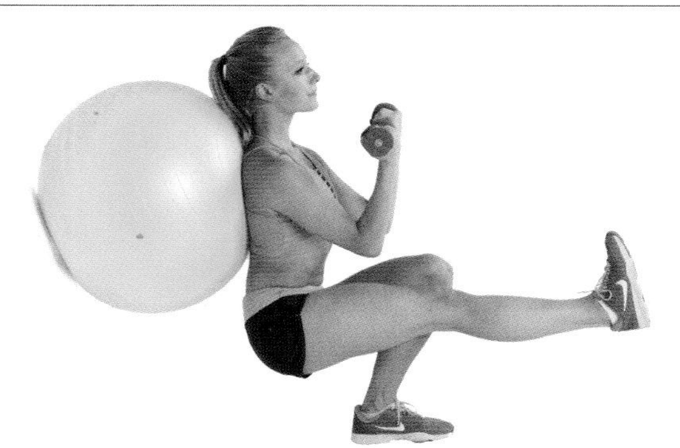

340 Weighted Ball Box Squat with Side Leg Lift

Start with both knees bent, holding a weighted ball into your chest. With your left foot on a box, take a deep Squat, straighten the left leg up, and kick the right leg out to the side. Return to your Squat starting position. Alternate sides, and repeat.

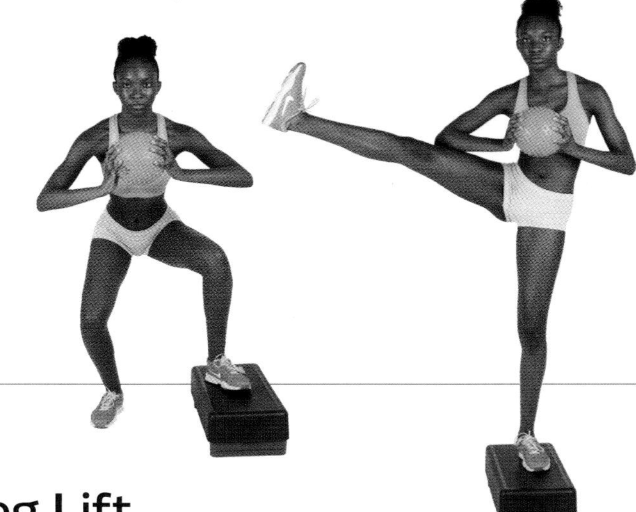

341 Dumbbell Box Squat with Side Leg Lift

Incorporating a box and a weighted dumbbell into this squat variation pinpoints the work into the hamstring and thighs. Keeping a tight core will help you balance while executing this dynamic move.

- Start with both knees bent, holding a dumbbell into your chest.
- With your left foot on the box, take a deep Squat, straighten the left leg up, and, kick the right leg out to the side.
- Return to your Squat starting position. Alternate sides, and repeat.

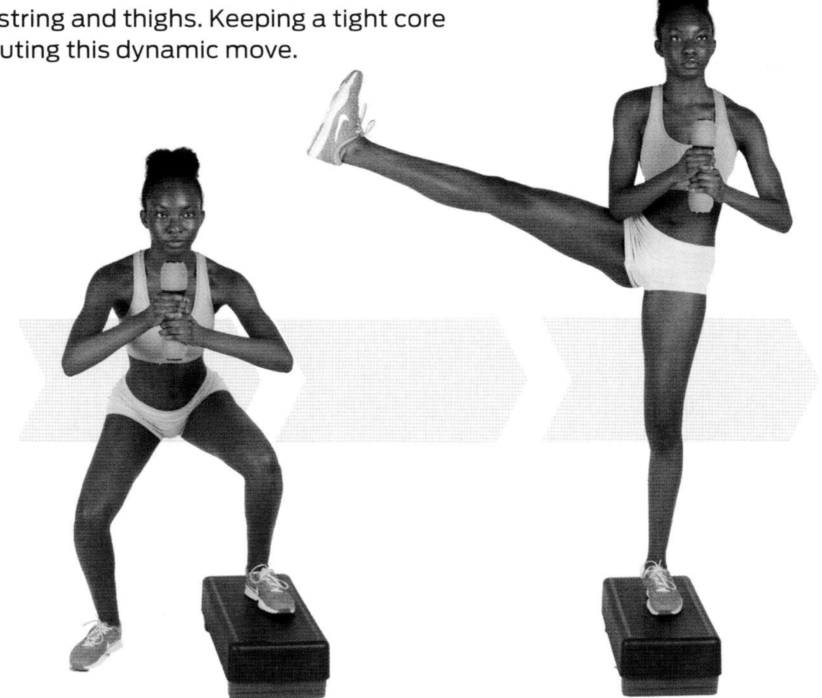

342

Barbell Squat

The Barbell Squat works your lower and upper body deeply while, simultaneously, stabilizing all of your back muscles. Working this move into your routine will give you the ability to keep your back straighter throughout your various daily activities. And, believe it or not, doing a few sets of Barbell Squats will also increase your cardio capacity.

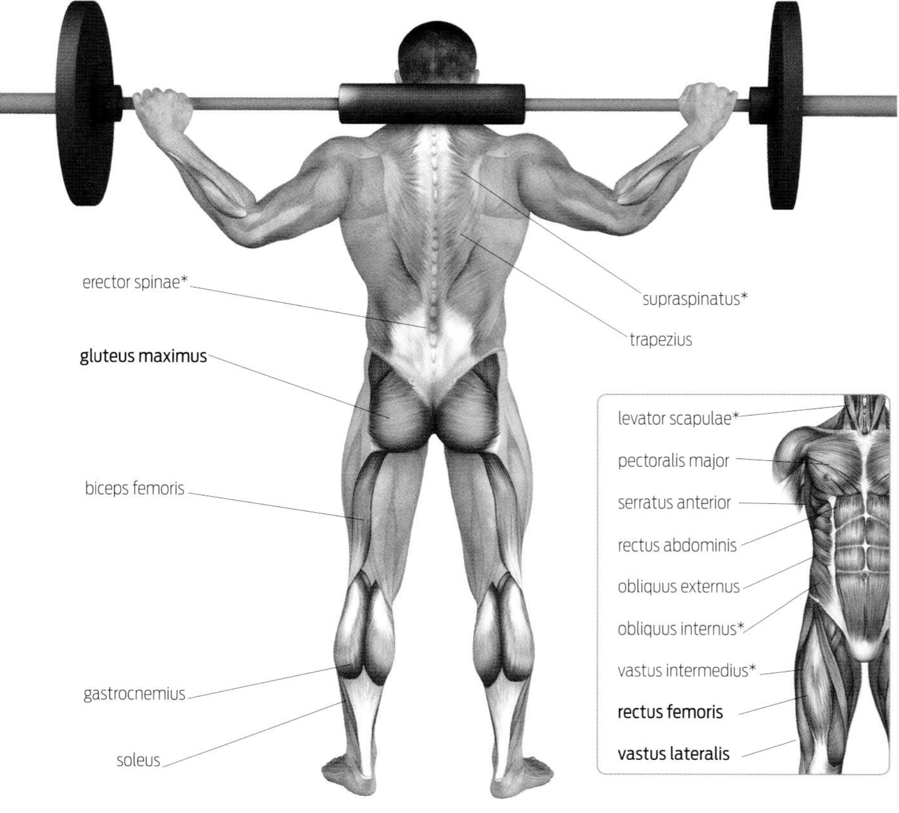

Correct form

Make sure you engage your back muscles as well as your core for this move. You will also need to have a strong rooted stance with both legs.

Avoid

Dont let the body bend forward more than you need to. It is important to keep your back up high so the barbell stays balanced.

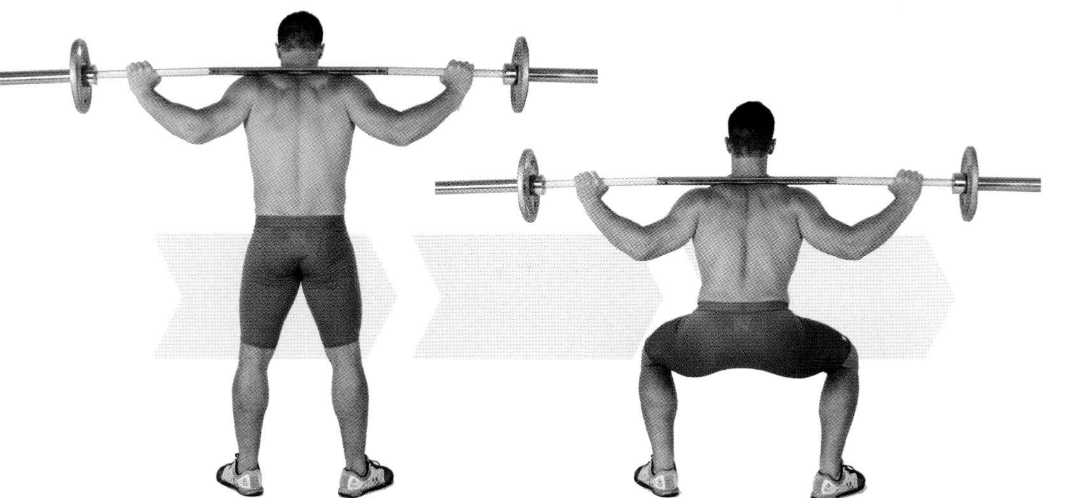

- Start in a shoulder-width stance with the barbell laid across the top of your shoulders.
- Hold the barbell safely, with both hands, pull in the core tightly, and bend the knees.
- Allow the hips to tip back, while keeping your back up as straight as you can. Come into your Squat position.

343 Front Barbell Squat

Open your legs into a shoulder-width stance. With an overgrip crossed-arm hold, secure your barbell in the front of the chest. Lengthen your spine, with the abdominals pulled up, bend deeply at the knees, and let the hips tip back into a static Squat.

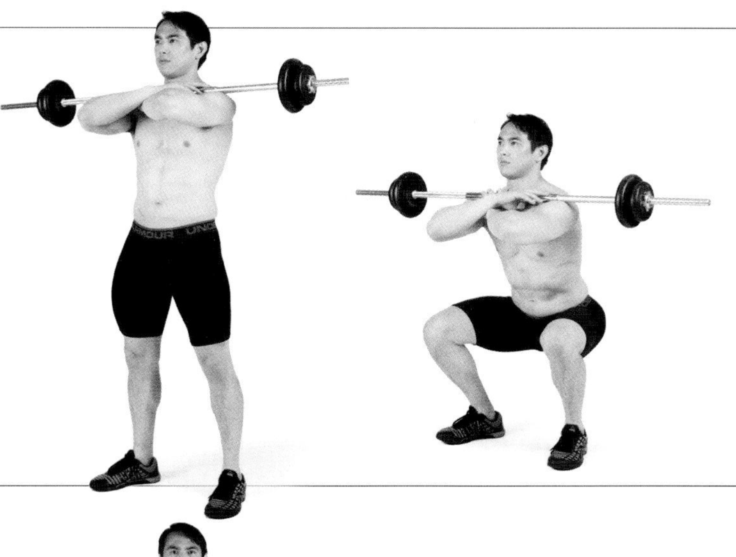

344 Barbell Sumo Squat

Open your legs wide and turn your feet out. Securely hold a barbell against the backs of your shoulders. Lengthen your spine, with the abdominals pulled up, and bend deeply at the knees. Once your thighs reach a 90-degree angle to the knees, return to standing.

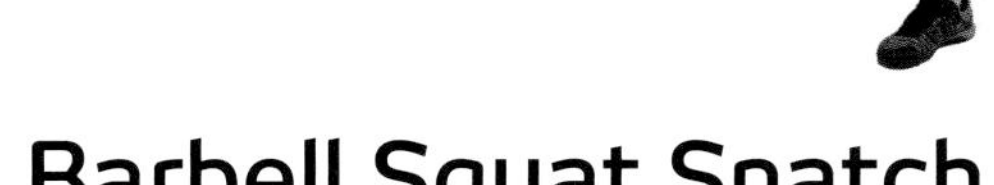

345 Barbell Squat Snatch

The Barbell Squat Snatch is a move that places the weight of your barbell directly in front of you. By lifting or snatching up the bar with a dynamic, quick count, you work on developing core strength as well as stability in the lower back and legs.

- Start in a deeply bent squat position, holding on tightly to your barbell.
- In one smooth move, with a "flip" movement, hinged at the elbows, pull the barbell up along the front of your body, high into your shoulders.
- Press the bar up high, directly overhead. Engage through the legs and core.

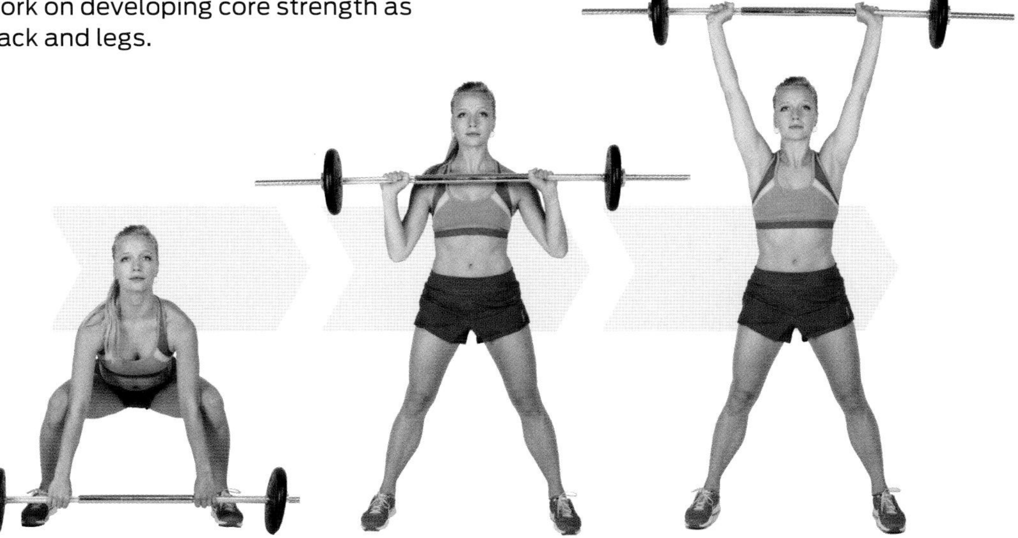

346 Overhead Barbell Split Squat

In a staggered stance, bend both knees into 90-degree angles, parallel to the ground. Press your barbell overhead, and keep the abdominals tucked into the spine and the front knee over the ankle. Straighten your front leg, coming to stand back up. Switch legs.

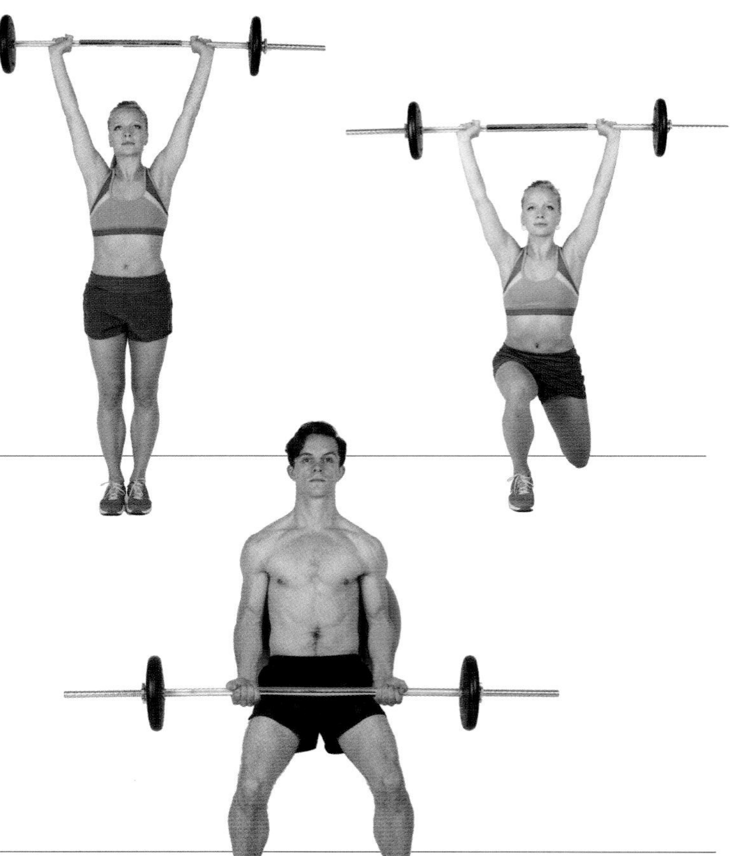

347 Swiss-Ball Squat with Barbell Curls

Place the Swiss ball between your upper spine and the wall behind you. Come into a Squat, securely gripping the barbell with each hand. Hug the elbows in and isolate the bend of your arm while you squat, bringing the bar into your chest.

348 Barbell Chair Squat

Performing this chair squat, especially, with the barbell, will greatly increase your core strength. This is also a great variation for those wanting to develop more stability in the knees and hips.

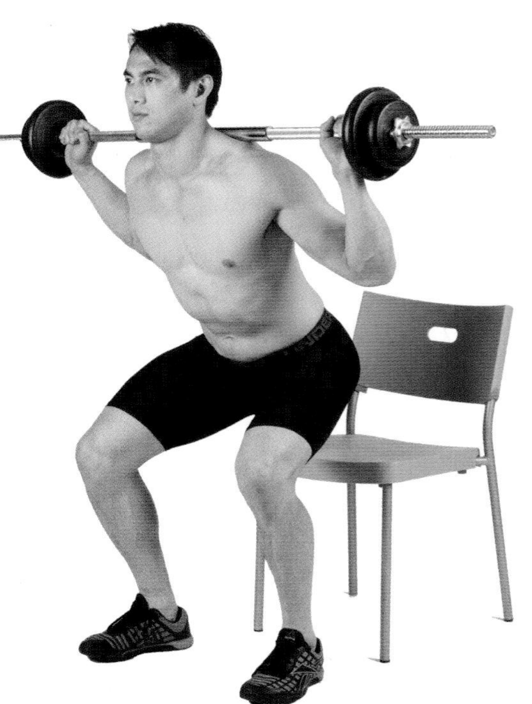

- Stabilize your feet hip-width apart in front of a chair and secure a barbell in both hands behind the shoulders.
- Keep your abdominals and core engaged, squeeze your legs, and come into your Squat, sitting onto the chair behind you.
- Quickly come to standing again, and repeat.

349 Barbell Alternating-Grip Squat

Open your legs into a shoulder-width stance. With an alternating grip hold a barbell securely in both hands. Lengthen your spine, with the abdominals pulled up, and bend deeply at the knees, touching the barbell to the floor out in front of you.

Prepare

You can give yourself a challenging leg and core workout in many different ways. Standing, sitting, or lying down are all great planes to work your movement in.

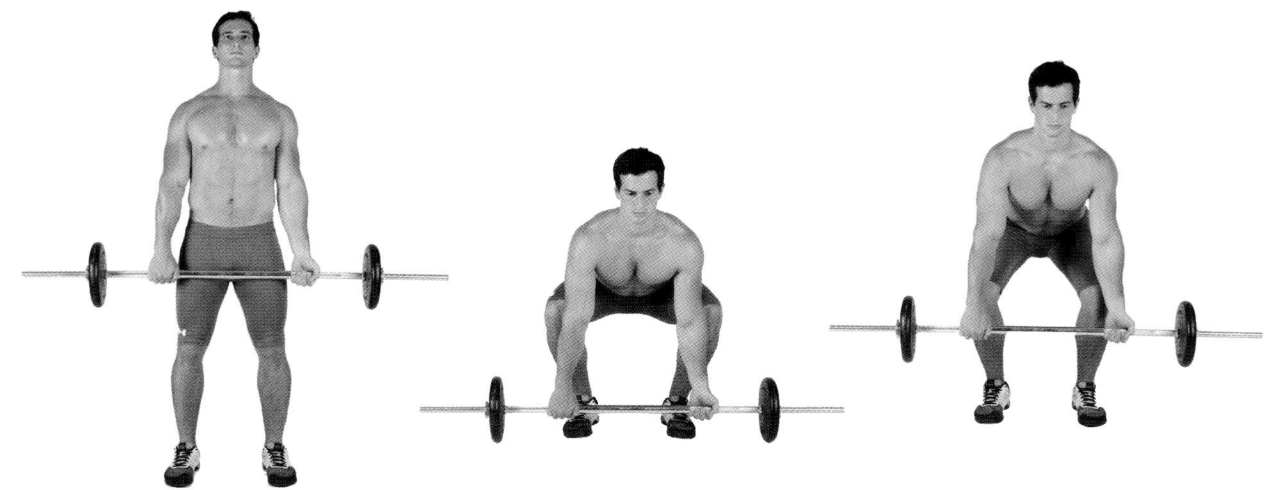

350 Bulgarian Split Squat and Barbell Overhead Press

Bulgarian Split Squats with weighted overhead presses are excellent for toning the upper body as well as the upper leg muscle groups. Working with dynamic levels, this variation also provides you with a stretch in the front of the hip, down through the quad.

- With one foot elevated behind the other, find your Bulgarian Split Squat (#328) stance.
- As you bend into the Squat, raise your arms overhead and hold there.
- Both knees should be at 90-degree angles to the floor. Squeeze your glutes here.

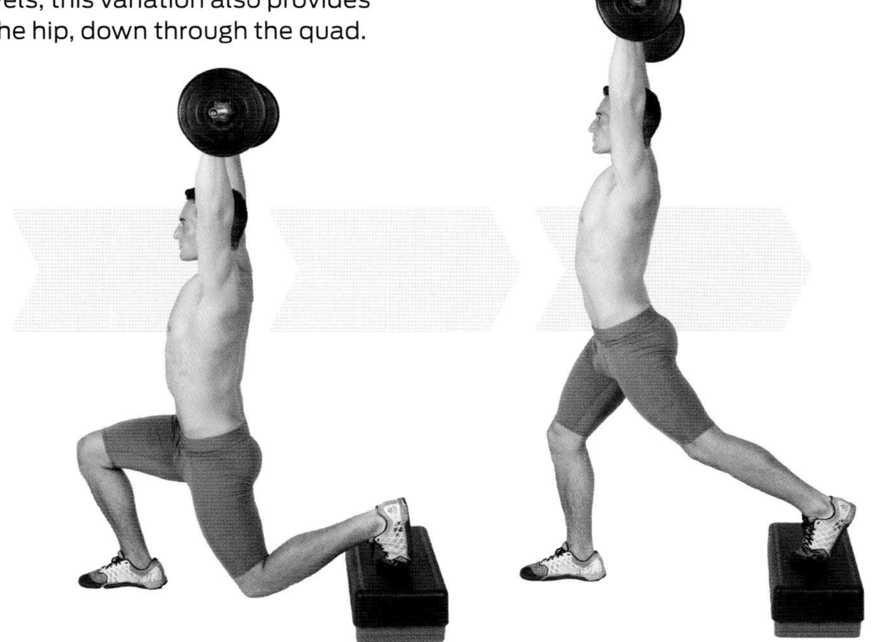

351

Dumbbell Foot Raise

Sitting with a weight held between your feet while bending and extending the knees may seem like a simple movement, but its benefits are great. In these exercises you will engage the quads and also stabilize the hip, knee, and ankle joints as your push and pull into and away from gravity with your shins.

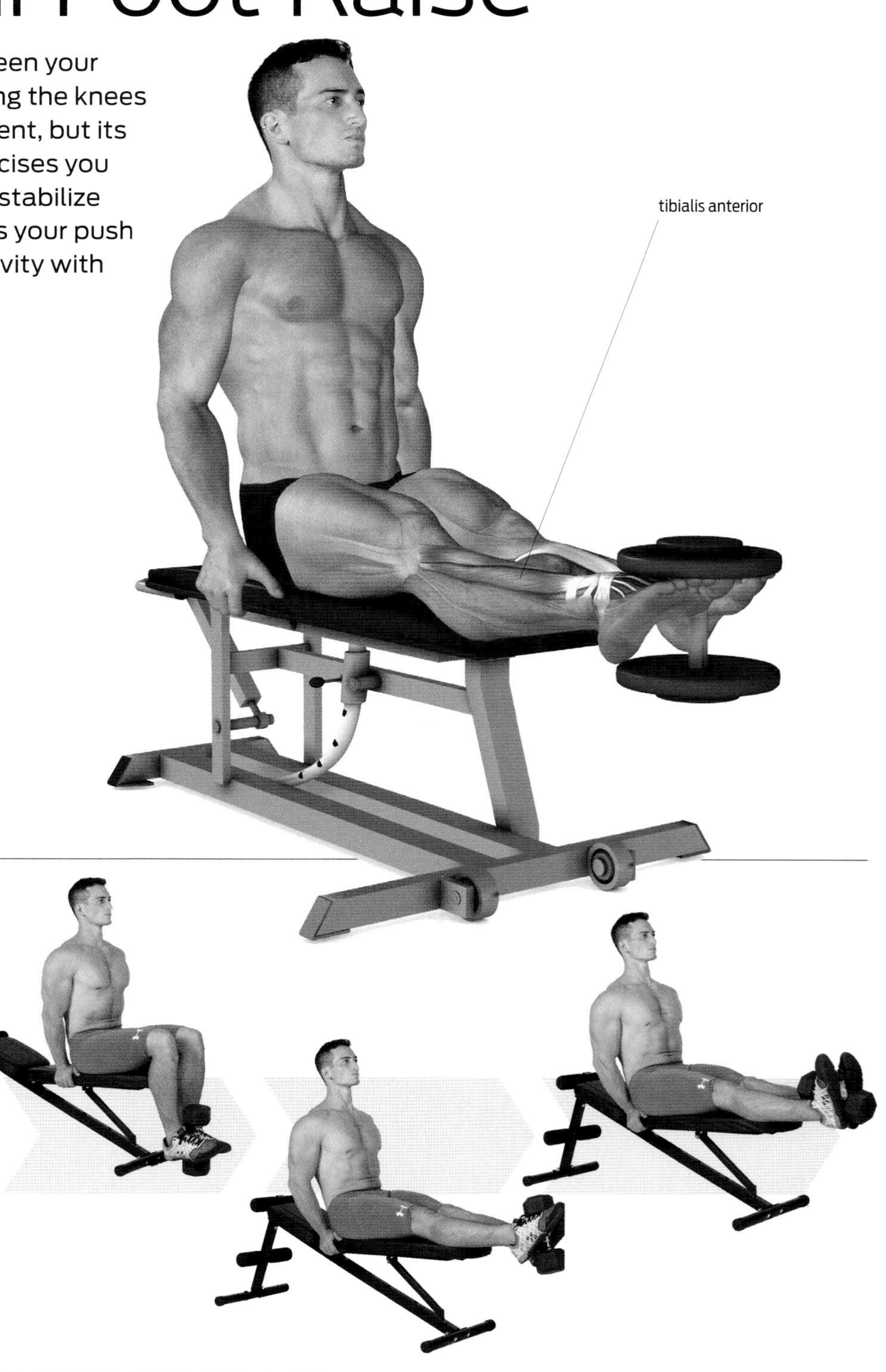

Correct form

Keep your chest open to the front. Try not to bend or arch the lower back while you isolate your legs.

Avoid

Do not use a weight for this variation if you have issues with your knees. You can move through this routine without weight.

Annotation Key
Bold text indicates target muscles
Black text indicates other working muscles
* indicates deep muscles

- Sit, with your back straight up, on an elevated surface or bench. Hold either side of the bench.
- Secure a weight or dumbbell between your feet, bringing your legs very close together.
- Alternate bending and extending the legs, putting the work into the fronts of your legs and shins.

352 Seated Leg Extension

Sitting while concentrating on extending your legs straight out in front of you is an intense workout for the lower extremities, as well as for your core. If you engage your core deeply, you will help to stabilize the lower back and pelvis so that the legs may work more efficiently.

- Sit, with your back straight up, on an elevated surface or bench. Hold either side of the bench.
- Secure a weight or dumbbell between your lower legs, bringing your legs very close together.
- Alternate bending and extending the legs, putting the work into the fronts of your legs.

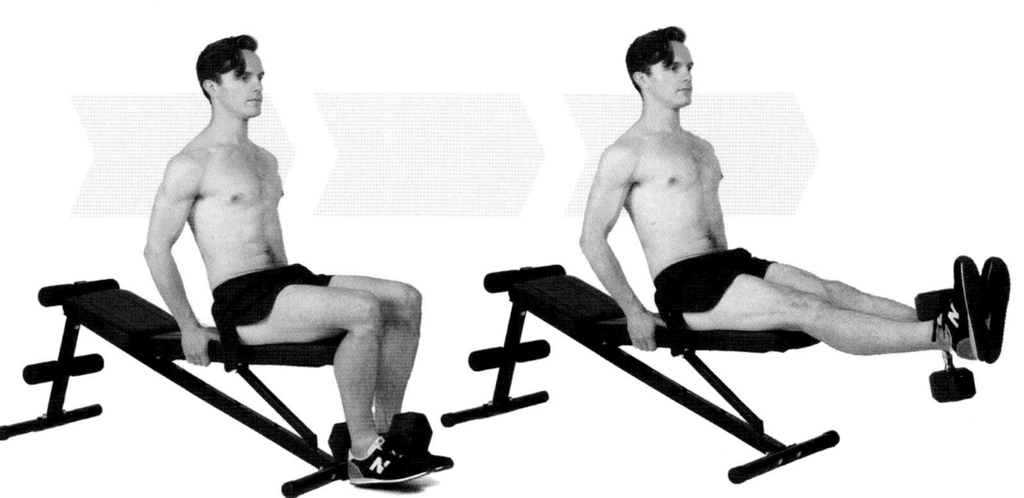

353 Lying Leg Curls

Lying leg curls are, essentially, pull-ups for the lower body. While lifting and lowering a weighted dumbbell toward and away from your body, you engage the backs of your legs, focusing the work into the hamstrings, glutes, and calves.

- Place a dumbbell between your feet and lie with your body extending long on a bench, grasping the front edges with your hands.
- Squeeze the legs together, activating your core, and isolate the knees, bending the weight into your hamstrings.
- Straighten the legs back to your starting position, and repeat.

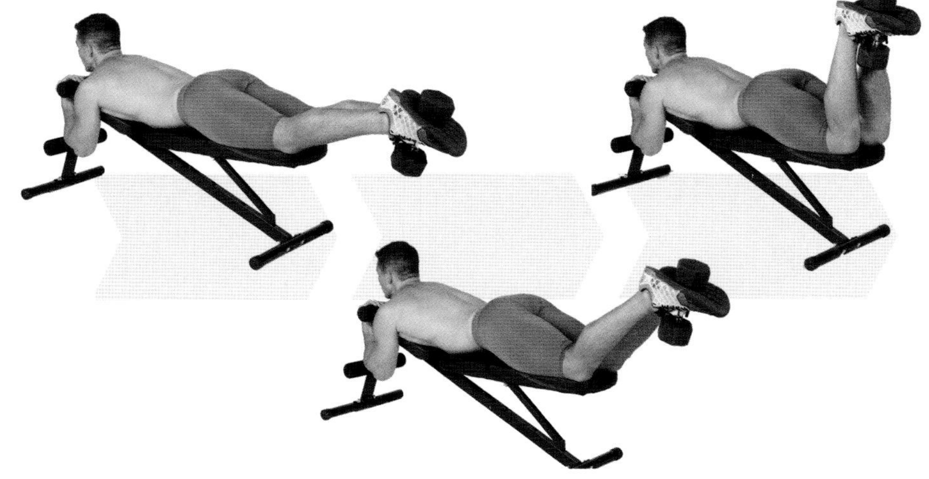

354 Standing One-Leg Curls

Performing these one-legged curls will activate the hamstring while also working your ability to balance on one leg at a time. Shifting the weight of the body from side to side, as you lift your leg, is a fine way to focus on also stabilizing the core.

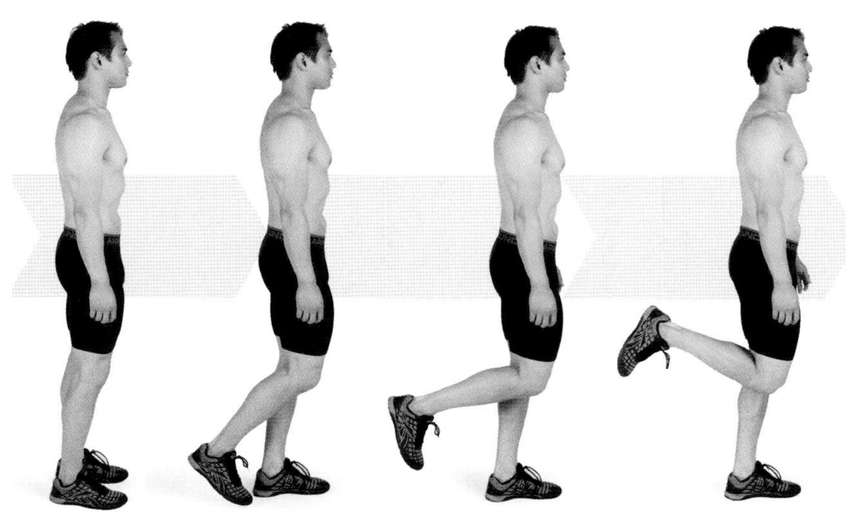

- Stand tall with a long spine, pull your abs up into your lower back, and shift your body weight into the balls of the feet.
- Slowly shift your body weight to your left side.
- Pick up the right foot, bending at the knee, and let the foot come up directly behind you.
- Once the knee flexes to 90 degrees, lower the foot back down. Alternate sides.

355 Hip Extension with Band

Secure a band at the center of left foot. Stand tall with a long spine, pull your abs up into your lower back, and shift your body weight into the balls of your feet. Pick up the left foot, bending at the knee, and push the foot away from you, then forward. Do the desired number of repetitions, then swap sides.

356 Butt Kicks with Leg Weights

Remove the leg weights, and this is a standard butt kick, but the addition of leg weight adds an extra element of difficulty. Either way, it is highly dynamic and plyometric. Working the body explosively in an attempt to jump and reach the foot to the back of your glute is challenging, and hugely strengthening at the same time!

- Start by securing a set of leg weights, one around each lower calf or ankle.
- Stand and squeeze the abs in very tightly.
- Bend into both knees and jump up quickly, extending your left leg and kicking your right foot back and up toward your hamstring.
- Alternate sides, and repeat.

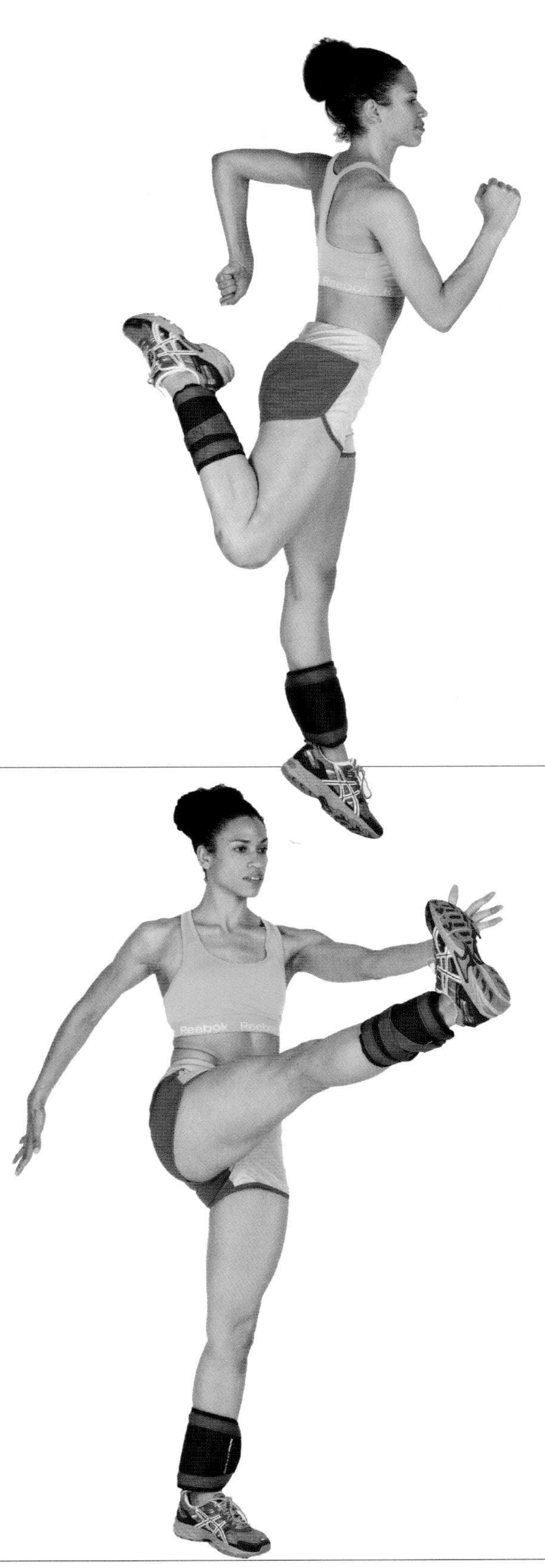

357 Monster Walk with Leg Weights

Stand tall with your leg weights tight around your lower calves. Engage your core and legs and swing the right leg out in front of you. Reach the left arm for your right leg and flex the right foot. Be sure to use a swinging motion in the legs and arms.

Boost your workout

Incorporating ankle weights into your workout routine is a great way to boost aerobic activity while also strengthening the legs. You can use these weights everyday while walking or jogging as well, to increase cardio and blood flow in the body.

358 Hip Adduction and Abduction

Anatomically speaking, the word "abduction" applies to the movement of one body part away from the midline of the body. Adduction infers the opposite–one part of the body moving in toward the body's midline. Focusing simultaneously on abduction and adduction, this exercise with a band puts the work into the pelvis. This simple movement facilitates mobility and stabilization for the outer and inner hip muscles, rotators, and tendons.

- Stand with a band securely around both feet, just at the upper ankle.
- Cross the right foot across the front of the left leg (adduction), flexing the foot.
- Bring the leg back to open to the right (abduction), slightly off the ground. Alternate sides, and repeat.

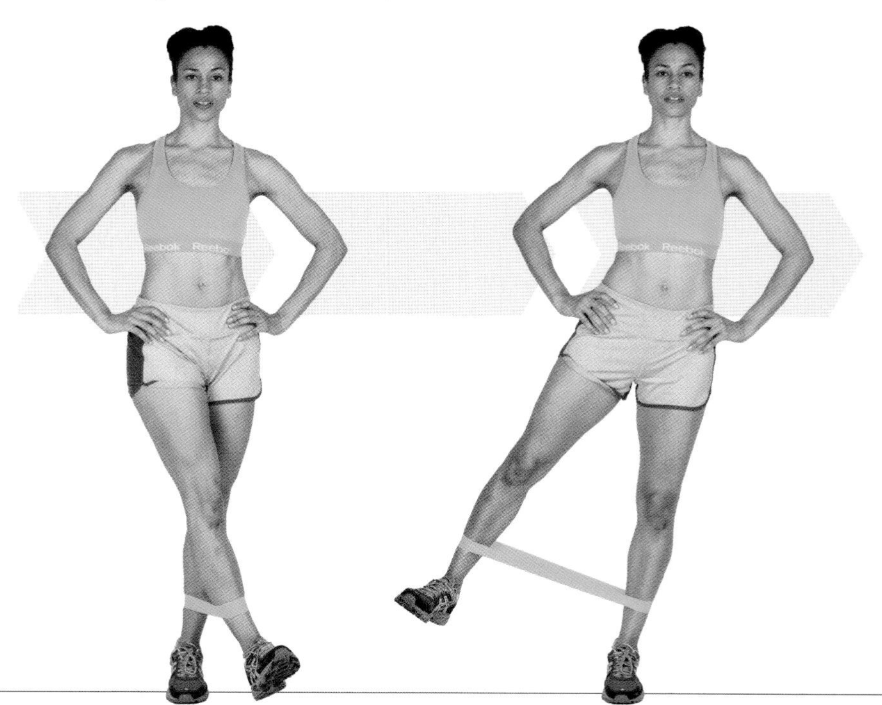

359 Resistance-Band Walk

Place a resistance band slightly below the knee joints. Stand tall and pull in the core, squeezing the abs into the lower spine and back. Take a step out to your left and come into your standard Squat. Stay in a Squat and continue moving to the left. Alternate sides.

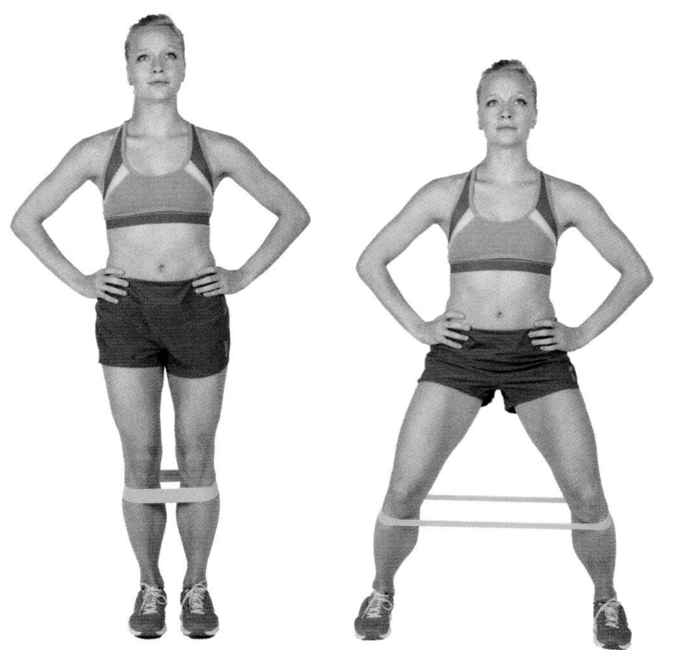

360 Side-to-Side Hop with Bands

In this exercise you will find another workout incorporating plyometric moves. Plyometric refers to the idea of "jump training." Using the body's own weight and agility, you move through routines that focus on enhancing speed and strength. If you wish, you can use a small object to hop over.

- Start upright, standing, with a secure resistance band under the lower calf.
- Open the legs to shoulder-width and take a quick, short bend on both legs.
- Explode up into the air, bringing both legs up and over to the side, moving about 1 foot (30 centimeters) from where you began. Use the arms to assist with your jumps.

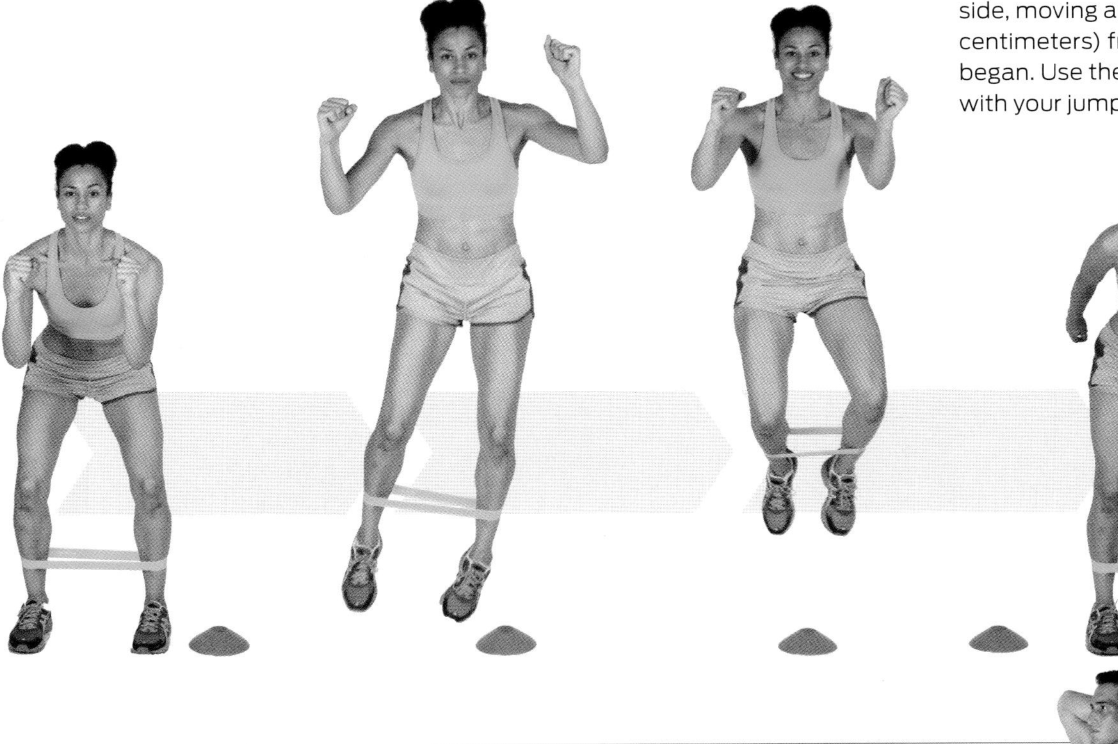

361 Band Good Morning

Start by standing tall with the legs wide apart. Take a band that is secured to a low base and bring the handles to either side of your upper shoulders. Engage the biceps strongly and pull the core up and in as you bend at the hips.

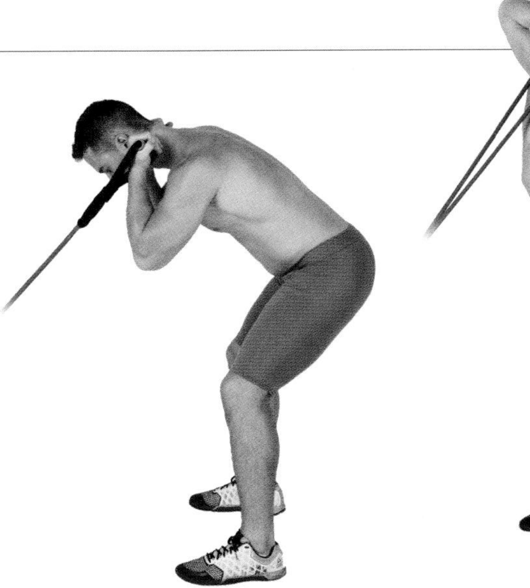

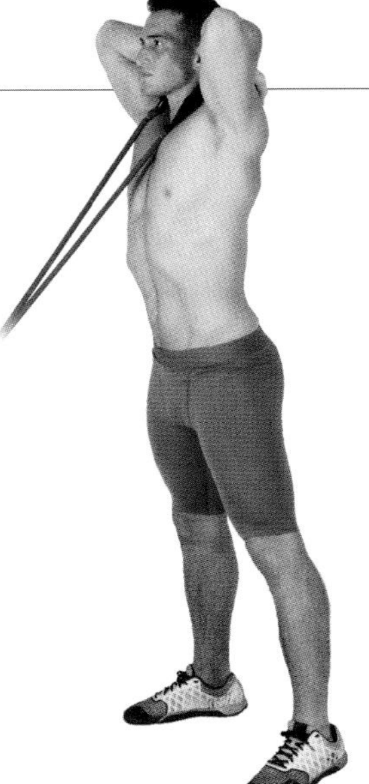

362

Forward Lunge

The Forward Lunge is a standard movement that allows you to work in the quads and larger muscle groups in the legs. Simultaneously, the Lunge requires you to control your core, keeping balanced between two legs. This movement will lengthen the front of the hip and the legs while stabilizing the core and lower extremities. Combining the Lunge with other exercises can create a powerful catalyst for body awareness and developing lower-body strength.

Annotation Key
Bold text indicates target muscles
Black text indicates other working muscles
* indicates deep muscles

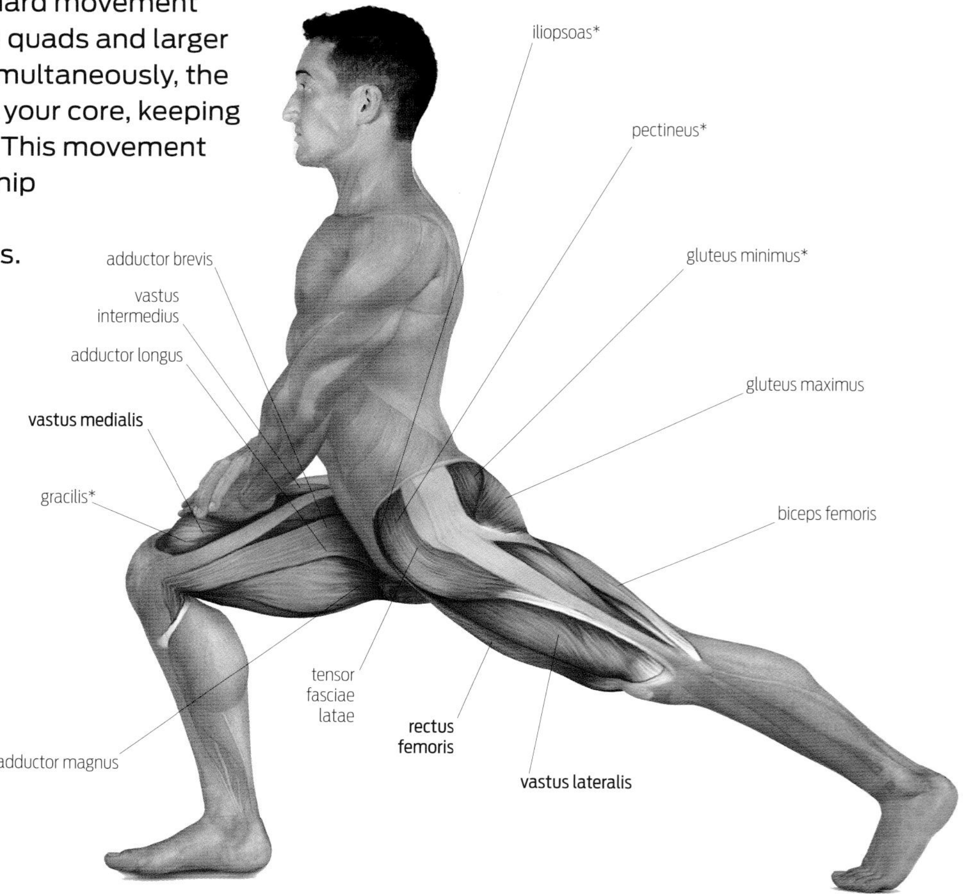

Correct form

The back leg should be extended straight behind you with the heel slightly off the ground.

Avoid

Do not let your back arch or sway. Instead, pull your lower abs up to support the stretch of the lower spine.

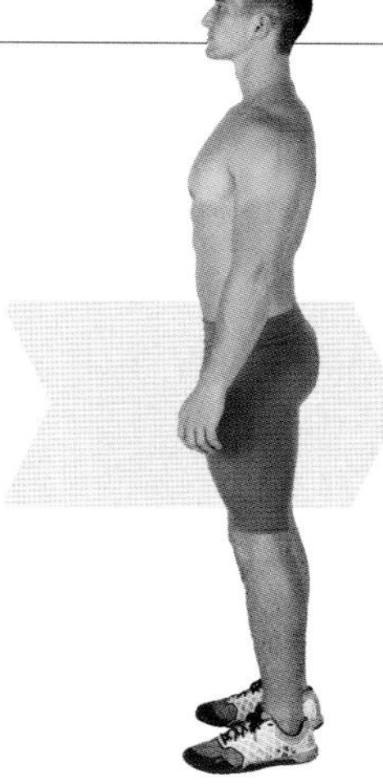

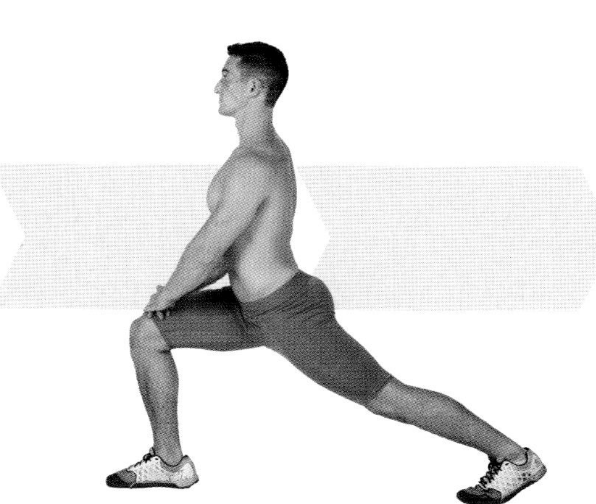

- Begin with your legs hip-width apart, arms hanging at your sides.
- Step forward generously with one leg into your Lunge and place your hands on the knee.
- Bring the front knee into a 90-degree angle to the floor with your knee directly over your ankle and both hips facing forward.

363 Lateral Lunge

With feet together and arms to the front, take a big step out to the left, bending the left knee deeply and lengthening the right leg. Keep the back straight up, the core tight, and twist your arms to the left. Push off the left foot to stand as you began. Repeat to the other side.

364 Forward Lunge with Twist

Stand tall and step forward generously with one leg into your Lunge. With one leg bent and the other straight, twist, reaching one hand to your outer ankle and the other up to the sky. Open the chest and breathe deeply.

365 Straight-Leg Lunge

Open your legs in a wide, staggered stance with the right leg forward. Bend at the hips, engage the core, and stretch the hamstrings. Place your hands on the right thigh and stretch the back out low on a diagonal to your left leg. Breathe and stretch.

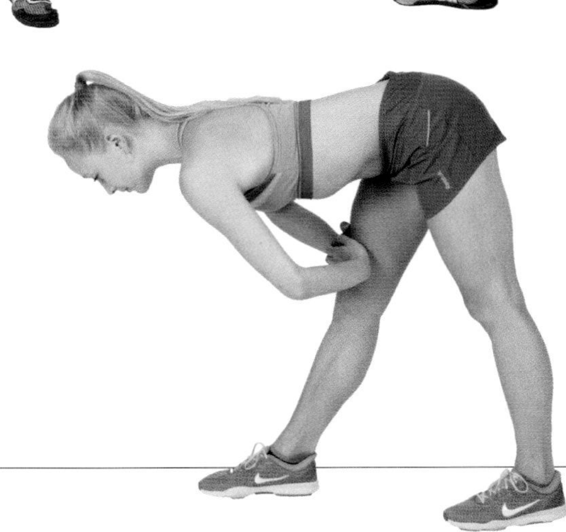

366 Straight-Leg Lunge with Floor Touch

Open your legs in a wide, staggered stance with the left leg forward. Bend at the hips, engage the core, and stretch the hamstrings. Place your hands on the floor on either side of your left foot. Breathe and stretch.

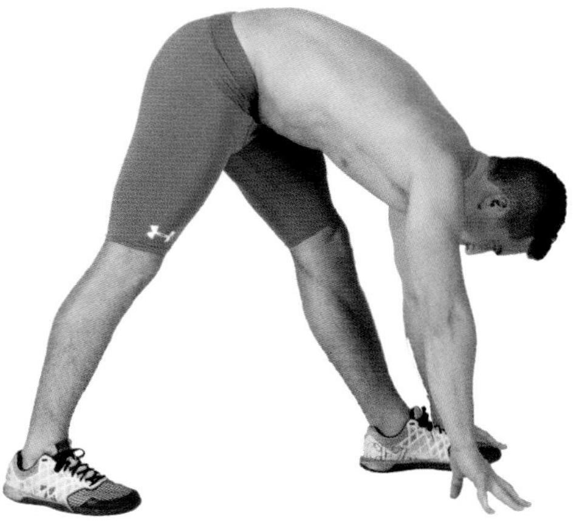

367 Forward Lunge Pass-Under

Step generously forward into a deep Lunge with both legs bent and holding a weighted ball at your chest. Hold in Lunge and quickly pass the ball under the forward leg, isolating the movement of the arms and working the core for balance.

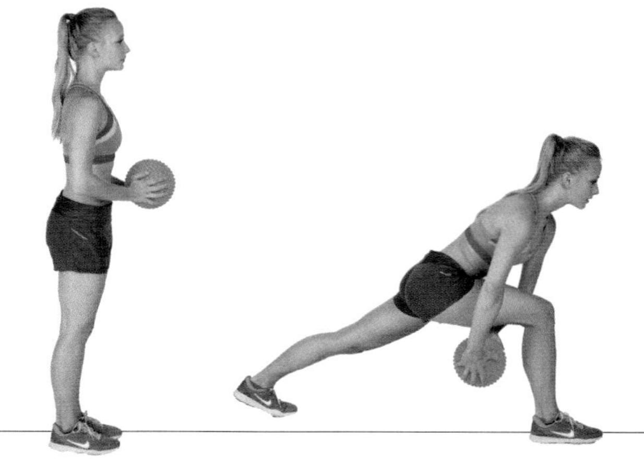

368 Forward Lunge and Rear Leg Raise

With hands on hips, step forward into a Lunge with both legs bent. Squeeze the core in deeply, move your body weight into the heel of your front foot, and, driving forcefully with the right glute, kick the back leg up. Extending the leg straight out behind you, land with both legs bent. Switch legs, and repeat. This is a great step for defining the legs.

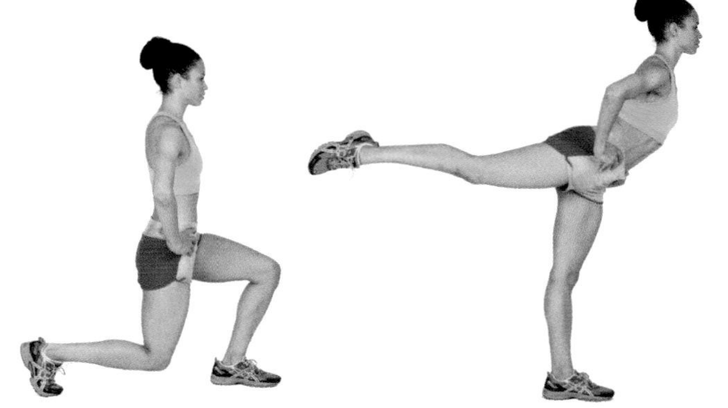

369 Tick Tock Lunge

Stand in a shoulder-width open-legged stance. Bend into Forward Lunge (#362) with both legs bent, quickly step back to stand, and switch legs, landing on the opposite leg in a bent Lunge position. Move quickly through this variation for explosive power.

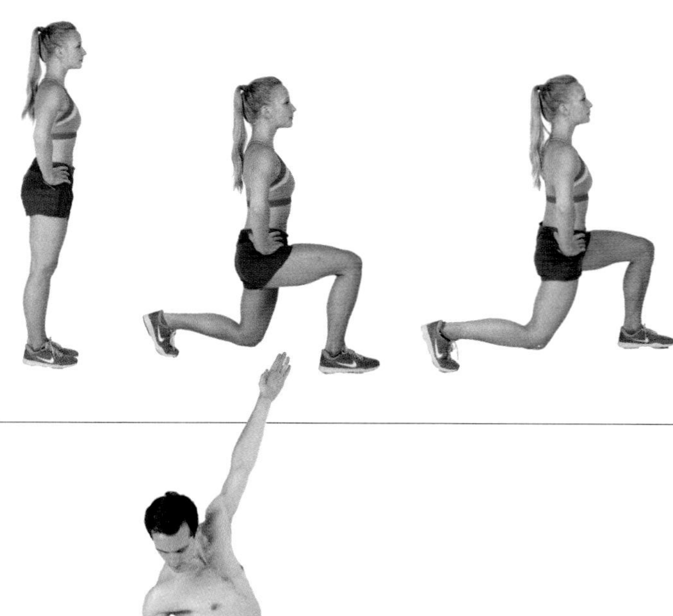

370 Twisting Lunge

This Twisting Lunge variation is similar to a yoga pose. Stand tall and step forward generously with one leg into your Lunge. With both legs bent, twist, reaching one hand to your inner ankle and the other up to the sky, open the chest, and breathe deeply.

371 Twisting Diagonal Lunge

Start upright with a long spine, feet together, and arms open at your sides. Pull in your core, pivot your feet to the diagonal, and take a large step out with your right leg. Reach the right arm back to the left heel. Return to standing and change sides.

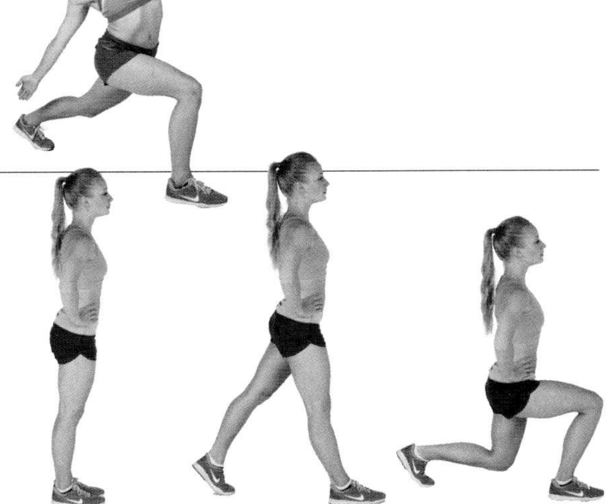

372 Walking Lunge

Stand tall and step forward generously with the right leg into your Lunge. With both legs bent and arms at your sides, spring up to extend both legs, and step with your left leg to lunge, again. Alternate sides, and repeat as if you were walking normally.

373 Reach and Twist Walking Lunge

Begin upright with a long spine. Step forward generously with the left leg into a Lunge, twisting the Medicine ball to your left side. Spring up to extend both legs, and step with your right leg to Lunge again, twisting the ball to the right.

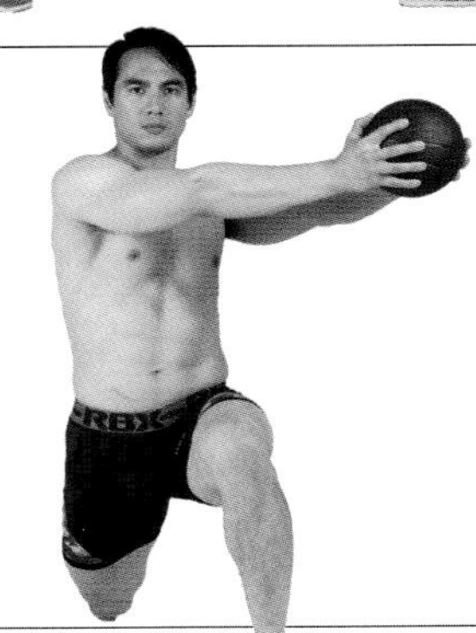

374 Reverse Lunge

The opposite of your Forward Lunge is the Reverse Lunge. Stand tall with your feet together, and step back into a Lunge with both legs bent. Keep your back straight and your body weight forward and balanced, engaging the legs strongly.

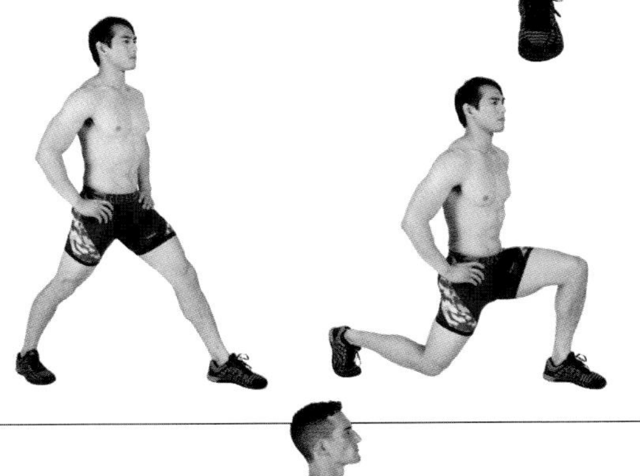

375 Jumping Lunge

Start with your feet slightly apart and arms to the front. In one move, step back into a Reverse Lunge with both legs bent, swinging your arms behind you, and then quickly explode up and forward into a jump. As you come down, change sides, landing into your opposite leg Lunge.

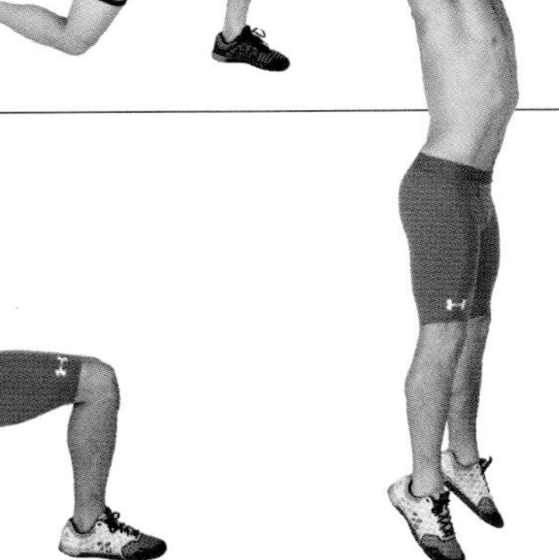

376 Reverse Lunge off a Box

Begin with the feet together, standing on a box. Deeply bend both knees and step back with your right leg into your Reverse Lunge, keeping the weight of your body in your front foot, on the box. Hold, breathe, and return to stand.

377 Lateral Raise and Reverse Lunge

Take a shoulder-width stance. From standing, open your arms wide to the side, and step into a Reverse Lunge with the left foot. Keep the front knee aligned over the ankles and your arms straight out and energized.

378 Reverse Lunge with Chest Fly

Take a shoulder-width stance. From standing, reach your arms forward with a dumbbell in each hand. Step into a Reverse Lunge with the right foot and open up the chest to the front and arms to the sides.

379 Reverse Lunge into Knee-Up

Standing with hands on hips, step back into a Reverse Lunge with both legs bent. Push off the back leg, bringing the knee forward and up into the chest. Swing the leg to land back with both legs bent. Repeat.

380 Reverse Lunge and Kick

Standing with your arms at your sides, step back into a Reverse Lunge with both legs bent. Kick off the back leg, extending that leg straight out in front of you, and swinging the arms in opposition. Land back in your Reverse Lunge. Alternate legs, and repeat.

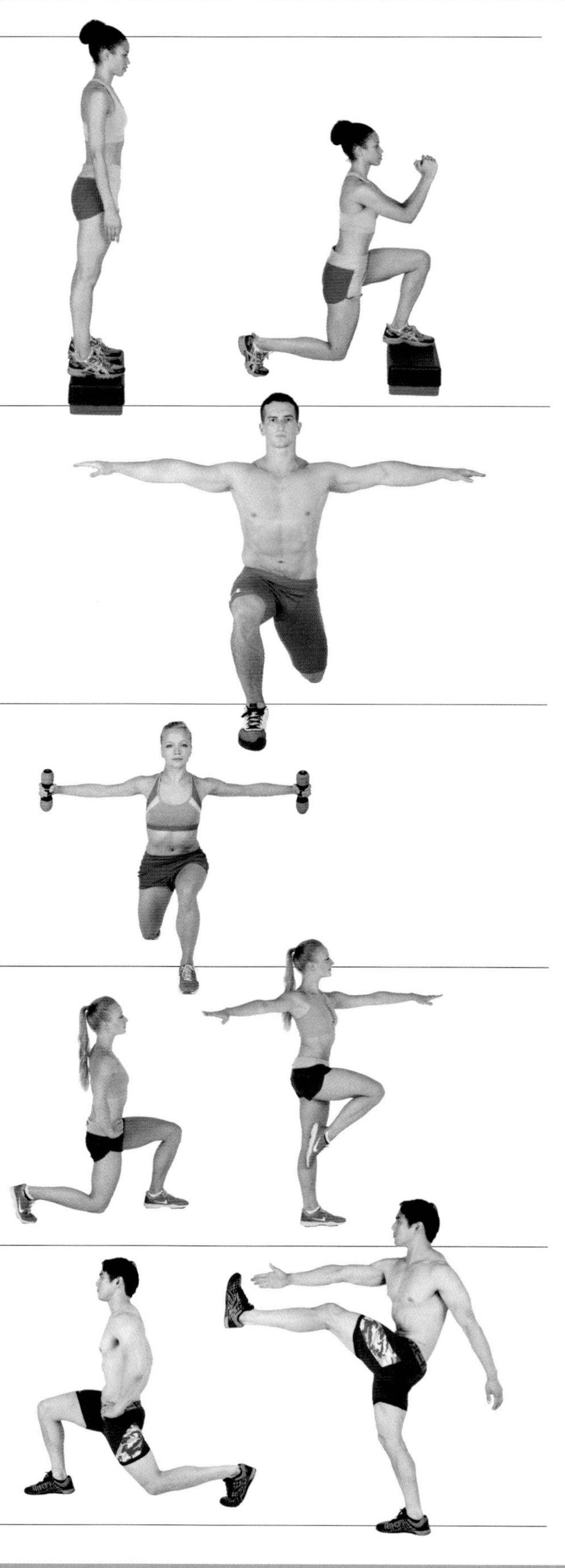

381 **Suspended Reverse Lunge**

Begin with the feet together, then place your left ankle into a supported band. Deeply bend both knees and push back with your left leg into your Reverse Lunge, keeping the weight of your body in your front foot. Hold, breathe, and return to standing.

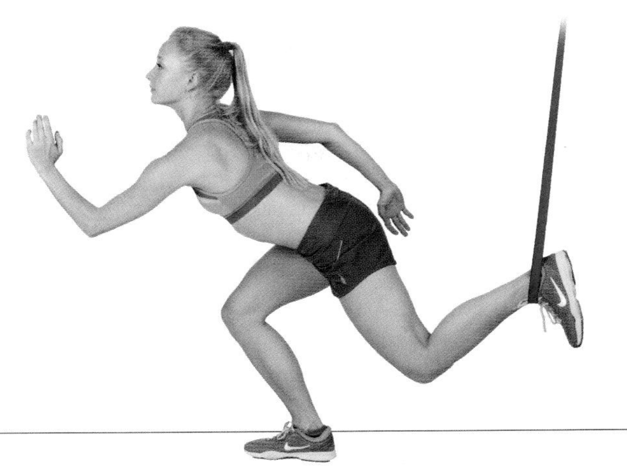

382 **Low Lunge**

Take your Forward Lunge (#362) and place your hands on the floor to either side of your bent knee. Look down at your hands, lower your leg, and push the back heel far back. Breathe—this is a deep leg and calf exercise! Stand, and repeat.

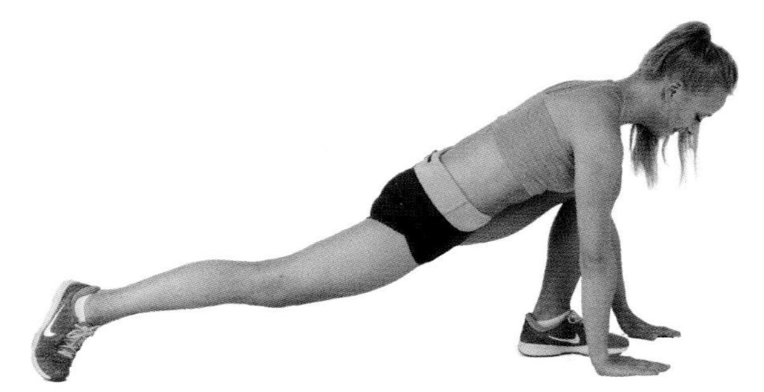

383 **Low Lunge, Arms to the Side**

Take your Forward Lunge and place your hands on the floor to either side of your 90-degree bent knee. Extending your arms straight and long, push the back heel far back. Change sides, and repeat.

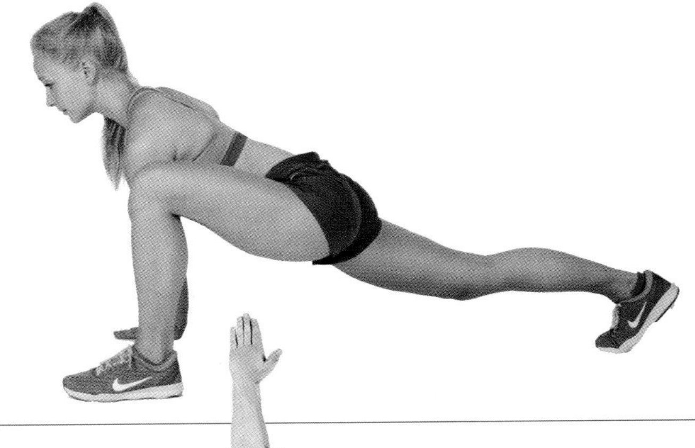

384 **Crescent Lunge**

Take your Forward Lunge and place your hands on the floor to either side of your bent knee. Reach your arms up and long overhead, bringing the palms together in a prayer position. Inhale and exhale here. Change sides, and repeat.

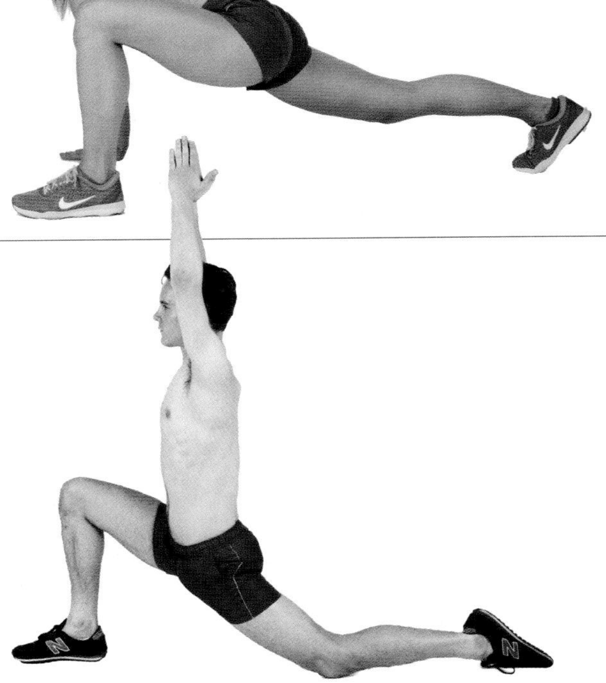

385 Low Lunge with Reach

Start by standing tall with the core engaged. Step forward with the right leg into a Forward Lunge. Reach both arms forward on the diagonal with the left leg long behind you. Breathe deeply and squeeze the core in to strengthen the lower back.

386 Lateral Low Lunge

Start by standing tall with your core engaged strongly into the lower back. Reach your arms out to the front, lift the weight into your toes, and move into your Lateral Lunge (#363). Breathe deeply and squeeze the core in to strengthen the back.

387 Dumbbell Lateral Raise and Lateral Lunge

Begin in a hip-width stance, holding dumbbells at your sides. Open your arms wide to the side with the dumbbells. Step open to your left side into a Lateral Lunge, bending the left knee and straightening the right leg. Keep the core squeezing in and the arms up to shoulder height.

388 Clock Lunge

Start with the feet together and a your hands on your hips. With your right foot, step into a Forward Lunge, spring off the right to stand, then lower into a Lateral Lunge with the left leg. Spring back into a Forward Lunge with the left leg. Keep the core tight.

389 Single-Leg Lateral Lunge with Lift

Take a Lateral Lunge onto the right leg. With your arms straight out in front of your chest, touch the fingers down to the floor, framing the right leg. Extend the right leg straight and lift the left leg off of the floor into a 90-degree angle.

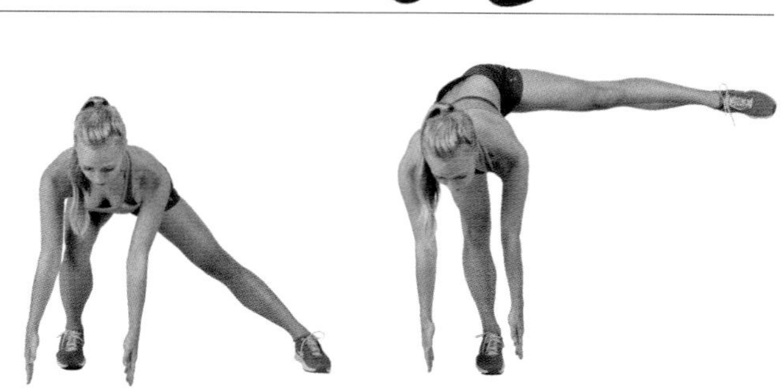

390 Alternating Touchdown Lunge

Start with the legs wide apart. Reach the left hand to the right foot, bending the right knee and lengthening the left leg. Keeping the back and core muscles engaged, bring the body to stand at center, and reach to the left.

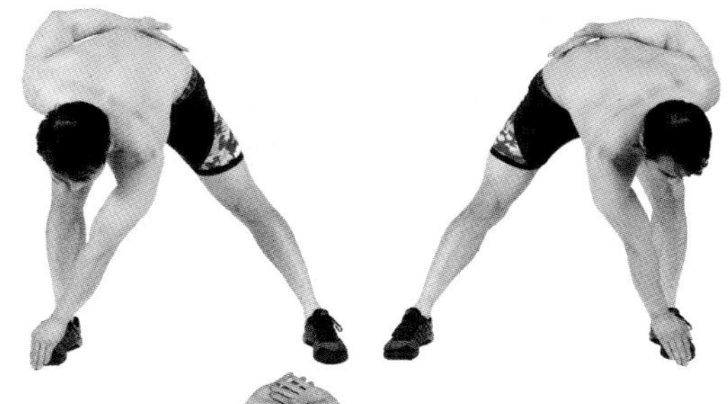

391 Plyo Touchdown Switch

Quickly move into your Lateral Lunge, bending the right knee and tapping the right toe with your left hand. Swing the arms up, into a jump, with your core and glutes engaged, and land to the left, tapping your left toe with the right hand.

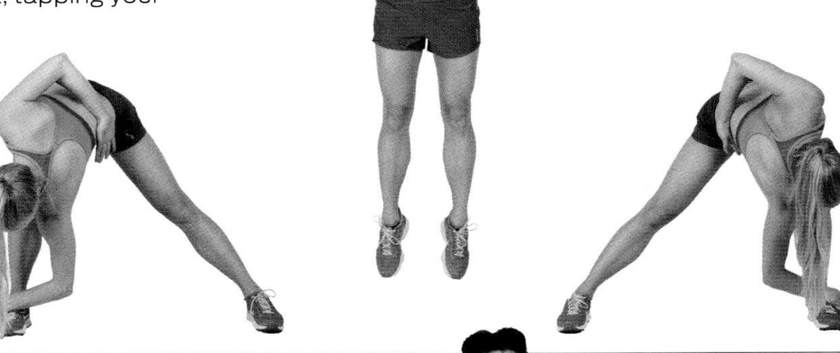

392 Straddle Adductor Lunge

With feet together and hands clasped together in front of your chest take a big step to the left, bending the left knee and lengthening the right leg. Keep the core tight and back supported. Spring off the left foot, using your adductors to stand, as you began.

393 Suspended Adductor Lunge

Standing tall with your feet together, place your left leg into a supported suspension strap. Hop your right foot out a bit, away from the strap and pointed forward. Clasping your hands at your chest, extend your left leg out long and bend the right knee deeply. Keep the core tight and back supported. Push off the right foot to stand as you began. Repeat for the desired number of repetitions, then switch sides.

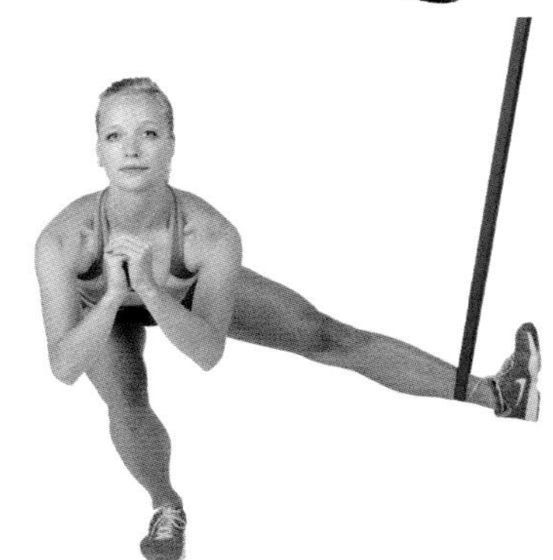

394

Dumbbell Lunge

The Lunge comes in many variations, shapes, and sizes. It is a powerful movement that allows you to push and pull, simultaneously, in a variety of directions: forward, backward, side, up, and down into gravity. When done in combination with weights, the Lunge can become a great tool for upper- and lower-body strengthening.

Correct form

Let the head float on top of the neck and put the weight of your feet forward into your toes.

Avoid

Do not let the front knee bend past a 90-degree angle. Keep the knee directly over your ankle and both hips facing forward.

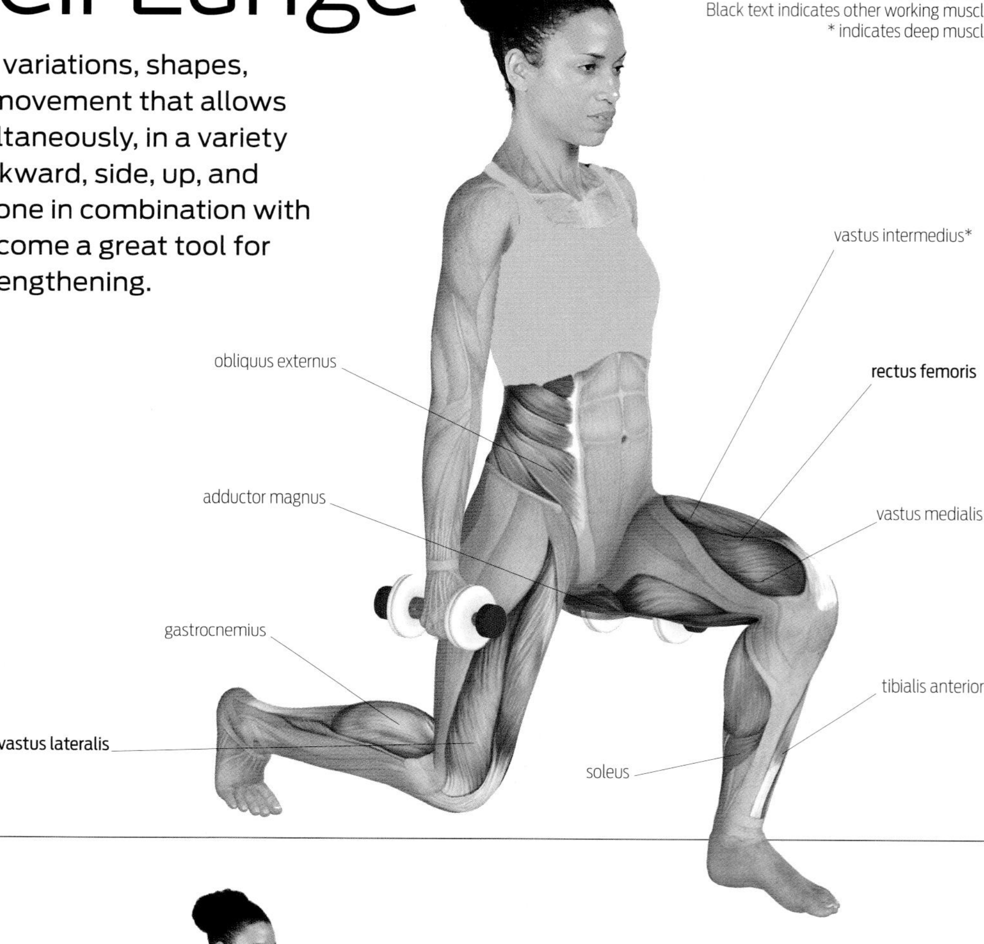

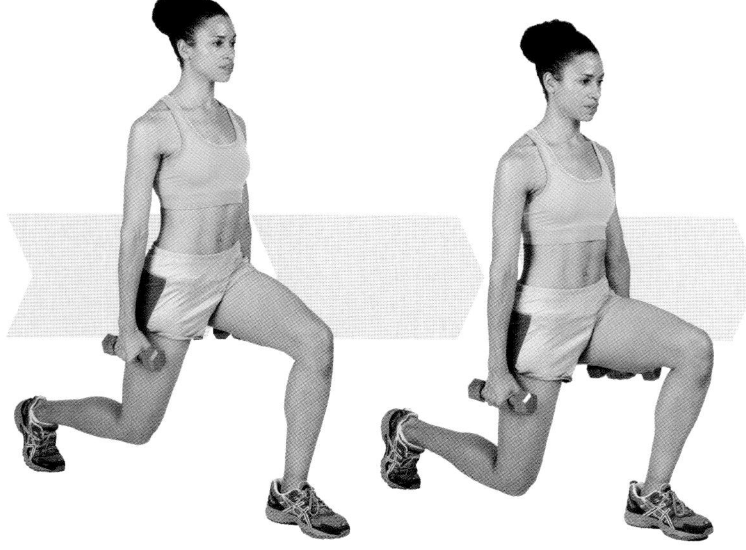

- Begin with the legs hip-width apart, hands holding dumbbells at your sides. Pull the core muscles up and in to lengthen them along the spine.
- Step forward generously with one leg into your Lunge.
- Your back leg knee should be at a 90-degree angle, with the shin parallel to the ground. Pull your lower abs up to support the stretch of the lower spine.

395 Barbell Forward Lunge

Executing the Forward Barbell Lunge correctly requires the ability to lengthen the front of the hip and the legs, meanwhile also stabilizing the core and lower extremities. Incorporating the barbell into your Lunge workout will develop a strong core and shoulder girdle.

- Begin with feet together, holding the barbell behind your head, balanced on your shoulders.
- Step forward with one foot and deeply bend into your Lunge, keeping the weight of your body on your front foot.
- Hold in your Lunge, breathe deeply, and return to standing.

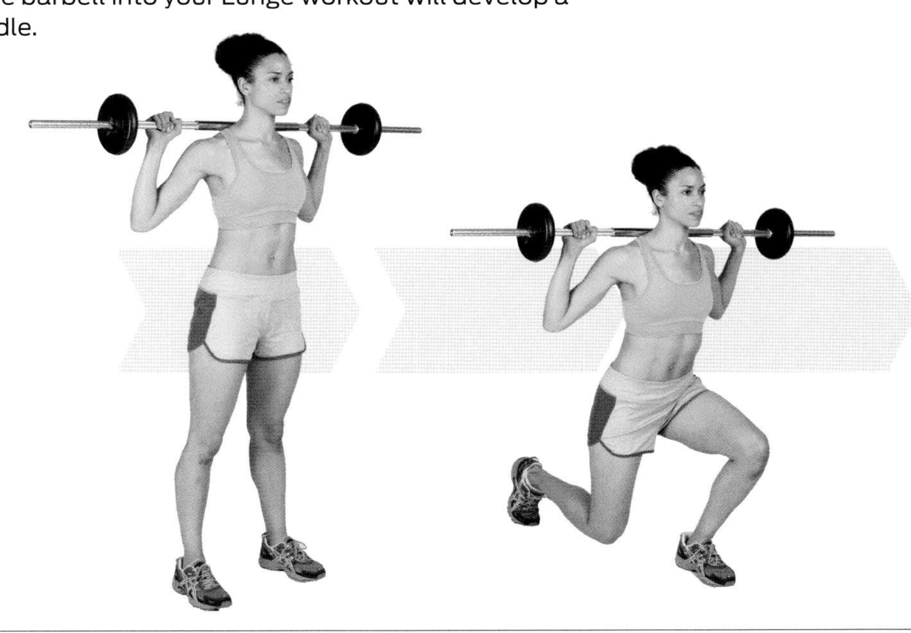

396 Barbell Forward Lunge and Rear Leg Raise

With the barbell secured at the shoulders, step forward into a Lunge with both legs bent. Move your body weight into the heel of your front foot and drive forcefully with the right glute to be able to kick the back leg up, extending the leg straight out behind you, and land with both legs bent. This is a great step for defining the legs.

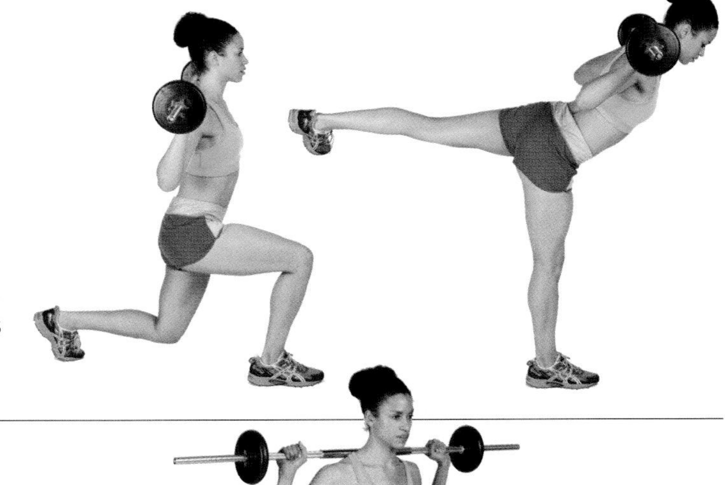

397 Barbell Diagonal Lunge

Start upright with a long spine, feet together, with the barbell at your shoulders. Tighten your core into your back, pivot your feet, and step out to the diagonal. Quickly return to stand, working the inner and outer legs.

398 Weighted Ball Jumping Forward Lunge

Performing this move requires great concentration and the ability to focus on keeping a solid core, coupled with isolated, quick, dynamic leg and upper arm movements. The benefits will include a strong set of abdominals, super-developed back and core muscles, and sleek shapely arms.

- Begin by standing tall. Step into a Forward Lunge with both legs bent, holding the ball at your chest.
- Quickly jump up high, swinging your arms overhead and bringing your legs together in the air.
- Land on the opposite leg in a bent Lunge position. Feel the burn.

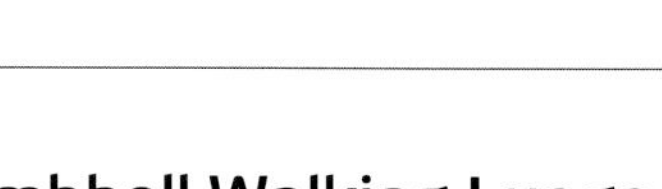

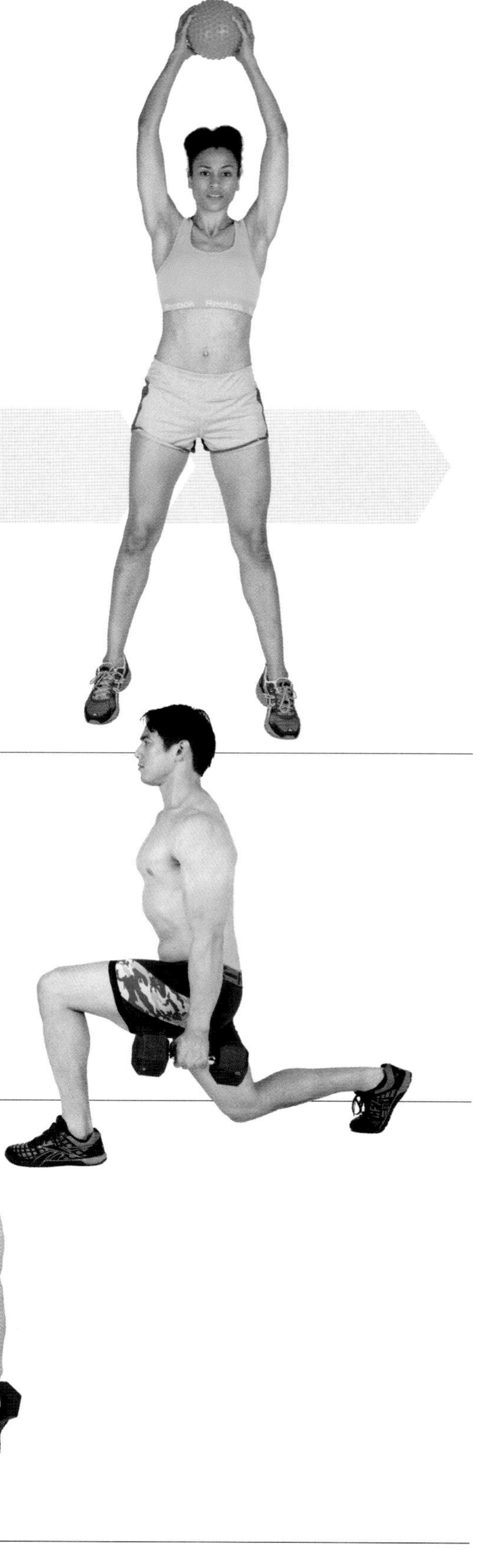

399 Dumbbell Walking Lunge

Stand tall with your dumbbells at your sides. Step forward generously with one leg into your Lunge. With both legs bent and arms at your sides, rise up to standing tall as you began. Repeat as if you were walking normally.

400 Dumbbell Reverse Lunge

The opposite of the Forward Lunge is the Reverse Lunge. Stand tall with feet together, and step back into a Lunge with both legs bent. Keep your back straight and your body weight forward and balanced, with the dumbbells at your sides.

401 Barbell Reverse Lunge

Executing the Barbell Reverse Lunge correctly requires the ability to work with balance in the space behind the body. Incorporating the barbell into your workout will develop a strong upper body and shoulder girdle, while also stabilizing the core and lower extremities.

- Begin with feet together, holding the barbell behind your head, balanced on your shoulders.
- Step the right leg back behind you, deeply bending into your Lunge and keeping the weight of your body in your front foot.
- Hold in your Lunge, breathe deeply, and return to standing.

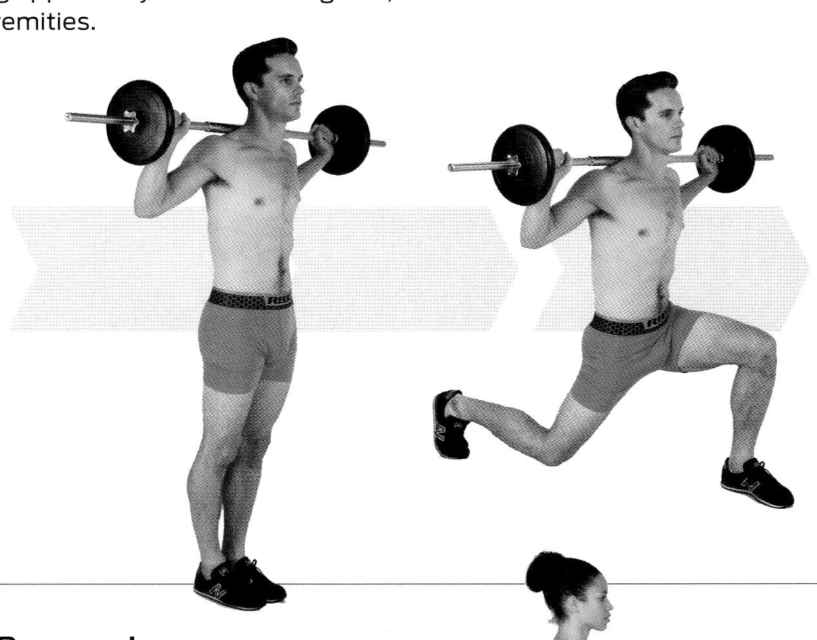

402 Weighted Ball Reverse Lunge

Stand with your legs hip-width apart. With a weighted ball at your chest, step back into a Lunge with both legs bent. Squeeze the core and the backs of your legs and push off the back leg, coming back to stand. Alternate sides, and repeat.

403 Kettlebell Overhead Reverse Lunge

Take a kettlebell into your right hand and open the left arm out to the side for balance. From standing, step into a Reverse Lunge with the left foot. Keep both knees aligned over the ankles and your arms energized as you raise the kettlebell straight up above your head.

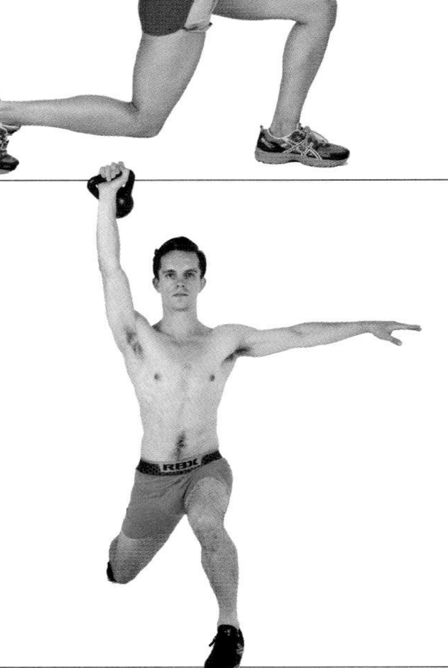

404 Dumbbell Lateral Raise Reverse Lunge

Stand tall with your feet together and dumbbells at your sides. Step back generously. Open your arms wide to the sides, keeping them in line with your shoulders. Keep your back straight and your body weight forward and balanced.

405 Barbell Reverse Lunge into Knee-Up

Stand tall with your barbell resting behind the head. Step back into a Reverse Lunge with both legs bent. Push off the back leg, bringing the knee forward and up into your chest. Swing the leg to land back with both legs bent. Repeat!

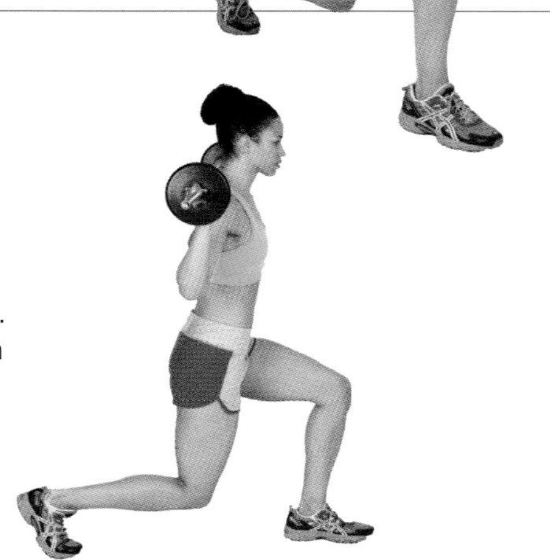

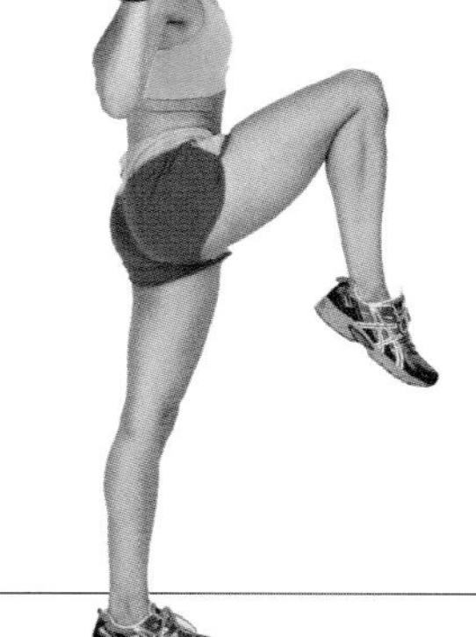

406 Clock Lunge with Body Bar

Start with the feet together and a body bar along your shoulders. With your left foot, step into a Forward Lunge, spring off the left foot to lower into a Lateral Lunge, and then spring back to the Forward Lunge. Keep the core tight.

407 Weighted Ball Plyo Touchdown Switch

Quickly move into your Lateral Lunge, bending the left knee and tapping the left toe with the weighted ball. Swing the arms up, into a jump, with your core and glutes engaged, and land to the right, tapping your right toe.

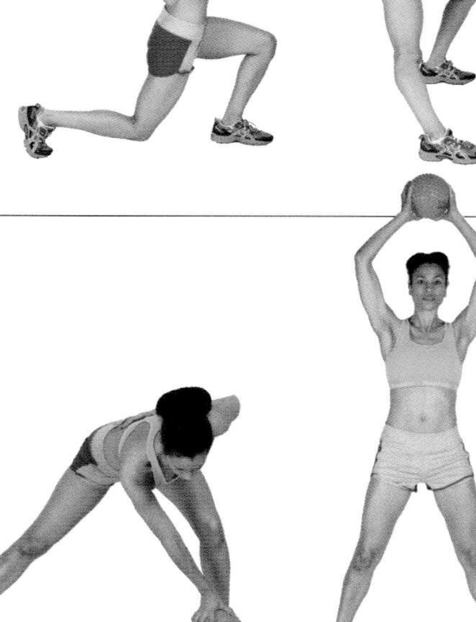

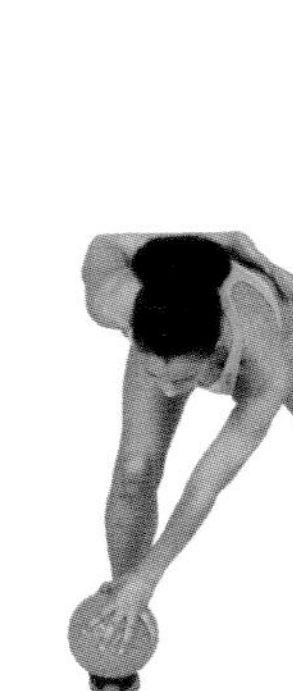

408 Dumbbell Alternating Touchdown Lunge

This variation is great for stretching the back out long on the diagonal while giving the hamstrings a stretch in opposition to the back. Also, switching the weight from side to side in this exercise aids in stabilizing the knee and ankle joints from the work of the core muscles.

- Start with your legs wide apart and arms out to your sides, holding the dumbbells firmly.
- Reach the right hand with dumbbell for the left foot, bending the left knee and lengthening the right leg.
- Keeping the back and core muscles engaged, bring the body to stand at center, and then reach to the right.

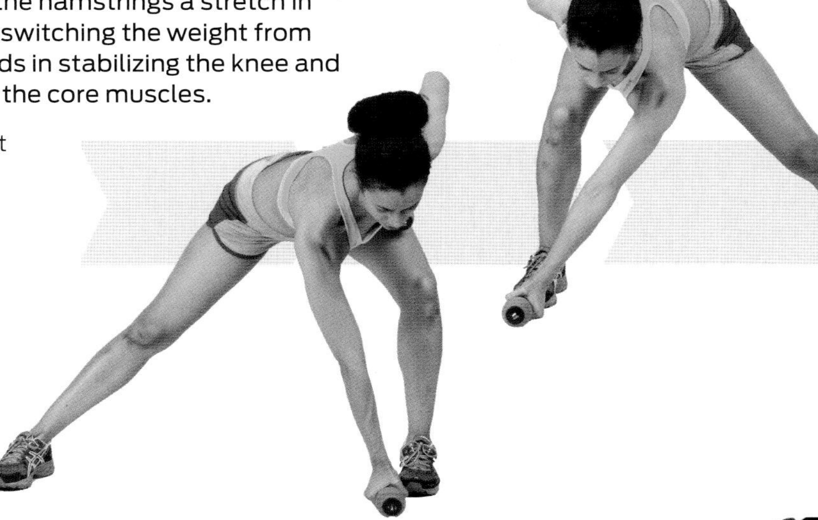

409 Weighted Ball Suspended Adductor Lunge

Standing tall with your feet together, place your right leg into a supported suspension strap. Hop your left foot out a bit, away from the strap and pointed forward. Squeeze your weighted ball into the chest, extend your right leg out long and bend the left knee deeply. Keep the core tight and the back supported. Push off the left foot to stand as you began. Repeat.

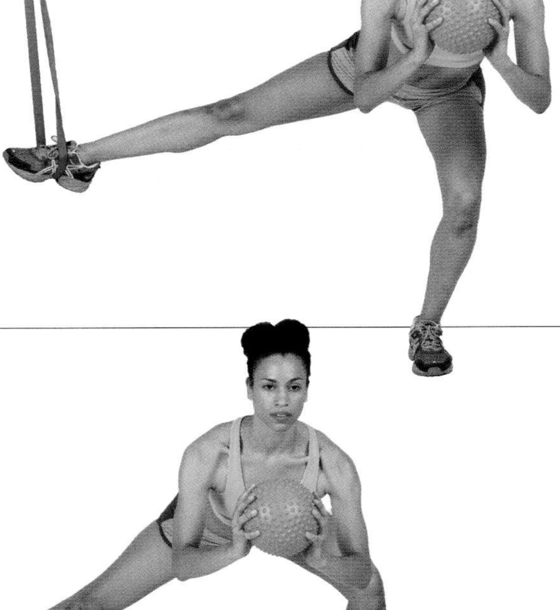

410 Weighted Ball Straddle Adductor Lunge

With feet together and arms in front holding your weighted ball, take a big step to the left, bending the left knee and lengthening the right leg. Keep the core tight and back supported. Spring off the left foot to stand as you began.

411

Side Kick

Static Side Kicks, in which you push the leg out from the midline and then bring it back in without moving any other part, are excellent for stabilizing the sides of the body. They also help with strengthening the core and enhancing balance.

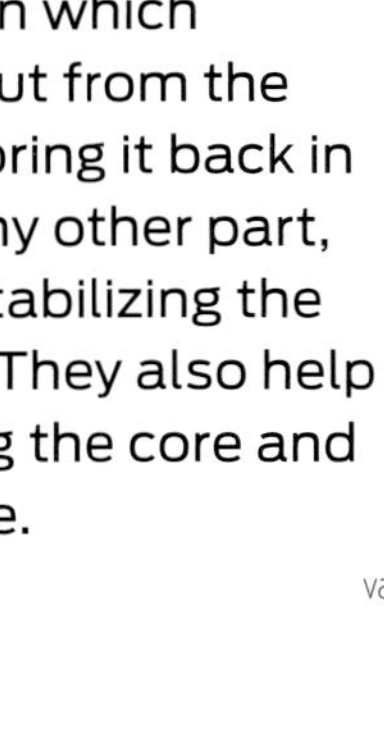

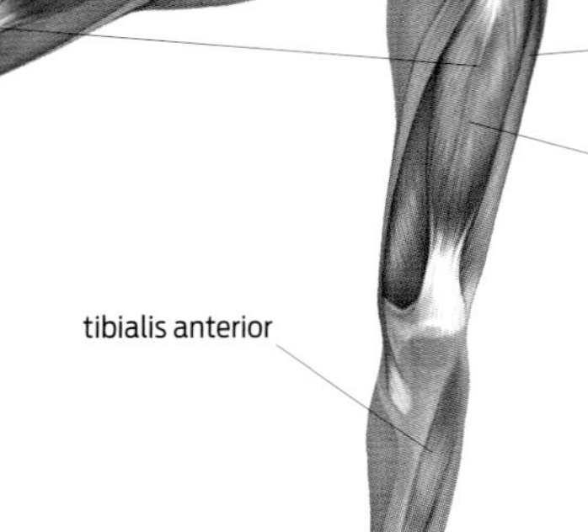

Annotation Key
Bold text indicates target muscles
Black text indicates other working muscles
* indicates deep muscles

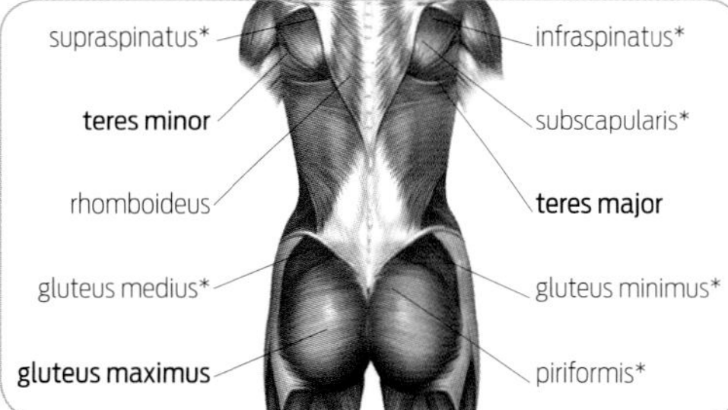

Correct form

Make sure when you kick the leg out to the side that you keep the hip of the moving leg down. Try not to hike the hip up in an unnatural way.

Avoid

Avoid kicking the leg with tons of force. The movement should be light and easy.

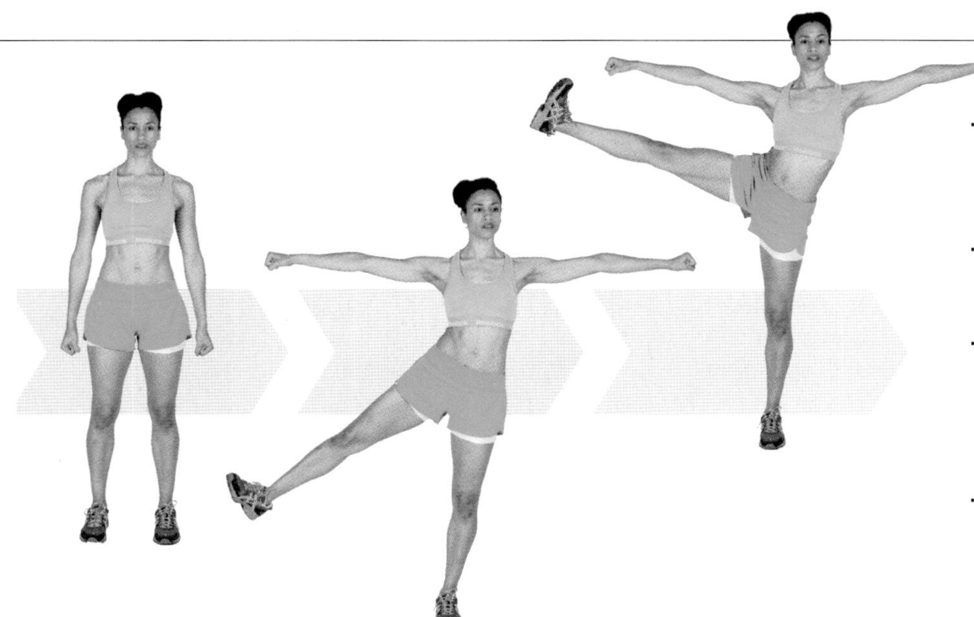

- Reach the arms long at your sides and open the legs to shoulder-width.
- Stand tall with your core engaged and the spine very long.
- In one movement, swing the right leg open to the side and open the arms up wide to help keep you balanced. Flex the right foot.
- Allow the weight of the leg to bring it back to the starting point, and change sides.

412 Low Round Kick

The Low Round Kick derives from mixed martial arts craft. This kick, also used throughout kickboxing practices, aims to deliver a strong thrust of momentum from the back of the legs by moving the hips dynamically forward.

- Start facing forward in a wide, open staggered stance with your right leg open behind the left.
- Turn your hips and feet toward your right, keeping your chest to the front. Bring your arms up in front of your chest and make two fists.
- In one move, strongly thrust the hips to the front, turning the left foot out to the left, and kicking your right leg out to the side and forward at hip height.

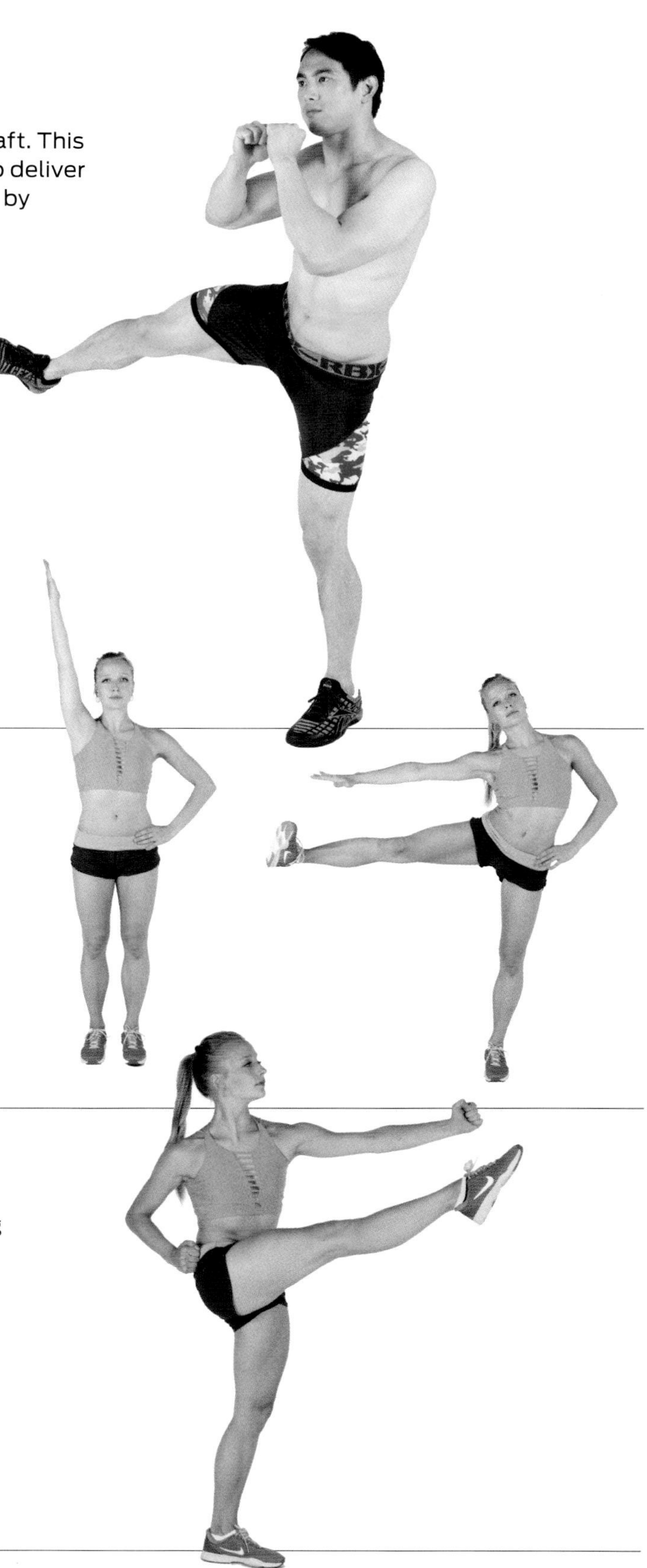

413 Side Kick Reach

Stand tall with your core engaged and the spine very long. Reach the right arm up to the sky. In one movement, swing the right leg open to the side and bring your right arm to meet it. Flex the right foot. Bring the leg back down to stand and switch sides.

414 Straight Kick

Stand tall with your legs open to shoulder-width. Engage your core and legs and swing the right leg out in front of you. Reach the left arm out in front of you and point the right foot. Be sure to use a swinging motion in the legs and arms.

415 Kick with Toe Touch

Kicks with Toe Touch are excellent for stabilizing the core and stretching the hamstring and hips. They also help with strengthening the lower body and enhancing balance. If you are not yet able to reach your toe to touch it, aim to reach as far forward as you can.

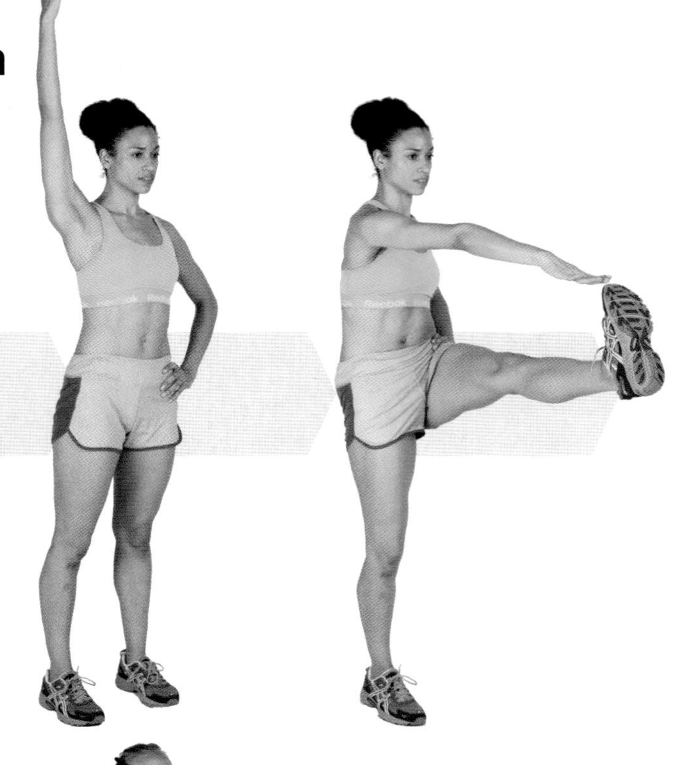

- Stand tall with your legs open to shoulder-width. Reach the right arm up.
- Engage your core and legs and swing the left leg out in front of you.
- Reach the right arm out in front of you to touch the right foot. Be sure to use a swinging motion in the legs and arms.

416 Kick with Arm Reach

Stand tall with your legs open to shoulder-width. Engage your core and legs and swing the right leg out in front of you. Reach the left arm out very far in front of you and flex the right foot. Be sure to keep your back straight.

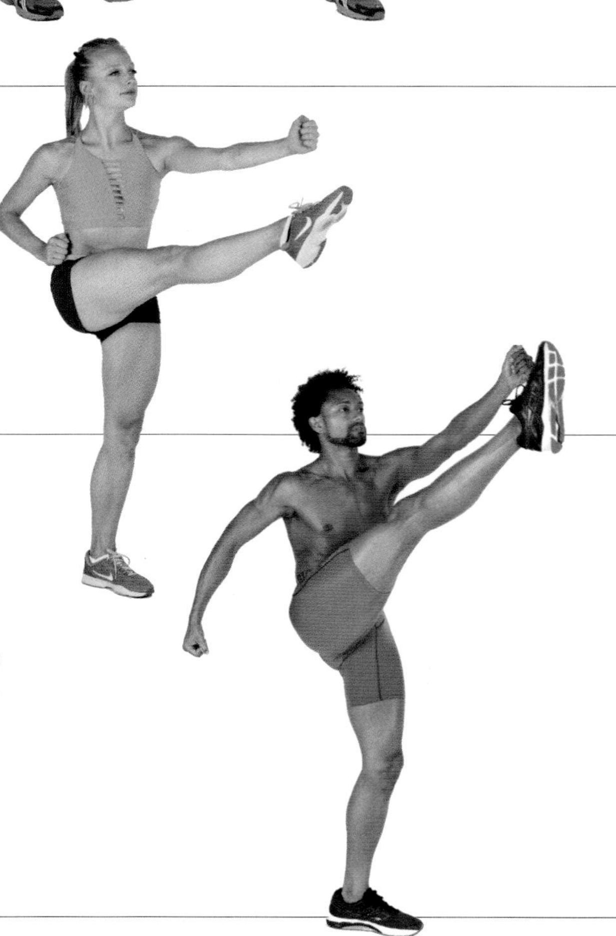

417 Switch Kick Reach

Stand tall with your legs open to shoulder-width. Engage your core and legs and swing the right leg out up high toward your chest in front of you. Reach the left arm to your right toes on the diagonal. Point the right foot in the air and feel the stretch in the back of your legs.

418 Martial-Arts Kick

Kicks found in martial arts have been performed for hundreds of centuries. The execution of these kicks begins with balance and power from the legs and core. The kicks should be performed in repetitive flowing movements.

- Standing with the knees slightly bent, bring your hands up to form fists at the chest.
- Pull the right knee into the body, engaging the core and hamstring deeply.
- Quickly kick the right leg out, turning the hips to face sideways and flexing the foot.

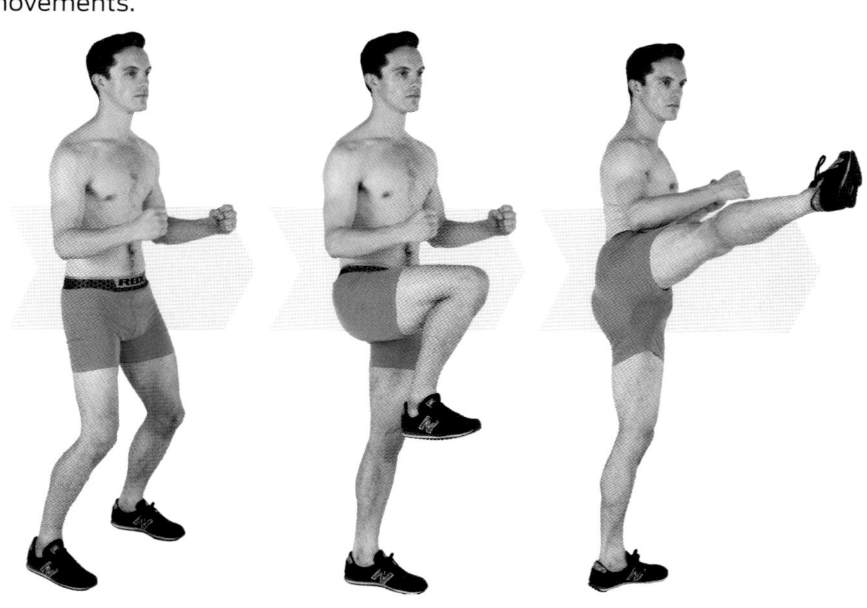

419 Roundhouse Kick

Face forward in a staggered stance with your right leg open behind the left. In one move, strongly thrust the hips to the left side and kick your right leg out to the side toward the front, bringing the leg up very high.

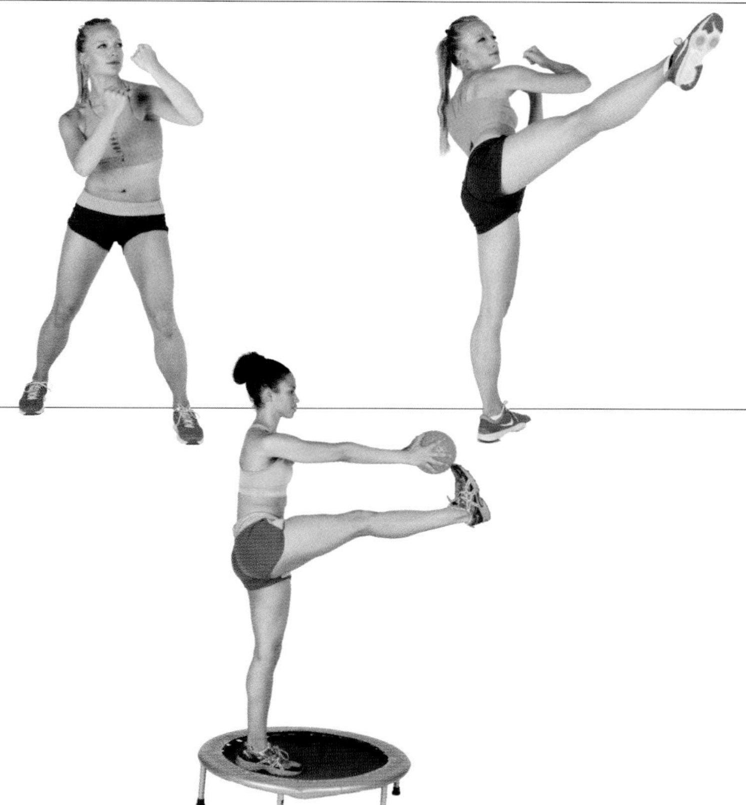

420 Toe Touch on Trampoline with Weighted Ball

Stand tall on a trampoline, holding a weighted ball out in front of your chest. Engage your core and legs and swing the right leg out in front of you. Reach the arms and ball for your right leg and flex the right foot.

421

Fire Hydrant

This core-exercise variation can be found in almost all abdominal-focused workouts like yoga, Pilates, ballet barre, and calisthenics. The focus is on keeping the core stabilized between two hands and one leg, while you lift and lower the other leg to the side, working the inner and outer muscles of the hip and glutes.

Correct form

Keep your back flat by pulling the abdominals deeply in toward the lower back.

Avoid

Do not position the knees in or out further than a 90-degree angle. Square alignment is key in this set of movements.

Annotation Key
Bold text indicates target muscles
Black text indicates other working muscles
* indicates deep muscles

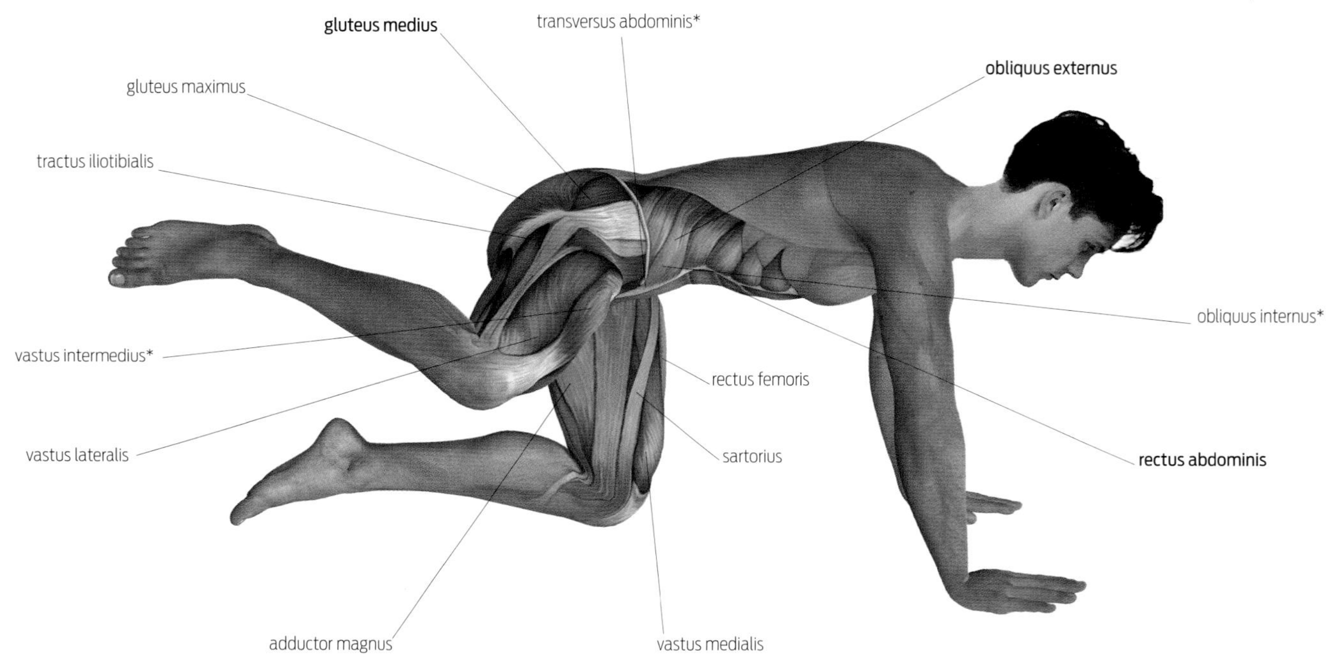

- Come to balance on your hands and knees (quadruped position).
- Strongly pull your abs up and into the back and squeeze the obliques along the sides of your torso.
- Lift your right leg out to the side, keeping the knee bent and your chest facing the ground.

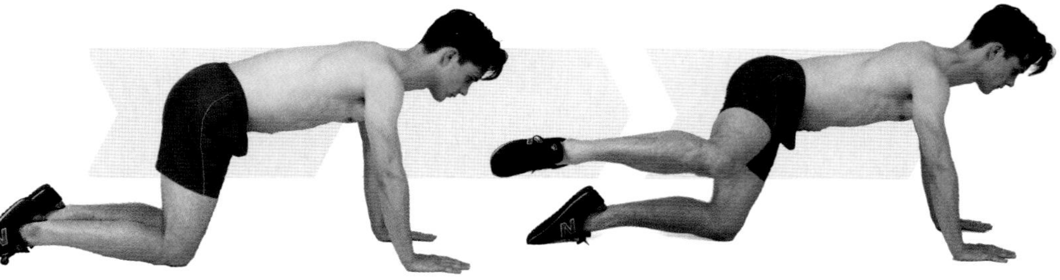

422 Fire Hydrant Push-Back

Isolating the work of one leg at a time from this four post position, on the hands and knees, is a great way to use the body's own weight in building core strength. You can do these leg isolations anywhere you see fit.

- Come to balance on your hands and knees.
- Strongly pull your abs up and into the back and squeeze the obliques along the sides of your torso.
- Lift your right leg out to the side, and push the leg so that it extends back behind you.

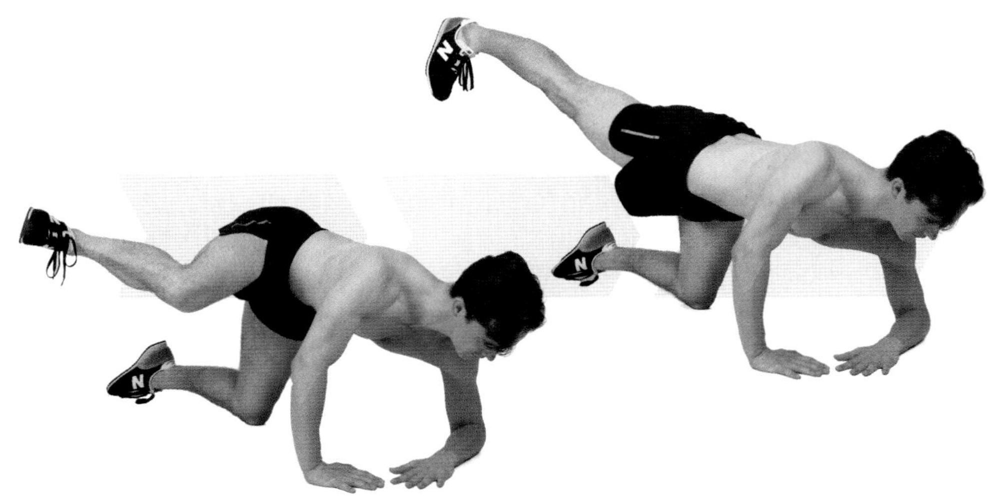

423 Straight-Leg Fire Hydrant

Begin with your body weight centered between your hands and knees. Engage your legs and abs, squeezing the obliques in along the sides of your torso. Lift your right leg out to the side, with the knee bent, then extend the leg to a straight position.

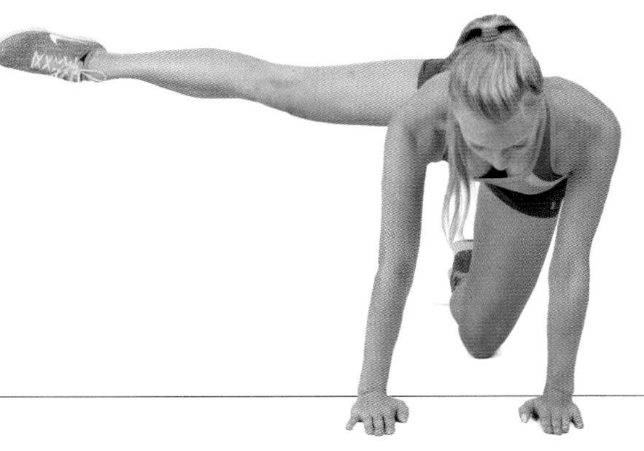

424 Straight-Leg Fire Hydrant with Leg Weights

Secure a leg weight at the upper ankle on your left leg. Begin with the weight centered between your hands and knees. Engage your abs, squeezing the obliques in along the sides of your torso. Lift your left leg out to the side with the knee bent, then extend the leg to a straight position.

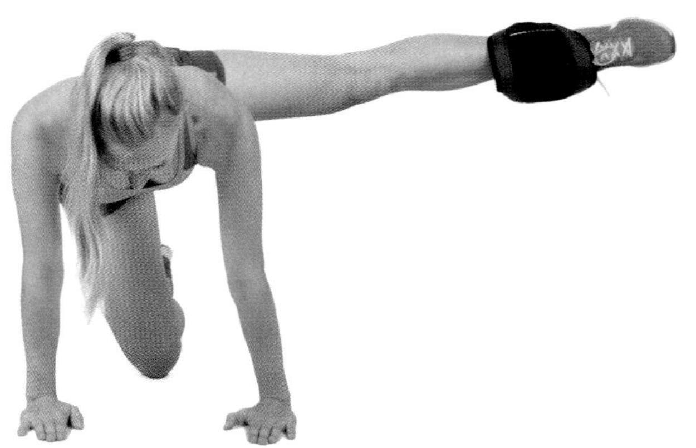

425 Clamshell

The Clamshell is another exercise that can be done almost anywhere. If you are looking to define the muscles around the hips and upper legs, this is a great exercise to do. Isolating the work into the outer hip, while keeping the feet raised, will give you long strong thighs.

- Begin by lying on the left side of your body. Place your left forearm down on the floor, propping up your upper body.
- Bring the knees into a right angle behind your hips and flex the feet. Squeeze the abs in, lift the heels up, and open the knees. Lower, and repeat.

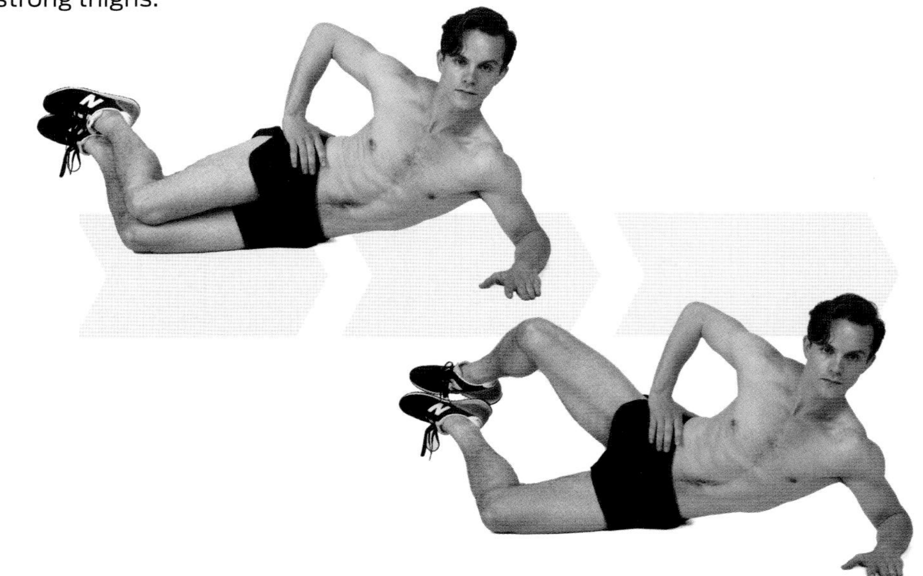

426 Clamshell with Resistance Bands

Resistance bands are a great way to work against the body's own power. They are virtually weightless and easy to use. Coming in a variety of thicknesses, bands range from very dense to very thin. Generally, the thicker the band, the stronger it is.

- Secure a band around the upper calves. Begin by lying on the left side of your body. Place your left forearm down on the floor, propping up your upper body.
- Bring the knees into a right angle behind your hips and flex the feet. Squeeze the abs in, and open the knees. Lower, and repeat.

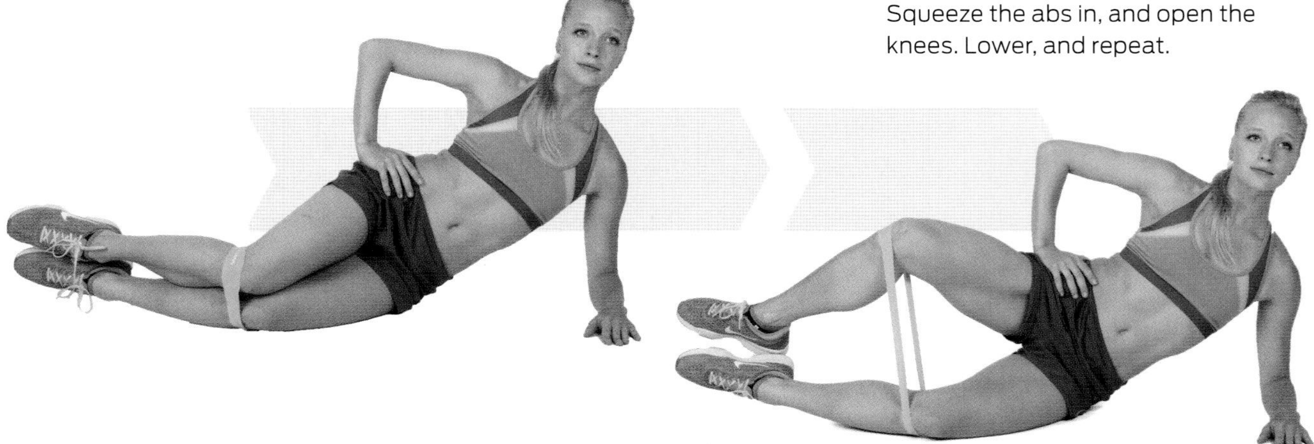

427 Gluteal Kick-Backs

This core exercise is done in conjunction with many different workout routines like yoga, Pilates, ballet barre, and calisthenics. The focus is on keeping the core stabilized between two hands and one leg, while you push and pull your leg out to the side and behind you.

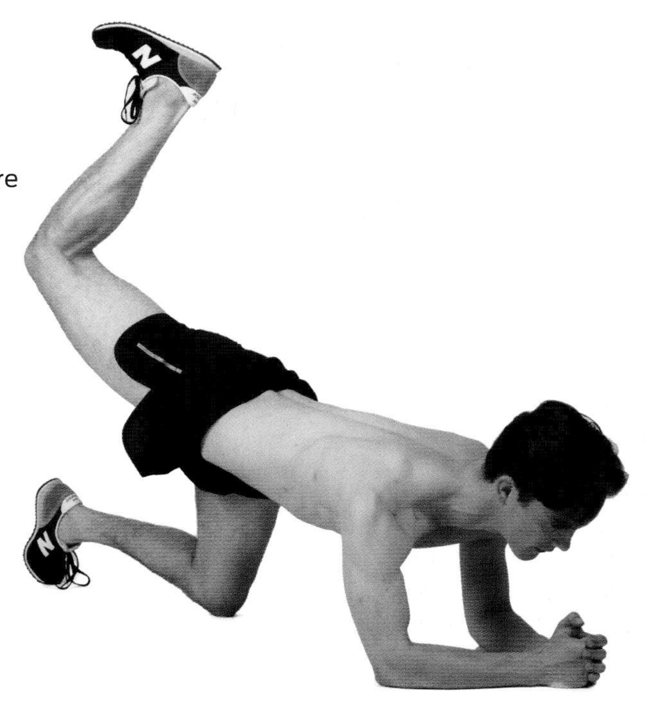

- Come to balance on your hands and knees.
- Strongly pull your abs up and into the back and squeeze the obliques along the sides of your torso.
- Push and lift your right leg up behind you, keeping the knee bent at a right angle and your chest toward the ground.

428 Gluteal Kick-Backs with Resistance Band

Putting a resistance band to use in this variation will enhance the stretch in your quad. The band will also create resistance between your hamstring and glute muscle.

- Start with your hands and knees apart and firmly planted into the floor. Loop a resistance band around the heel of your right foot.
- Strongly pull your abs up and into the back and squeeze the obliques along the sides of your torso.
- Push your right leg up against the band, keeping the knee bent at a right angle and your chest toward the ground.

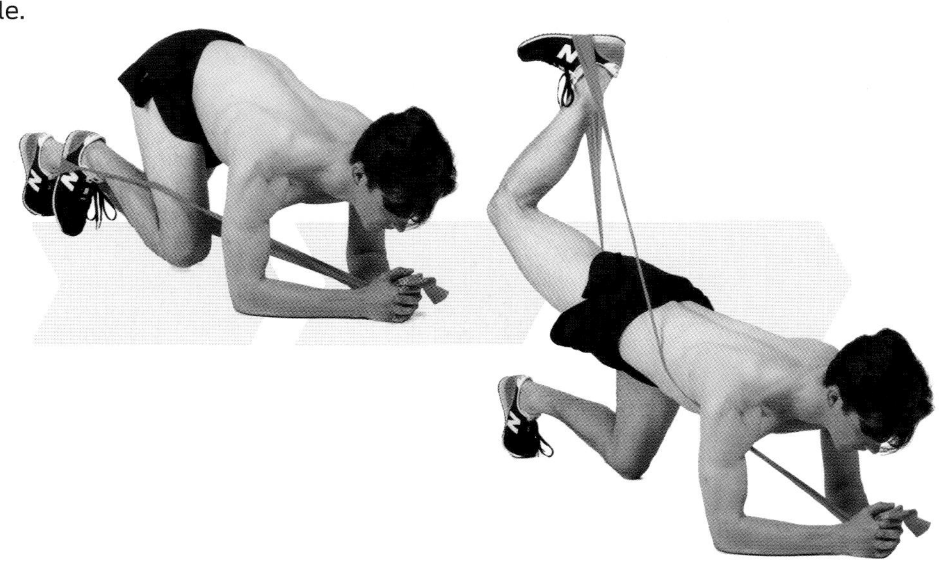

429

High Knees

When you bring your knee up past hip height you are engaging your core deeply, and also giving the lower back a stretch down through the hamstring. Alternating the knees up into the chest in this exercise will increase your balance, agility, and core strength.

Correct form

Keep the back long and upright. Keep the abs glued into the lower back to support the core.

Avoid

Do not let the shoulders hunch forward, or open too far behind you. Keep your abdominals engaged for proper alignment.

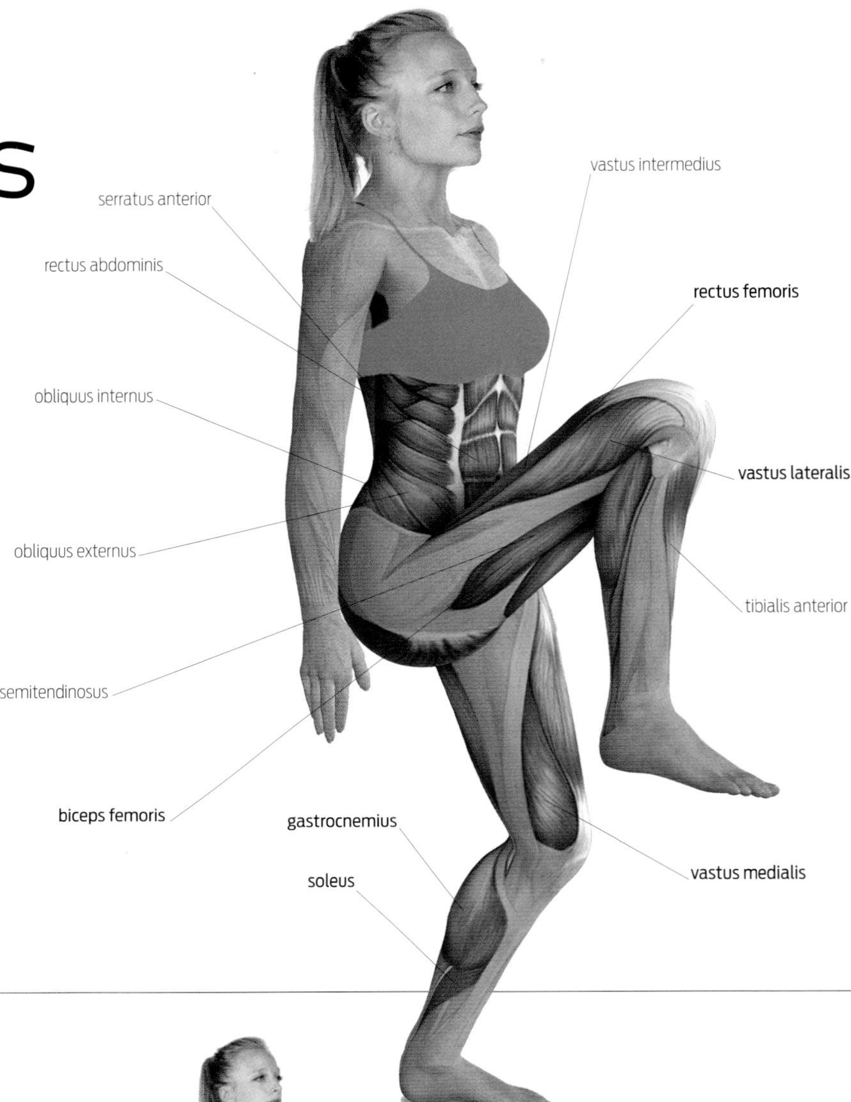

Annotation Key
Bold text indicates target muscles
Black text indicates other working muscles
* indicates deep muscles

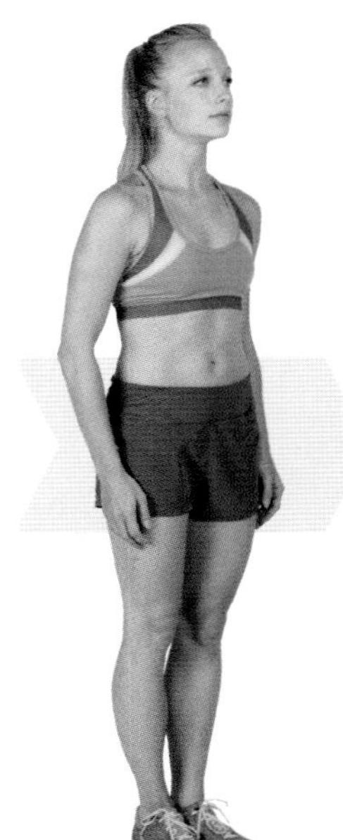

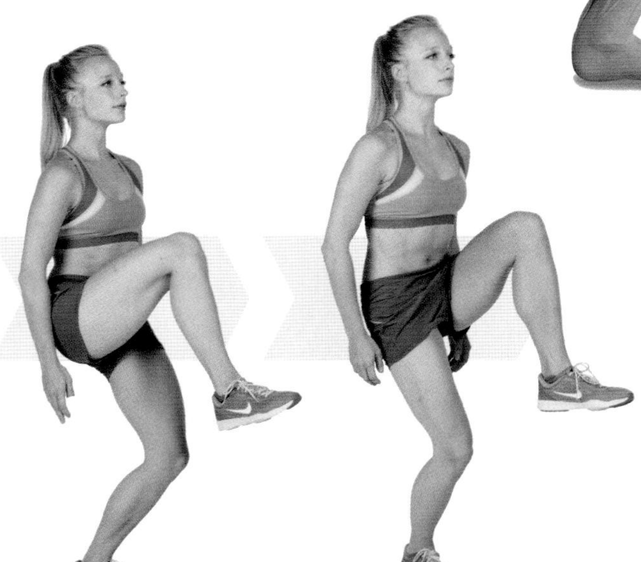

- Stand tall with your arms long at your sides.
- Engage the core and the backs of your legs and lift the right knee high into the chest.
- In one quick move, step the right leg down and bring the left leg up. Allow both legs to bend as you move through the exercise.

430

High Knees March

Stand tall with your forearms reaching out from the elbows in front of you. Engage the core and the backs of your legs and pull your right knee up to touch the right hand. Alternate, and bring the left knee up to touch the left hand.

431

High Knees with Leg Weights

Stand tall with your arms reaching long at your sides. Engage the core and the backs of your legs and bring your right knee up into the chest. Alternate, and bring the left knee up. Allow the knees to bend gently from side to side.

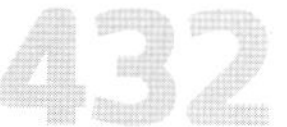

Dumbbell Lateral Raise and Knee Raise

Take a narrow-width stance. From standing, open your arms wide to the sides with dumbbells in hand. Bring the right knee up and extend it out to the side. Take care to keep your arms out to your sides and energized.

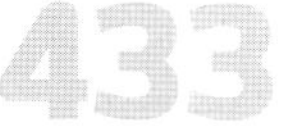

Lateral Bounding with a Medicine Ball

Start with your feet slightly apart and arms holding a Medicine ball in front of your chest. In one move, jump up and to the side into a lateral moving lunge with both legs bent, and then quickly jump up and to the side again. Keep changing sides.

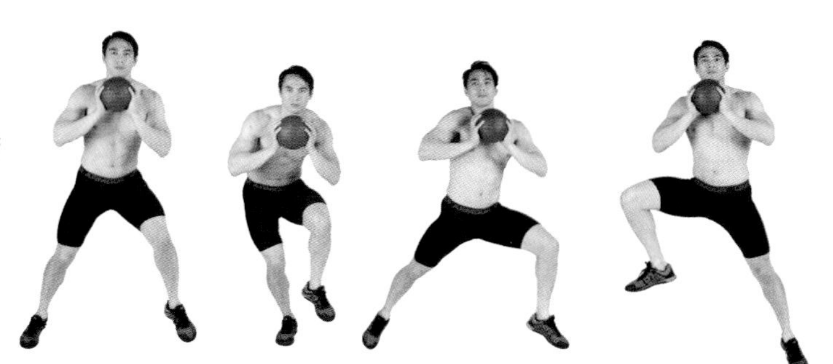

434

Double Leg Lifts

This double-leg, beautifully simple, exercise gives you the opportunity to work the deep inner core muscles, which can sometimes be hard to reach. By keeping the legs elevated in the air and stabilizing from deep inside your core, you will strengthen both the internal and external abdominal groups.

Correct form

You should aim to have your entire upper, middle, and lower back flush with the floor underneath you.

Avoid

Avoid dropping the legs so low past the point of being able to keep the abdominals pulling into the body.

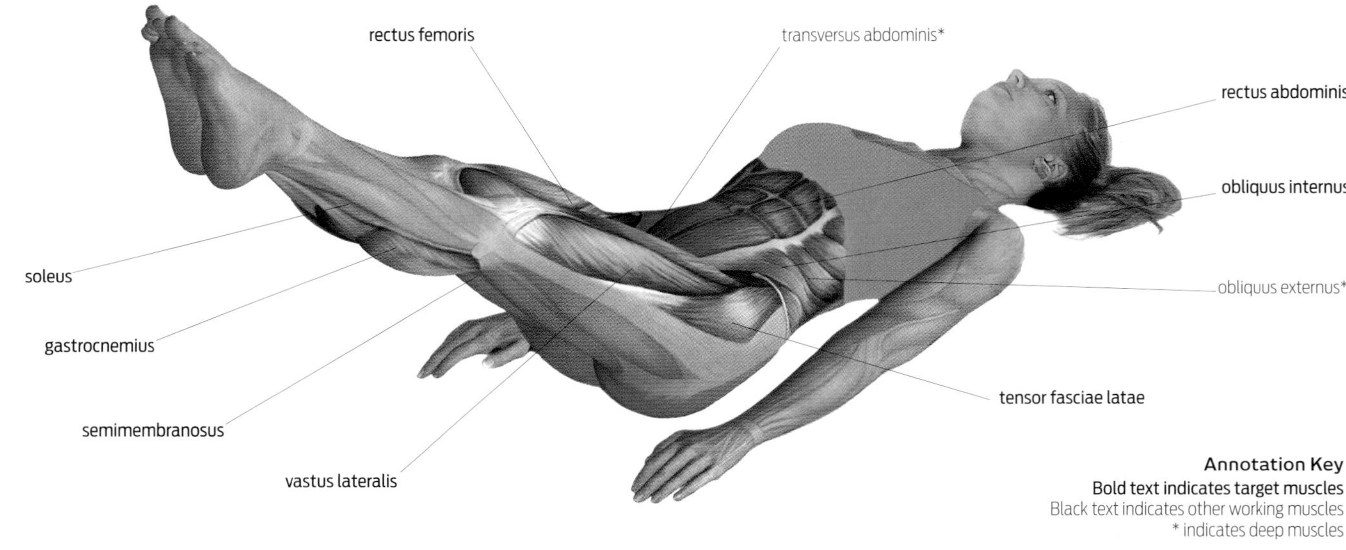

- Lie down with your legs extended above you, long out from the hips.
- Scoop the lower abdominals and lower the legs down into the air with your feet pointed.
- Keeping your back flat along the floor, pull the abs in again and lift the legs back up.

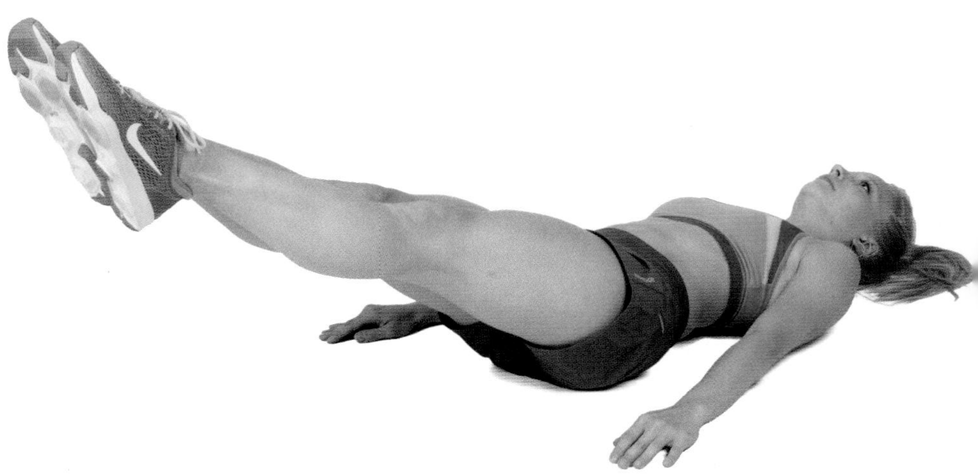

435 Foam-Roller Double Leg Lift Alternative

Lie down with your hips supported by the foam roller. Extend the legs above you, out long from the hips. Scoop the lower abdominals and lower the legs down with your feet flexed. Keeping your chest hips still, pull the abs in again and lift the legs back up.

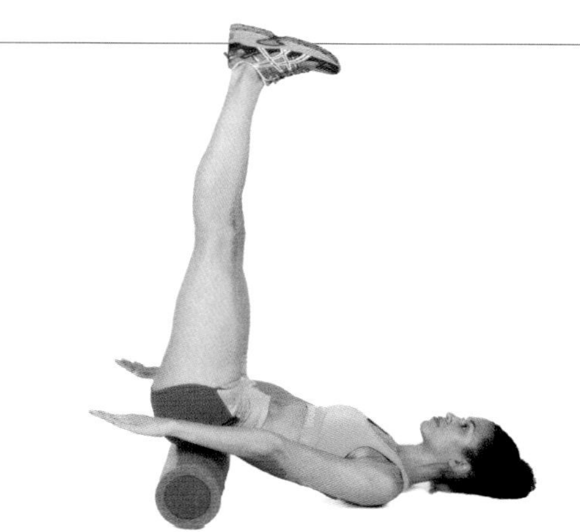

436 Isometric Oblique Hand-to-Knee Presses

With your spine along the foam roller and your arms at your sides, bring your arms flat on the floor out in front of your body. As you pull your left knee in, squeeze the abs tightly and lift your right arm off the floor to touch your left knee. Alternate sides.

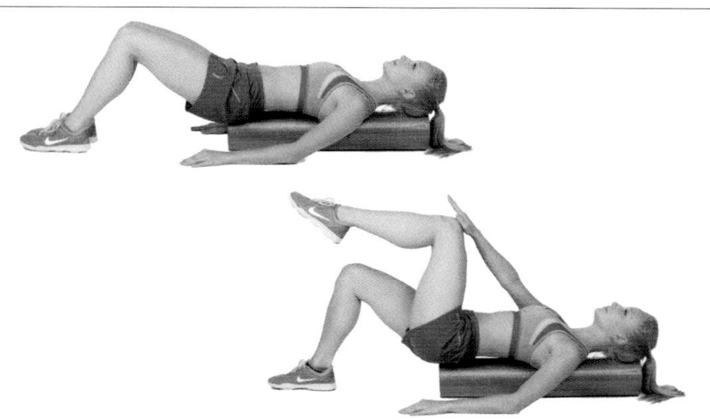

437 Foam-Roller Knee Lifts

Lie back on your roller with your arms at your sides. Place your feet flat on the ground with knees bent. Squeeze the abs and legs together tightly and take your Crunch (#167), bringing your chest to meet your knees.

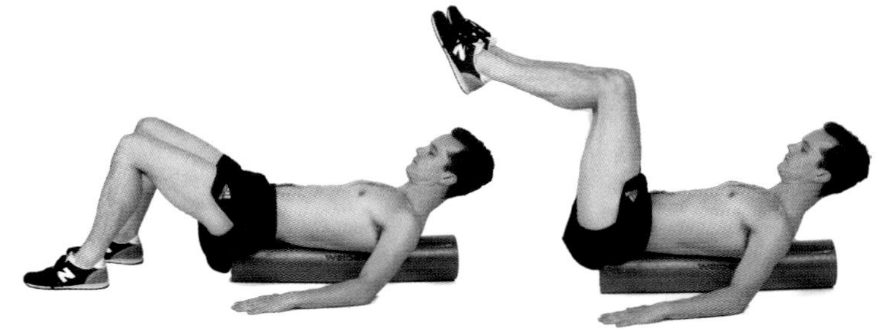

438 Foam-Roller Straight-Leg Bicycle

Lie with the roller supporting your spine. Bend your legs and bring them together at a 90-degree angle from your hips. Extend your right leg out, bring it in, and then extend the left leg. Squeeze your abs in strongly to support your core.

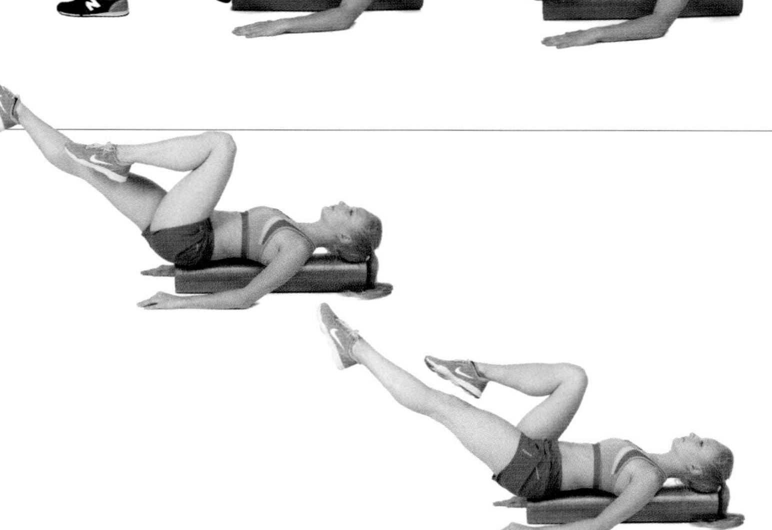

439

Step-Up

Incorporating a step creates muscle confusion in this exercise, and pinpoints the work into the hamstring and thighs. Keeping a tight core will help you balance while executing this standard Step-Up move.

Correct form

Keep your body's weight forward into the fronts of your legs and away from your heels.

Avoid

Be careful not to rush when stepping on and off the bench. Moving slowly will help you stabilize the core and create better balance.

- Begin with your feet together behind an elevated surface. Let your arms rest at your sides.
- Lift your right leg up onto the top of the bench, shift your weight into your right leg, and step up.
- Bring both feet together on top of the bench. Switch legs and step back down to stand.

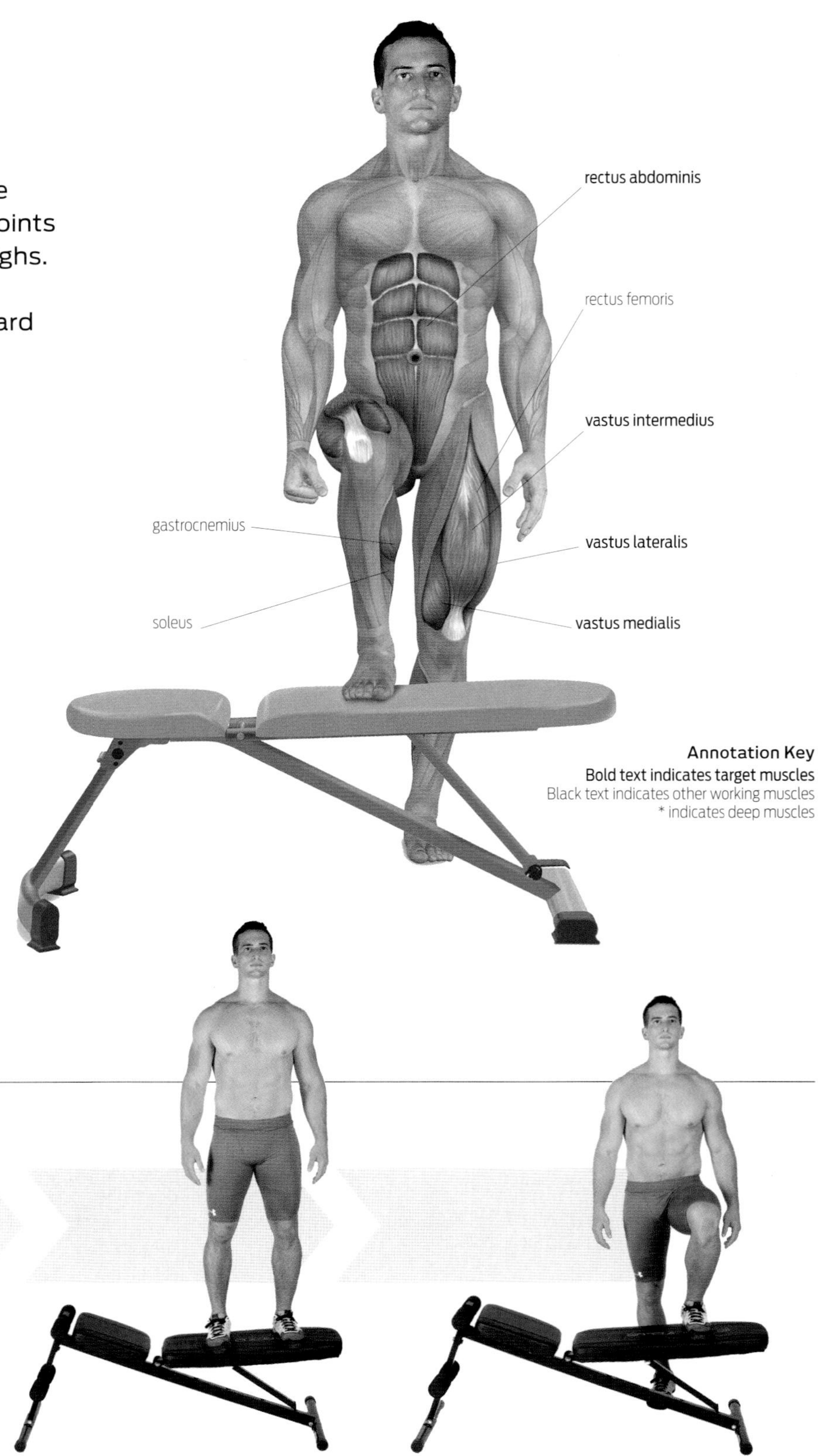

440 Alternating Step-Ups with Knee Lift

Alternating-leg Step-Ups with the lift of each knee is a basic aerobic workout move that helps facilitate better balance and strengthen the calves. By engaging the core and the backs of the legs on an elevated surface, you will create stability throughout the body.

- Stand tall with your hands resting on each hip, behind your box.
- Engage the core and the backs of your legs and step up onto the box with the left leg, bringing the right knee into the chest.
- Swing the right leg back to land standing, with both legs straight. Repeat.

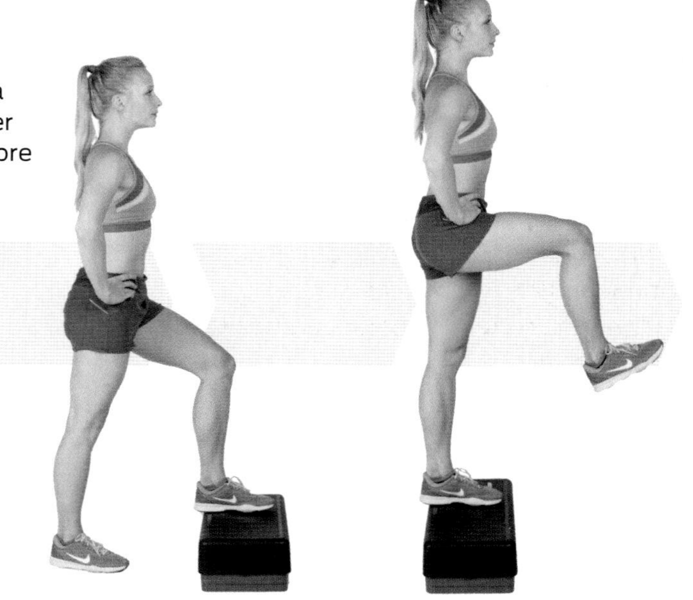

441

Box Jumps

Begin by standing tall behind your box. Take a standard Squat (#297) with both legs bent, quickly jump up high in the air, and land on top of the box with both knees bent. Extend the legs straight up, bend again, and jump back down. Use the arms as needed.

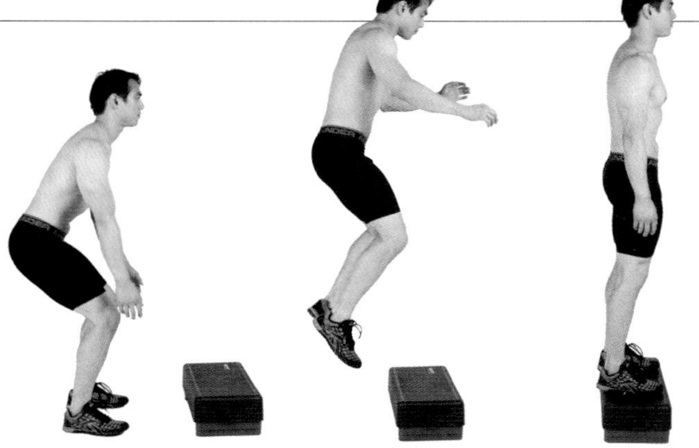

442

Medicine Ball Box Jumps

Begin by standing tall behind your box, holding a Medicine ball with both hands at the chest. Take a standard Squat with both legs bent, squeeze the core and legs, then quickly jump up high in the air, and land on top of the box with both knees bent.

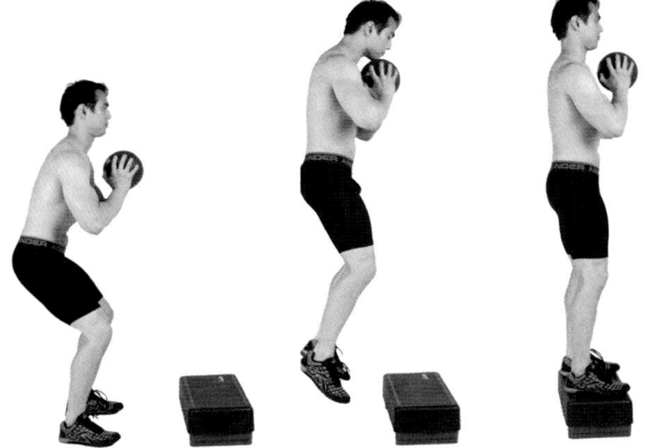

443 Burpees

The Burpee is said to be one of the best exercises in the world! It is not an easy move to perform but, if you can master it, the results are astounding. Performing Burpees correctly can benefit you in many areas: aerobic endurance, dynamic explosive power, core strength, and cardiovascular health.

- Start with your feet in a shoulder-width position.
- In one move, crouch down, placing your hands to the floor.
- Explode out into a Plank position (#213). Then, quickly, return to the crouched position.
- Last, fling your arms up to the air, leaping high with energy.

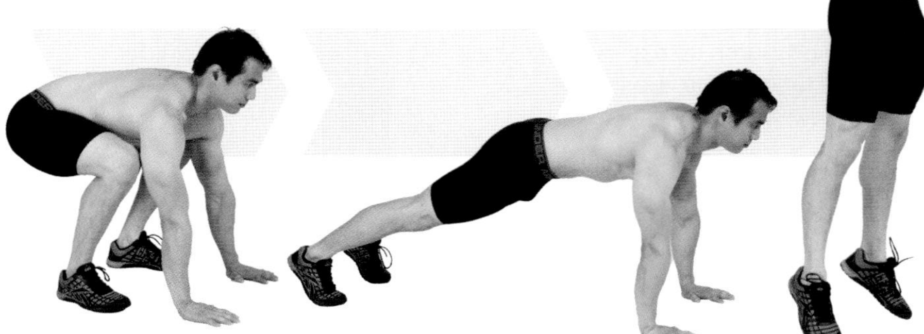

444 Balance Ball Burpee

Start with your feet in a shoulder-width position. In one move, crouch down, hands to either side of the balance ball (rounded side down). Explode out into a Plank (#213). Quickly return to the crouched position, lifting the balance ball. Last, leap up into the air, pushing the balancing ball overhead.

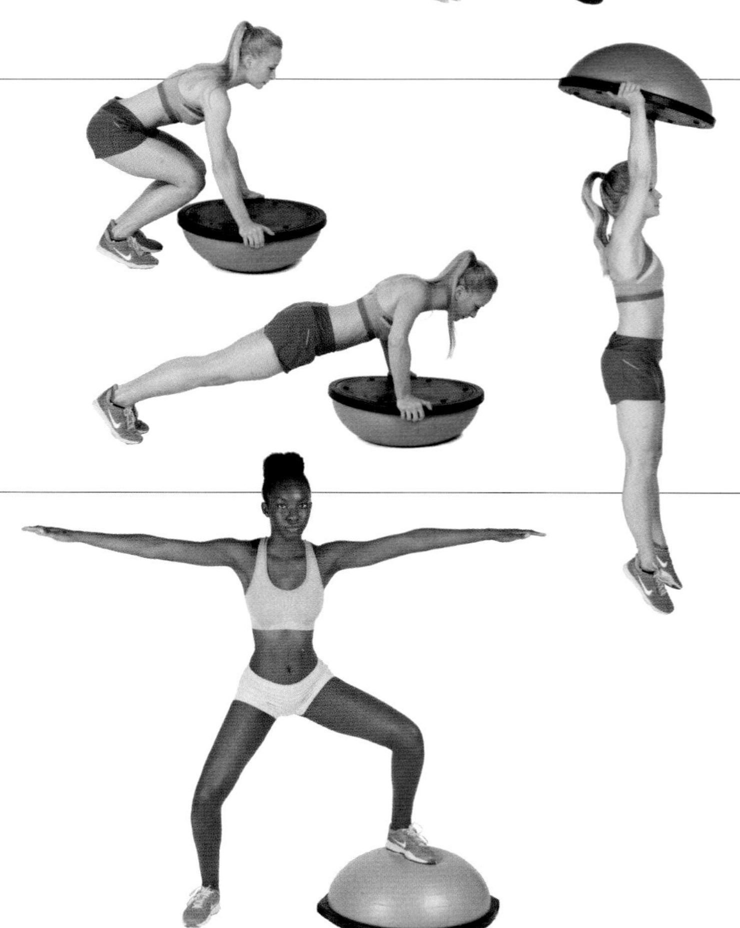

445 Balance Ball Squat Lateral Step-Up

Flip your balance ball so the rounded side is up. With your knees, and your arms open, put your left leg on the center of the balance ball. Take a Squat (#297), step the right foot up to meet the left, stabilize both feet, step off with the right foot to the right, then change sides.

446 Depth Jumps

Depth-jump or (box-jump) circuit training is another form of plyometric workout. Incorporating a set of low boxes, along with jumping movements between the floor and elevated levels, you enhance your speed and power.

- Begin by standing tall on top of one box in a series.
- Take a standard Squat with both legs bent, quickly jump up high in the air, and land on the floor in front of the next box with both knees bent.
- As soon as you land, extend the legs straight up, bend again, and jump up onto the next box. Use the arms as needed.

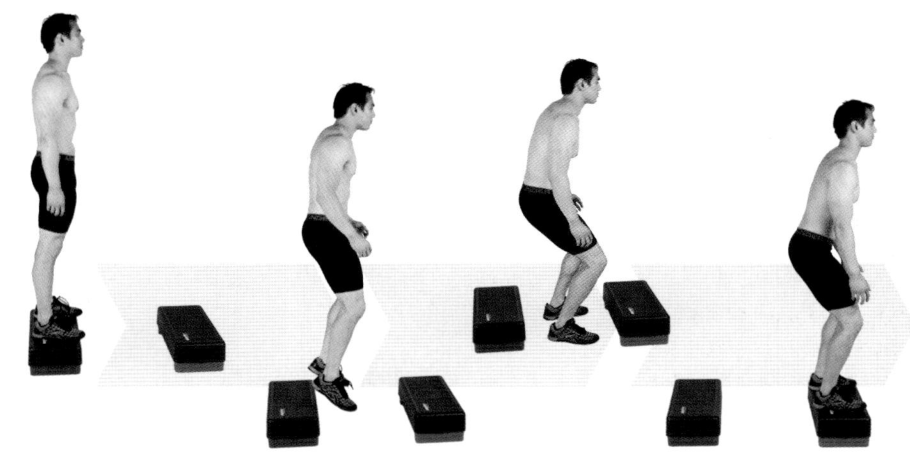

447 Medicine Ball Depth Jumps

Start on top of one box in a series. Take a Squat, holding your weighted ball, and quickly jump up high in the air, landing on the floor in front of the next box with both knees bent. As soon as you land, extend the legs straight up, bend again, and jump up onto the next box.

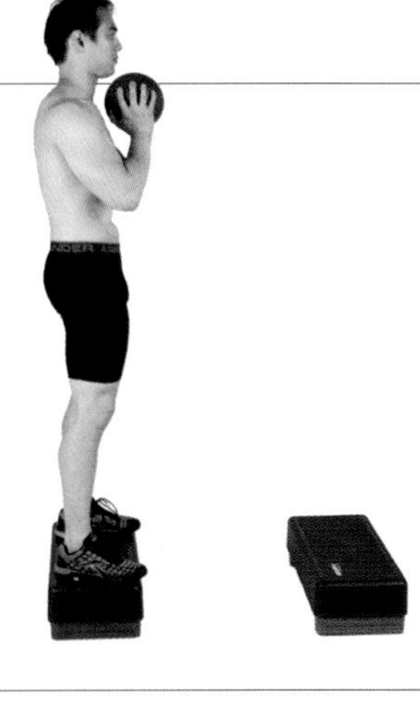

448 Step-Ups with Knee Lift and Overhead Extension

Stand tall with your hands at your sides. Engage the core and the backs of your legs and step up onto the box with the left leg. Swing the right knee up and extend the left arm overhead in opposition.

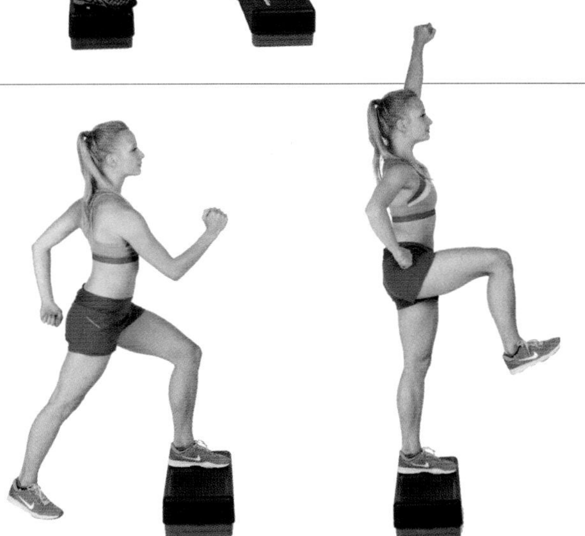

449 Dumbbell Step-Up

Begin with your feet together behind an elevated surface. Bring the arms into your chest, holding the dumbbells securely. Lift your left leg up onto the top of the box, shift your weight onto your leg, and extend the right leg behind the box. Switch legs, and repeat.

450 Dumbell Curl and Lateral Step

Standing parallel alongside a box, bring your arms into your shoulders, holding the dumbbells securely, and lift your left leg up onto the top of the box. Shift your weight onto your left leg.

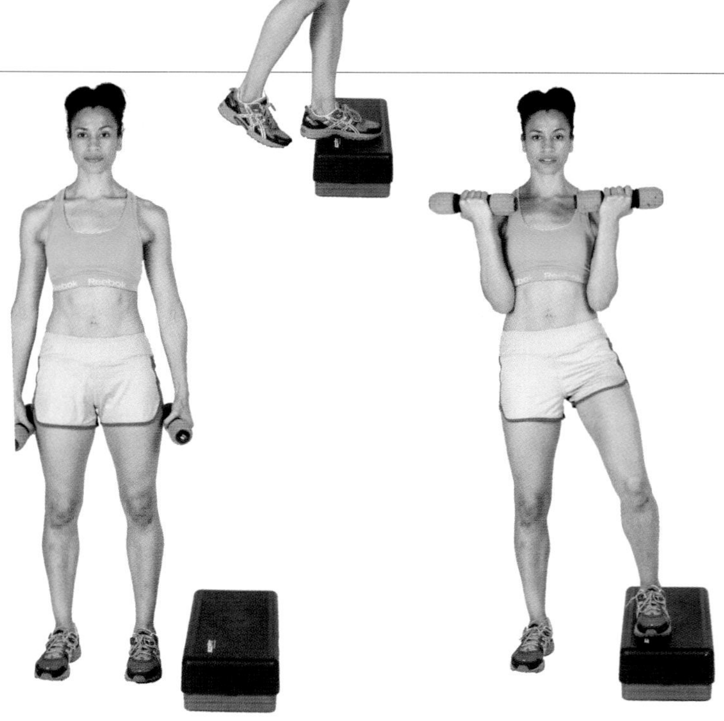

451 Curling Lateral Step and Raise

Standing parallel alongside a box, bring your arms into your shoulders, holding the dumbbells securely, and lift your left leg up onto the top of the box. Shift your weight onto your left leg, and raise the right knee.

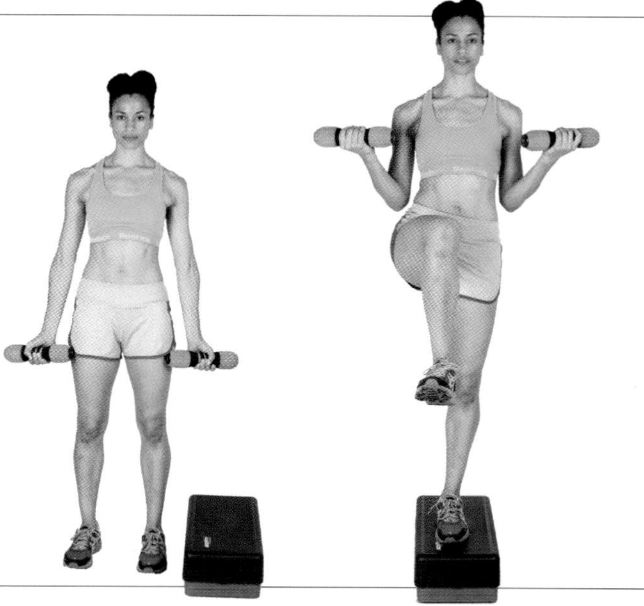

452 **Medicine Ball Crossover Step-Up**

Holding the ball at your center, lift your right leg across your body, placing it up onto the top of the box. Stand tall on your right leg, and step up. Bring the left foot to the second box. Cross the right leg down to the floor.

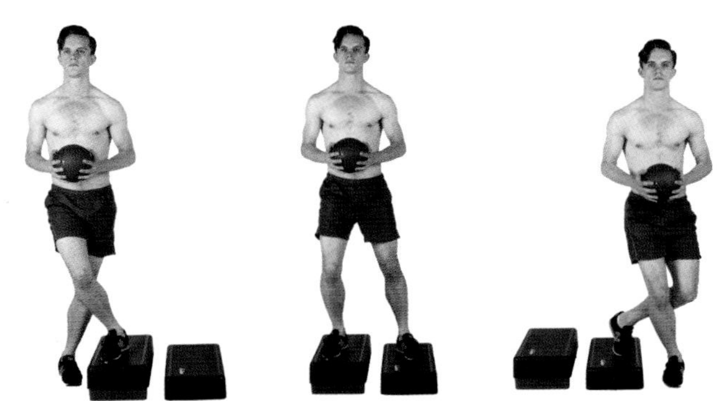

453 **Crossover Bench Step-Up**

Begin with your feet together alongside your bench. Let your arms rest at your sides. Lift your right leg across your body, placing it up onto the top of the bench. Stand tall on your right leg, and step up. Bring both feet together on top of the bench. Switch legs and step back down to stand.

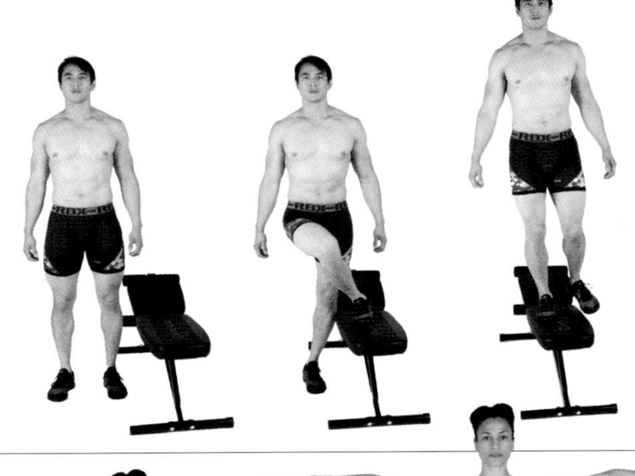

454 **Side Step with Lateral Leg Raise**

Stand tall with your core engaged and the spine very long. Reach your arms long at your sides. In one movement, step the left leg up onto a box and open your arms up wide to help keep you balanced. Flex the right foot.

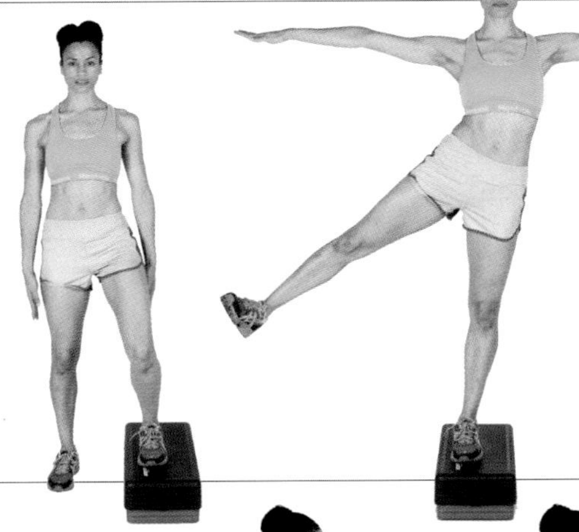

455 **Step-Down**

Begin with your feet together on an elevated surface. Bring your hands to your hips. Bend your left knee and lower your right heel forward of the front of the box, then extend the left leg back up and start again. Switch legs, and repeat.

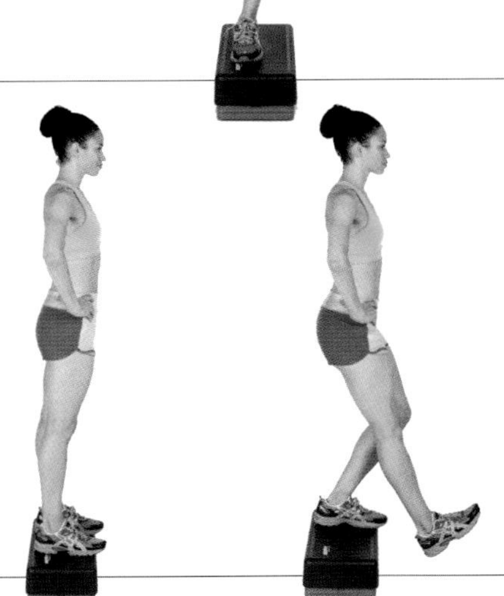

456 Weighted Ball Step-Down

Begin with your feet together on an elevated surface. Bend your left knee, lower your right heel forward and down in front of the box, and raise your weighted ball overhead. Straighten the left leg back up and start again. Switch legs, and repeat.

457 Lateral Step-Down

Begin with your feet together on top of and parallel to your box. Reach your arms out in front of you. Bend your left knee and lower your right heel down outside and along the side of the box. Extend the left leg back up and start again. Switch legs, and repeat.

458 Weighted Ball Lateral Step Down

Standing parallel alongside your box, bring your hands to your chest, holding the weighted ball securely. Lift your left leg up onto the top of the box, shift your weight onto your left leg, and extend the right leg.

459 Lateral Step-Over

Start by standing tall, with your arms relaxed at your sides. Visualize that there is a high bench on your left side that you must step over. Pick up your left knee and extend it to the left. Then, straighten your right leg out and pick it up to meet your left foot.

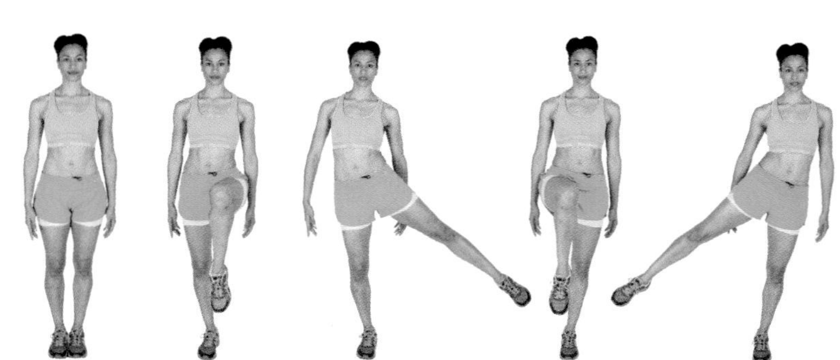

460 Crossover Step-Up

Begin with your feet hip-width apart alongside your box. Let your arms rest at your sides. Lift your right leg across your body, placing it up onto the top of the box. Stand tall on your right leg, and step up. Bring both feet together on top of the box. Switch legs and step back down to stand.

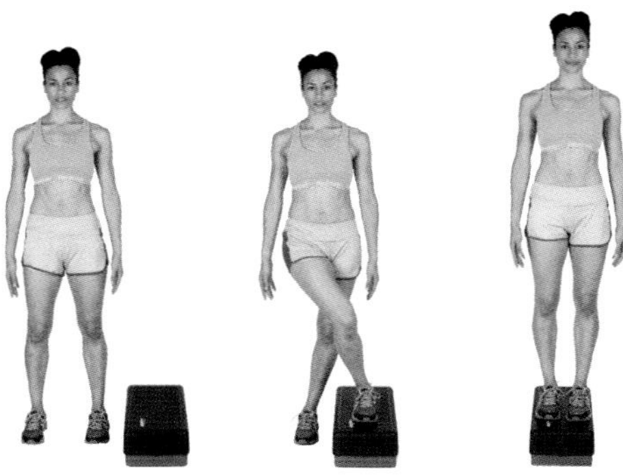

461 Dumbbell Crossover Step-Up

Begin with your feet hip-width apart alongside your box. Hold dumbbells in your hands at your sides. Lift your right leg across the body, placing it up onto the top of your box. Stand tall on your right leg, and step up. Bring both feet together on top of the box.

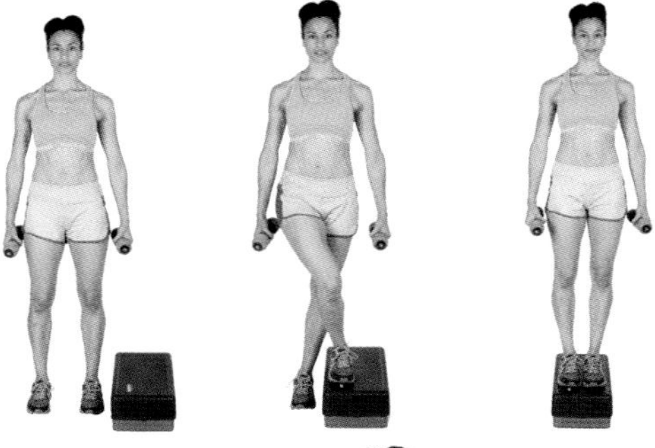

462 Dumbbell Skater

With your feet together and hands holding dumbbells, step to the left, bending the left knee and curling your weights into the shoulders. Angle your back over the bent knee with a straight spine. Spring off the left foot to stand as you began.

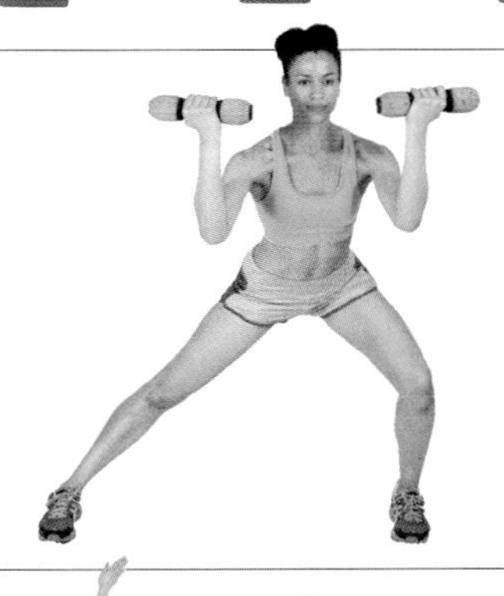

463 Step Skater

Start with your feet together alongside a box and your arms open at your sides. Step to the right, coming onto the box with a bent knee. Angle your back over the bent knee with a long spine. Reach for the right foot with your left arm and extend the right knee straight. Change sides.

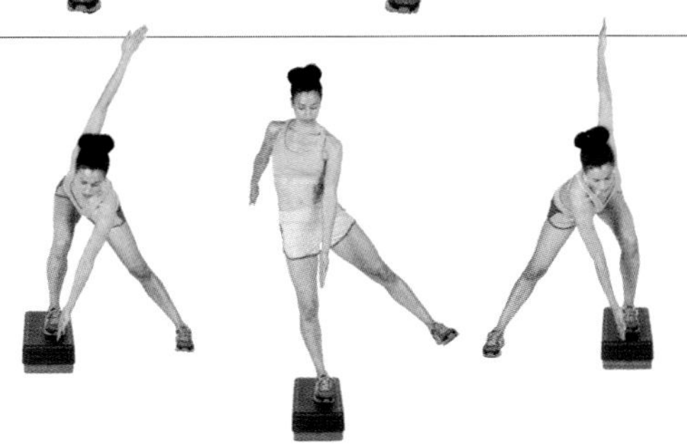

464 Dumbbell Step Skater

Start with your feet together alongside a box and your hands at your sides, holding dumbbells. Step to the right, coming onto the box with a bent knee. Angle your back over the bent knee with a long spine. As you step on and off the box with alternating feet, swing the opposite arm forward and back in turn.

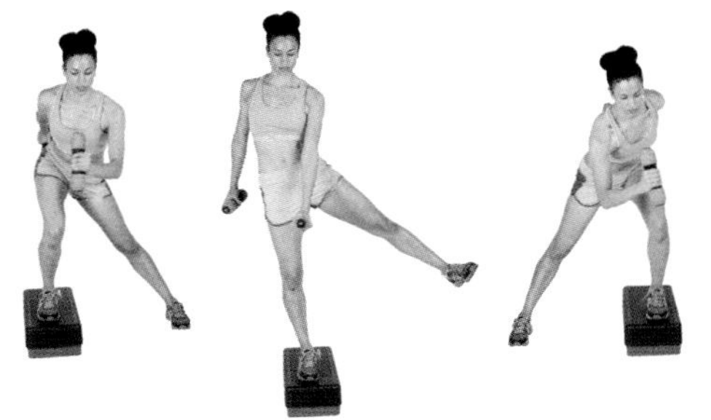

465 Balance Ball Leg Scissors

Lie with a balance ball supporting your back. Extend your legs and bring them together at a 90-degree angle from your hips. Come up into your Crunch position (#167) and hold there. Move your right leg forward and back, and then your left.

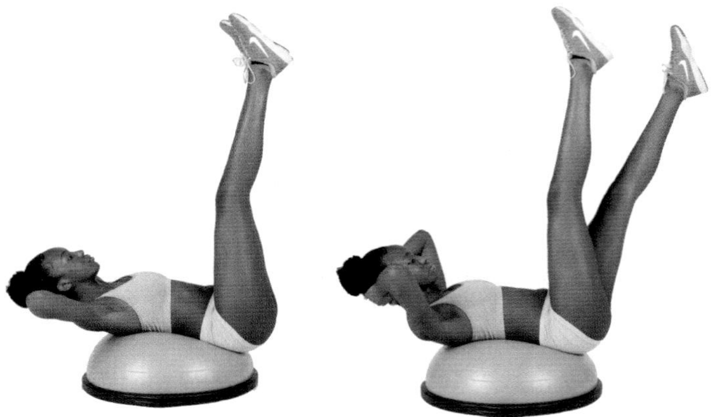

466 Balance Ball Seated Leg Tucks

Sit down on a balance ball with your legs bent in front of you. Lean back, putting some weight into the hands. Scoop the lower abdominals and lift the legs up into the air with your feet flexed. Keeping your chest open to the front, bend your legs back in.

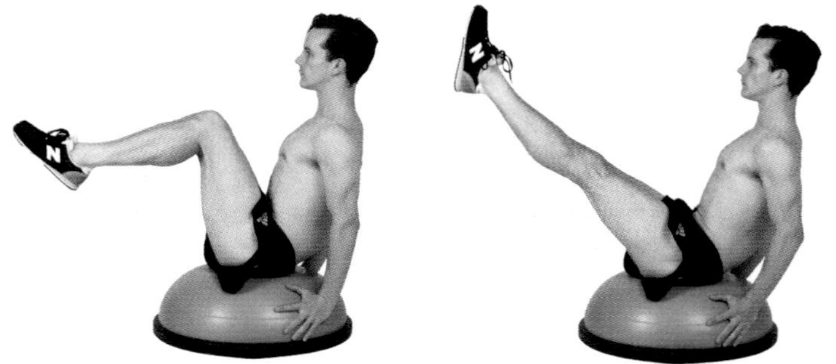

467 Foam-Roller Raised Leg Curl

With your spine along the foam roller and your arms at your sides, bring your legs together out in front of your body. Pull your knees into a right angle, squeeze the abs tightly, and lift your head off the foam roller to look forward through the knees.

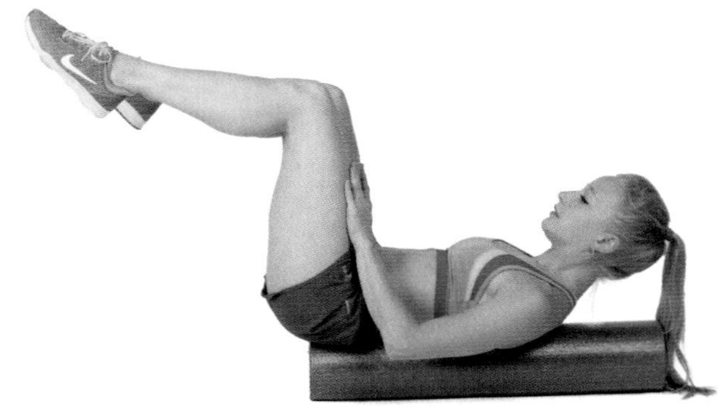

468 Foam-Roller Opposite Hand to Leg

Lie with your head and spine supported on the roller. With long legs, pull the abs in and sit up slightly. Simultaneously, lift the left leg, and bring the right arm up overhead. Diagonally cross your right arm to meet your left foot. Repeat with your left arm and right leg.

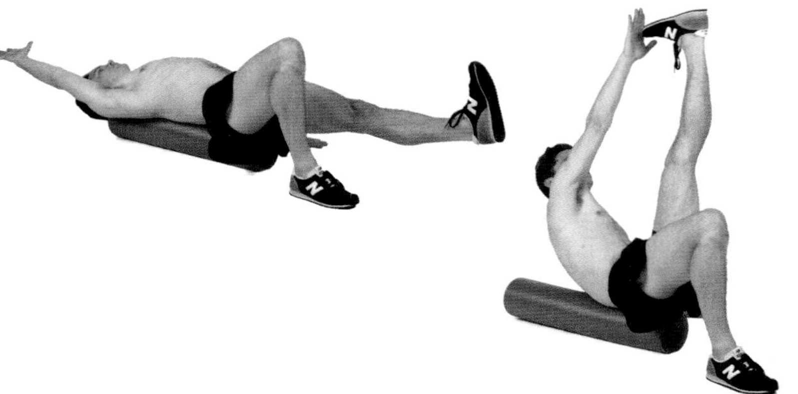

469 Kneeling Side Lift

Come to a kneel, with the weight balanced on both knees. Place your hands behind your head and shift your weight onto the right side. Extend your left leg long out from the hip. Press the hips forward, lift the abdominals up and kick the left leg up off the ground.

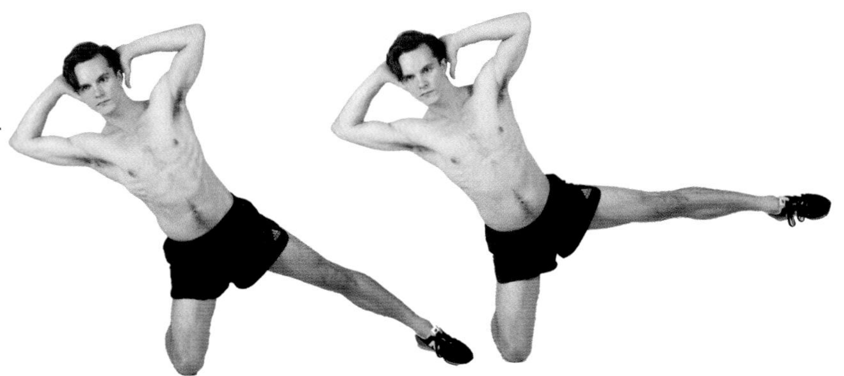

470 Kneeling Side Kick

Come to a kneel, with the weight balanced on both knees. Place your left hand behind your head and the right hand down to support you. Shift your weight onto the right side. Extend your left leg long out from the hip. Swing your left leg forward and then to the back.

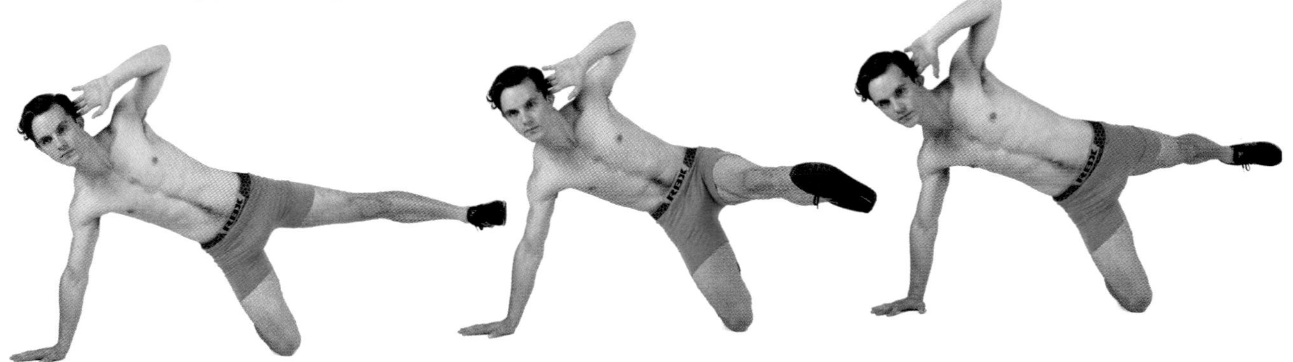

471 Straight-Leg Raise

Lie down with your hips flat. Extend your legs out long above you from the hips. Scoop the lower abdominals and lower the legs down with your feet flexed. Keeping your hips still, pull the abs in again and lift the legs back up.

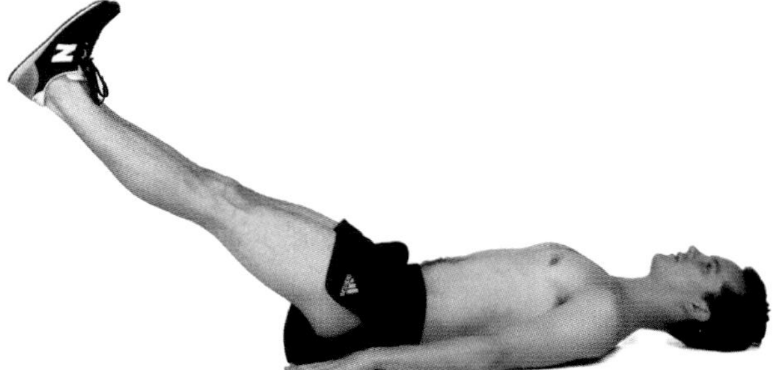

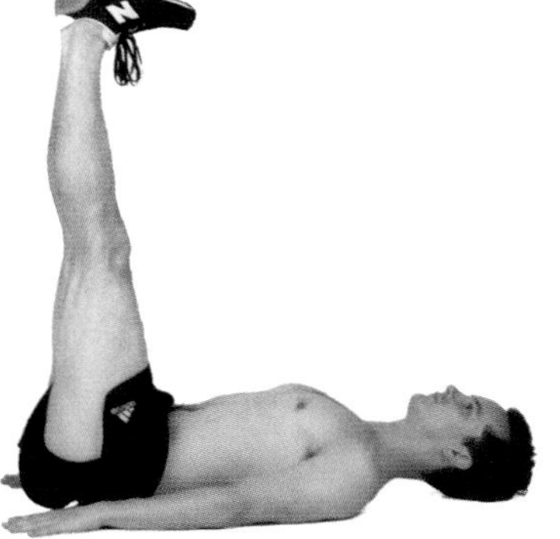

472

Bridge

Bridging activates all of the muscles in the lower and upper legs. In order to achieve your maximum Bridge, you must squeeze the abs in to support the lower back and hamstrings. Bridges can be made more challenging by adding weight onto the front of the hips and/or lifting one leg off the floor.

Annotation Key
Bold text indicates target muscles
Black text indicates other working muscles
* indicates deep muscles

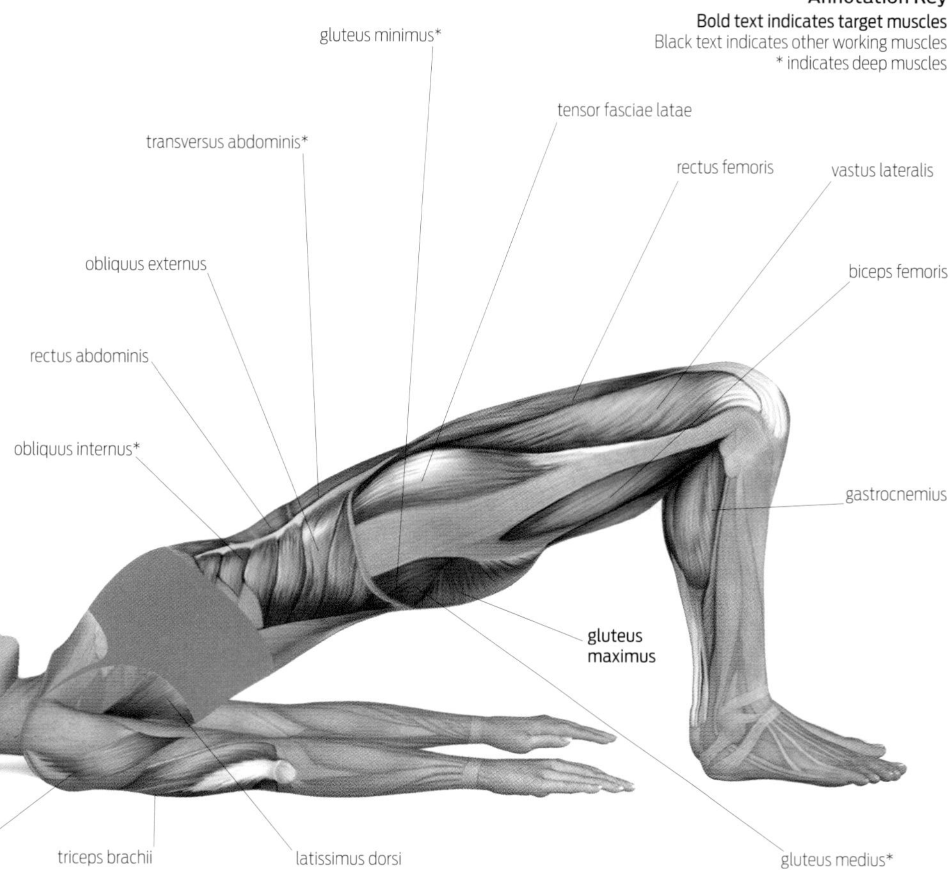

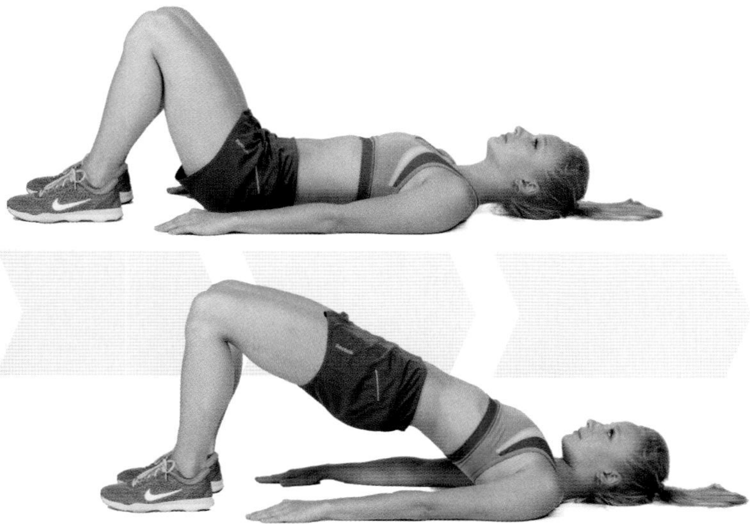

Correct form

Your body should be in a straight line from head to knee when you are at the top of your Bridge.

Avoid

Avoid bringing the feet in to close the bottom. Make sure there is enough space to bridge up and down with ease.

- Lie with your back long against the floor. Engage the abs so that they are pulled deeply into the lower back.
- Bring the soles of your feet flat to the floor and squeeze your inner thighs together.
- Press into your arms along the sides of your body and lift the hips high into the air. Engage the core and hamstrings at the top of your Bridge.

473 **Single-Leg Bridge**

Lie with your back long against the floor. Bring your feet to the floor and squeeze your inner thighs together. Press into your arms along the sides of your body and lift the hips high into the air. Extend your right leg out alongside your left knee. Repeat on the other side.

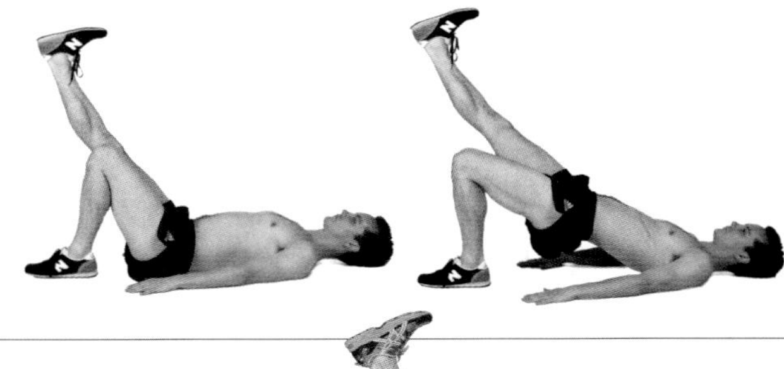

474 **Single-Leg Bridge with Weight Plate**

Lie with your back long on the floor. Bring the soles of your feet to the floor and squeeze your inner thighs together. Place a weight on top of the hips. Lift the hips high into the air. Extend your right leg out alongside your left knee. Repeat on the other side.

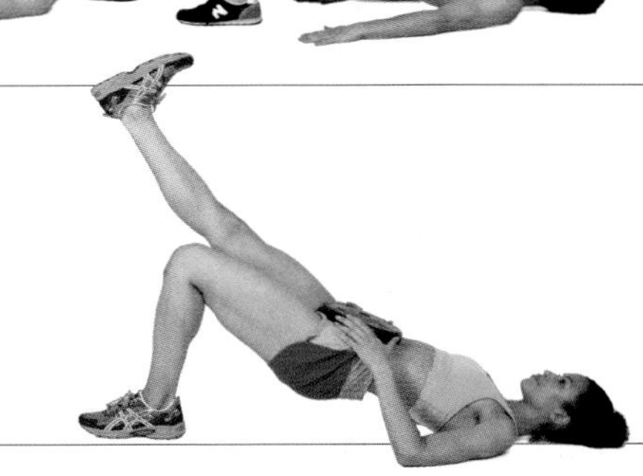

475 **Hip Bridge with Weight Plate**

Lie with your back long on the floor. Bring the soles of your feet to the floor and squeeze your inner thighs together. Place a weight on top of the hips. Lift the hips high into the air. Engage the core deeply.

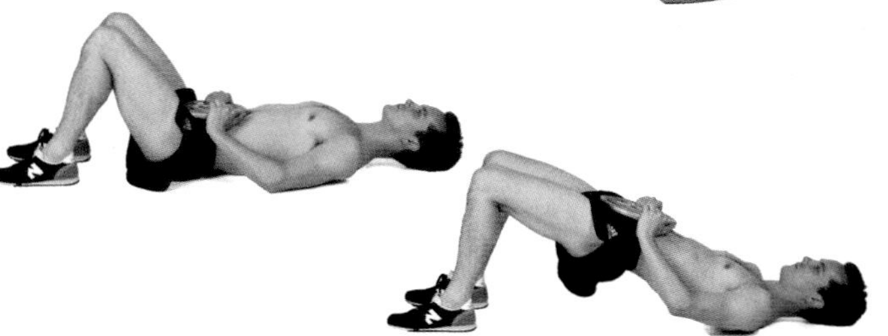

476 **Hip Bridge on Bench with Barbell**

Sit with your back supported by a bench, on the floor. Bring the soles of your feet to the floor and squeeze your inner thighs together. Hold your barbell at the hips and press it up high into the air, bringing your shoulders onto the bench.

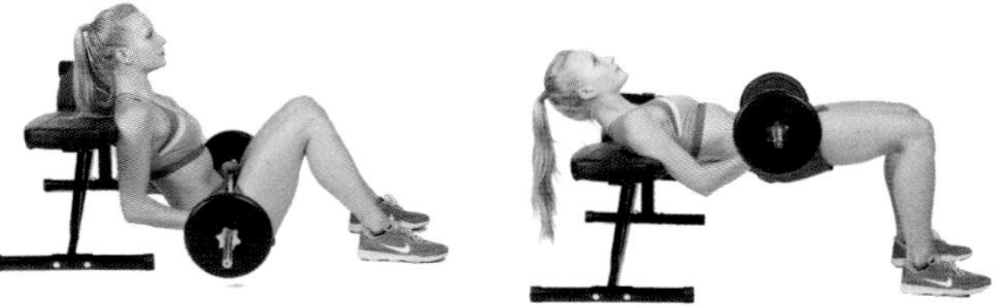

477 **Box or Bench Hip Bridge**

Lie with your back long on the floor and the backs of your upper arms against the floor, elbows bent at 90-degrees so the hands are pointing toward the sky. Bring your heels onto a bench or box. Lift the hips high into the air. Press down firmly into your shoulders and upper arms.

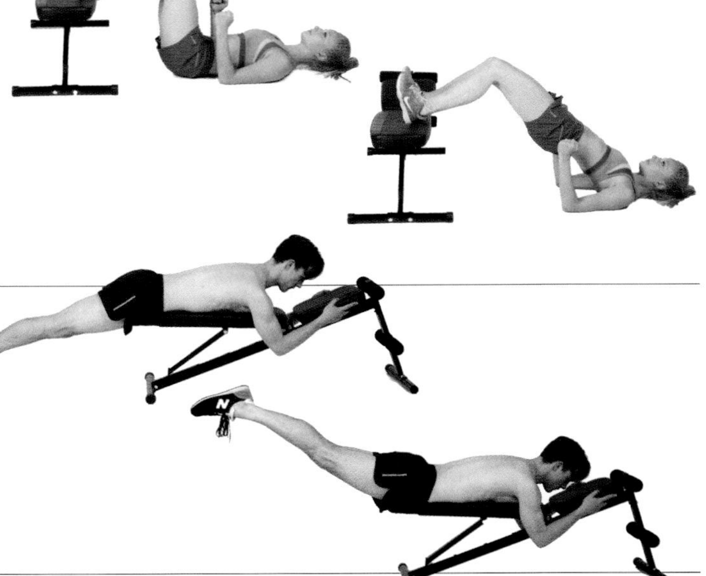

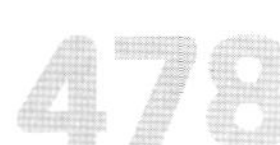

478 **Reverse Hip Raise**

Extend your body long on top of a bench. Bring your arms close together under the bench and bring your legs to touch, squeezing the inner thighs tightly. Engage the abs strongly, and in one move, lift your legs up into the air.

479

Mountain Climber

Mountain Climbers are coined so because they mimic the act of climbing, and because of the similar challenge they pose in alternating the legs up and into the chest while keeping the core and leg muscles fully engaged and flat to the floor. This move will create stability in the core and the arms, and deliver the ability to produce explosive movement.

Correct form

Be sure to keep your body in good alignment. You should be in a low Plank with the body flat to the floor. It should be a challenge to bring the knees in.

Avoid

Avoid swaying the lower back or hunching the shoulders. Keep the abs engaged strongly, with the arms pushing away from the floor.

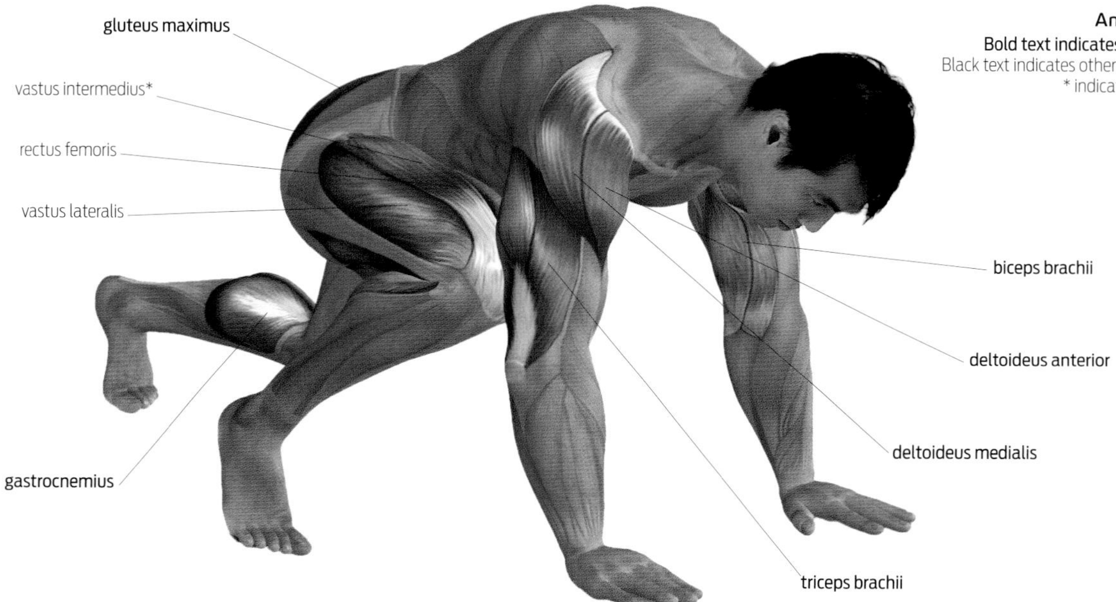

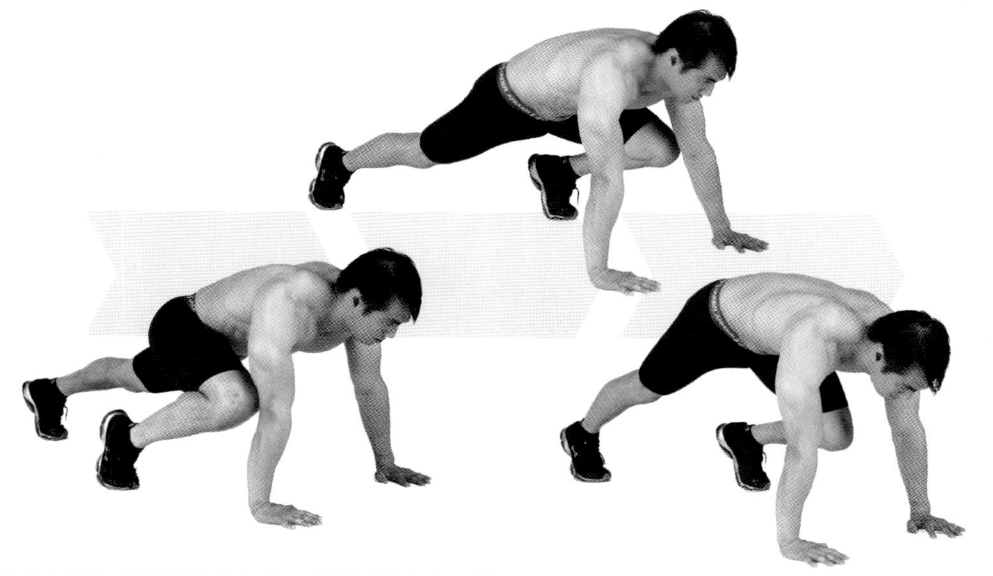

- Balance in your standard Plank (#213), with your palms down.
- Squeeze the core deeply and bend your right knee into your chest.
- Stay low in the Plank and alternate sides, bringing the left knee into the chest.

480 Balance Ball Mountain Climber

Balance in your standard Plank, with your palms down at the center of a balance ball. Squeeze the core deeply and bend your right knee into your chest. Stay low in the Plank and alternate sides, bringing the left knee into the chest.

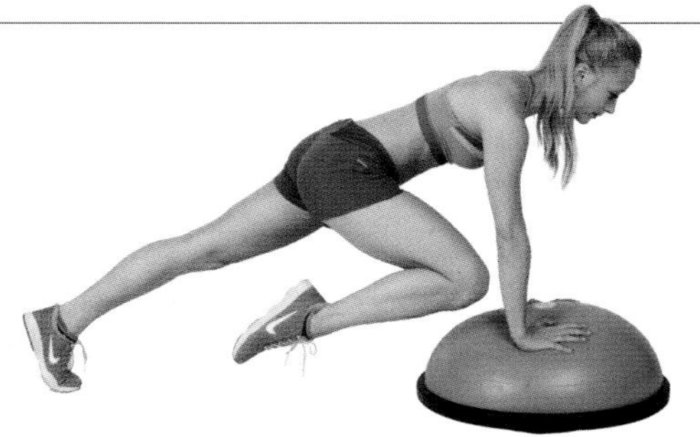

481 Foam-Roller Mountain Climber

Balance in your standard Plank, with your palms down on the floor. Walk your feet up onto a foam roller. Squeeze the core deeply and bend your right knee into your chest. Stay low in the Plank and alternate sides, bringing the left knee into the chest.

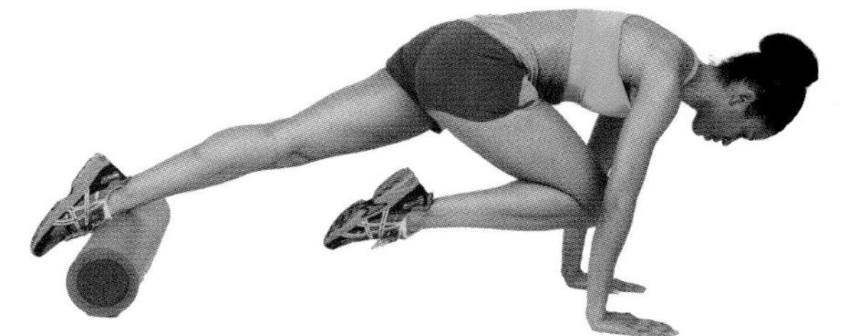

482 Swiss Ball Mountain Climber

Balance in your standard Plank, with your palms down at the center of your Swiss ball. Squeeze the core deeply and bend your right knee into your chest. Stay low in the Plank and alternate sides, bringing the left knee into the chest.

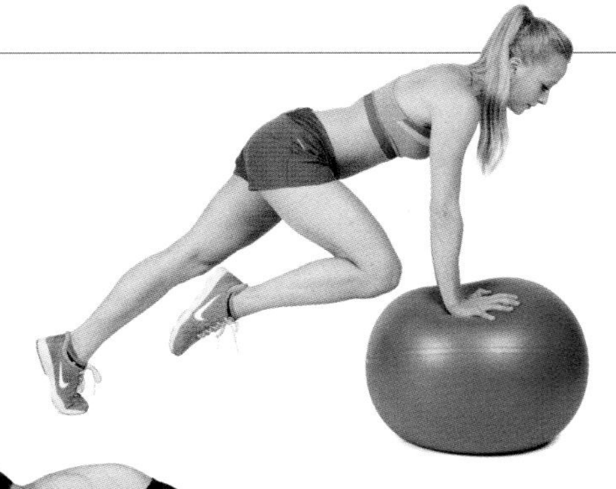

483 Medicine Ball Mountain Climbers

Balance in your standard Plank, with your palms down over the top of a Medicine ball. Squeeze the core deeply and bend your right knee into your chest. Stay low in the Plank and alternate sides, bringing the left knee into the chest.

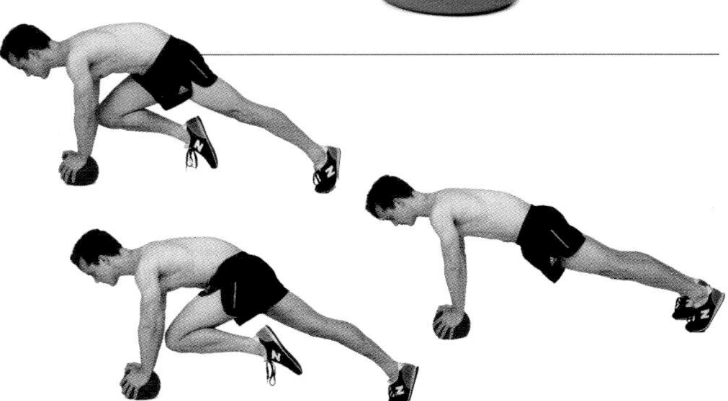

484 Cross-Body Mountain Climber

Come into your standard Plank. Squeeze the core deeply and bend your left knee into the right shoulder, across the torso. Stay low in the Plank and alternate sides, bringing the right knee across the body to the left shoulder.

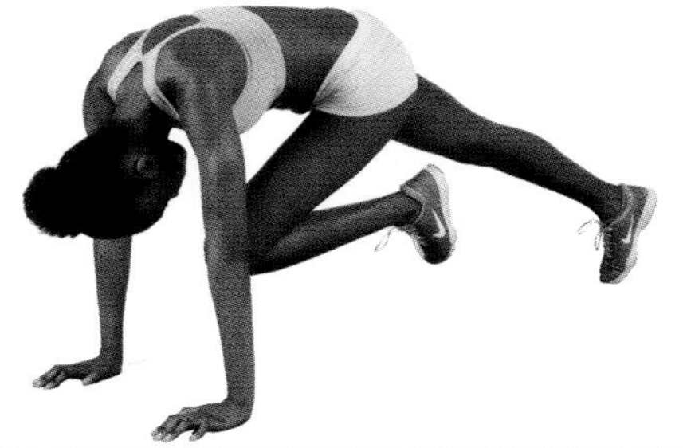

485

Stiff-Legged Barbell Deadlift

Correct form

The deadlift targets the lower-back muscles and the hamstrings. Be sure to keep both parts of the body straight and long.

Avoid

Avoid letting the barbell swing or alter at all during this movement. Keep the weight center at your body. Avoid rounding the back as you lower the weight.

Deadlifting a barbell targets all of the muscles responsible in creating good posture. You will be able to keep your back straighter throughout your various daily activities, too! It works all the body's muscles, all at once, and if you are looking to do only one magical exercise, this is the one to do. With any Deadlift, and especially this stiff-legged version, be careful not to lift too heavy a weight so as to protect your lower back. Push the hips back, and lower the weight with control until you feel a deep stretch in the hamstrings. There is no need to go to the floor.

Annotation Key
Bold text indicates target muscles
Black text indicates other working muscles
* indicates deep muscles

levator scapulae
trapezius
rhomboideus
erector spinae*
latissimus dorsi
obliquus internus
obliquus externus
rectus abdominis
gluteus maximus
biceps femoris

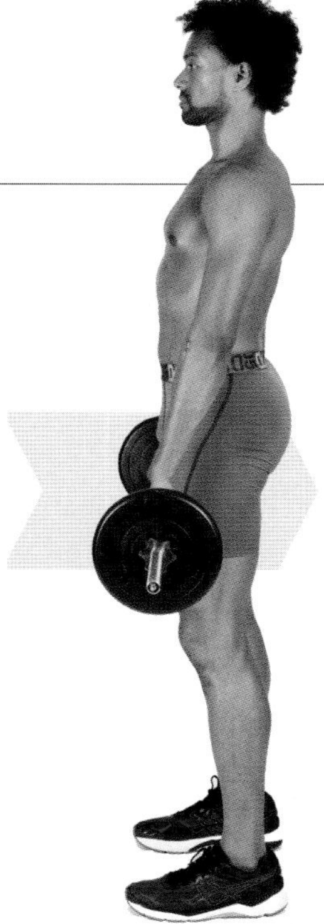

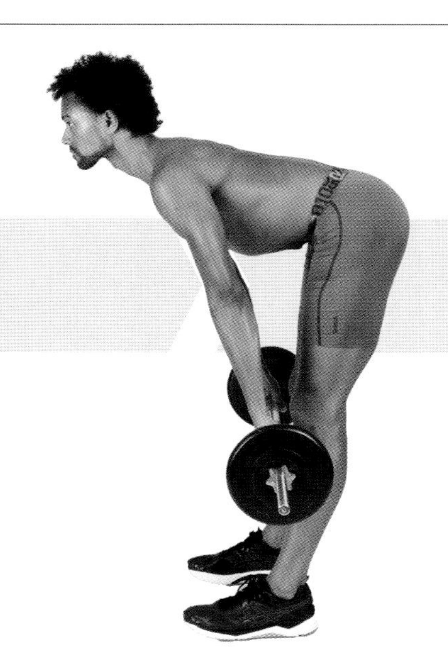

- Stand tall with your barbell directly held out in front of your thighs.
- Bend forward generously at the hips. Bring both legs to straighten and your barbell to meet your shins.
- Extend the back up to standing tall as you began. Repeat, and keep your back flat as you move forward and back.

486 Barbell Power Clean

The Barbell Power Clean is a move that places the weight of your barbell directly in front of you. By lifting or snatching up the bar with a dynamic quick count, you work on developing core strength as well as stability in the lower back and legs.

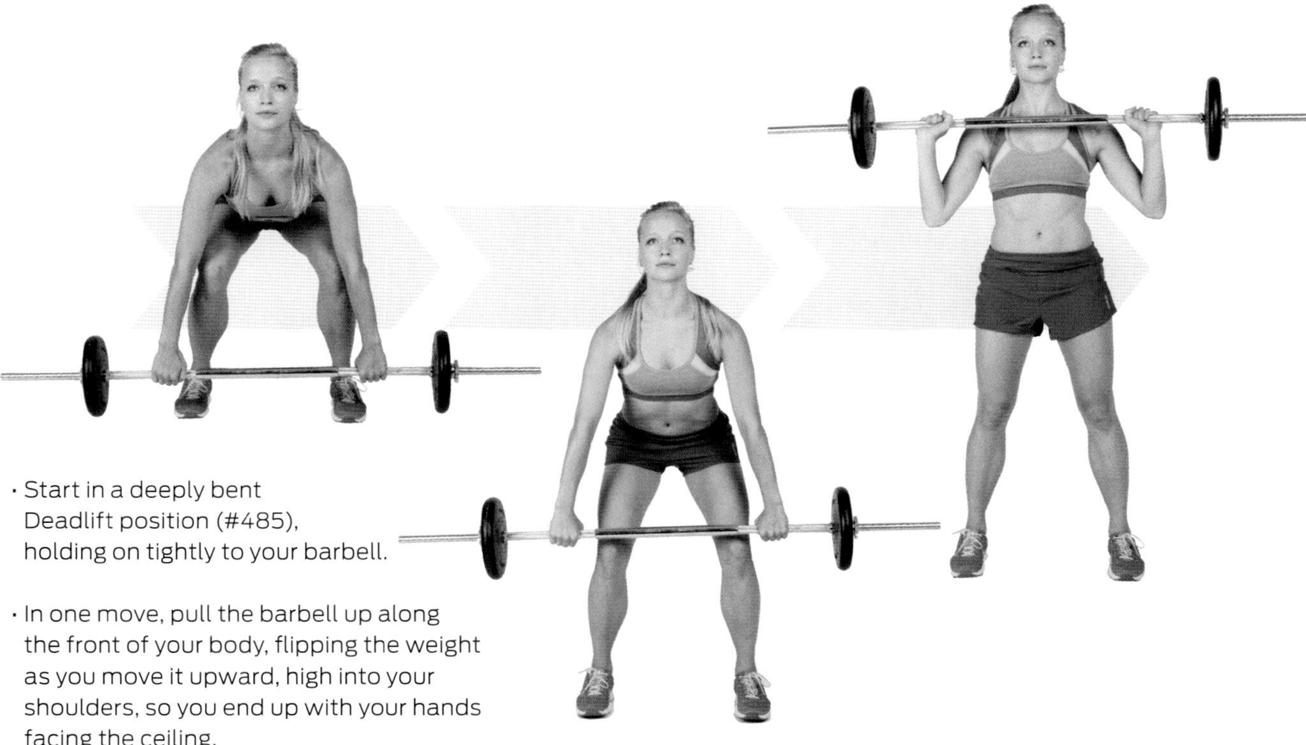

- Start in a deeply bent Deadlift position (#485), holding on tightly to your barbell.
- In one move, pull the barbell up along the front of your body, flipping the weight as you move it upward, high into your shoulders, so you end up with your hands facing the ceiling.
- Engage through the legs and core, and lower the bar back down again.

487 Barbell Power Clean and Jerk

Start in a deeply bent Deadlift position, holding on tightly to your barbell. In one move, pull the barbell up along the front of your body, flipping the weight as you move it upward, high into your shoulders, so you end up with your hands facing the ceiling.

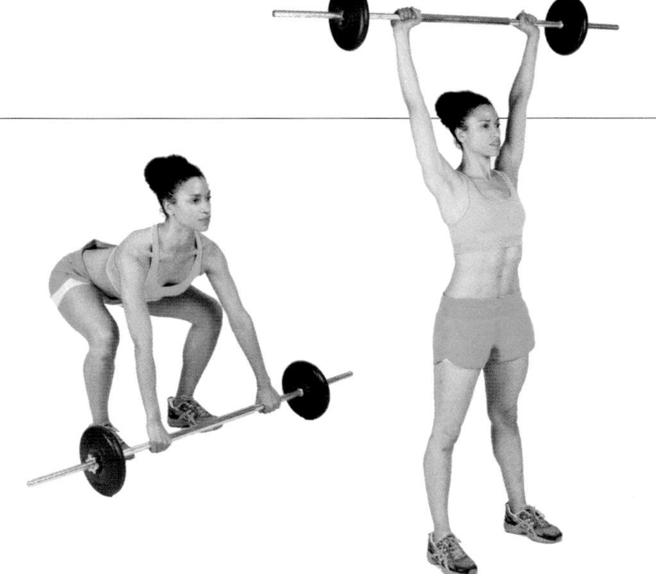

488 Power Clean and Jerk Modification with Bar

Start in a deeply bent Deadlift position, holding on tightly to your body bar. Engage the abs deeply and squeeze the backs of the legs. In one move, pull the barbell up along the front of your body, flipping the weight as you move it upward, high into your shoulders, so you end up with your hands facing the ceiling.

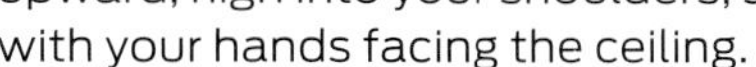

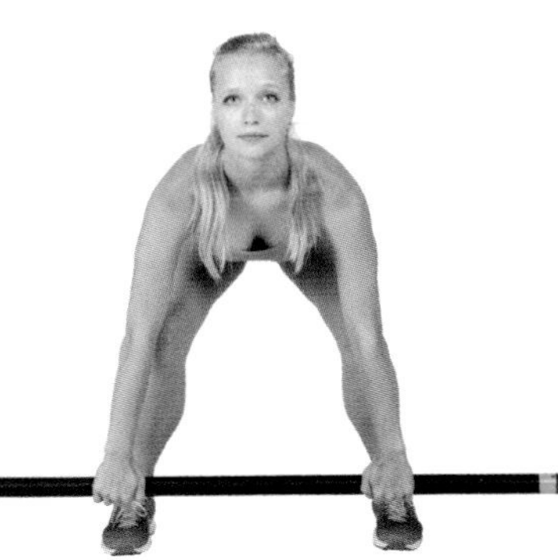

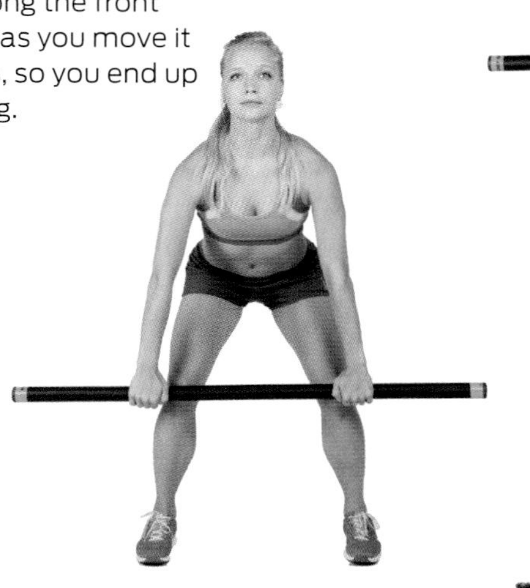

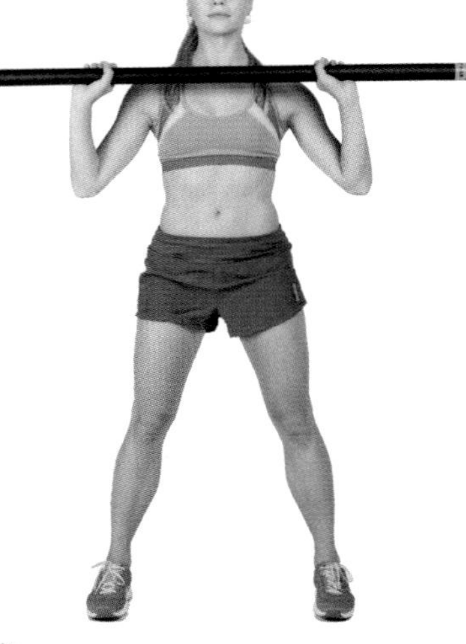

489 Stiff-Legged Dumbbell Deadlift

Stand tall with your dumbbells at your sides. Bend forward generously at the hips, keeping the dumbbells close to the body as you lower. Stiffen both legs and bring your weights to meet in front of you. Extend the back up to standing tall. Repeat, and keep your back flat as you move forward and back.

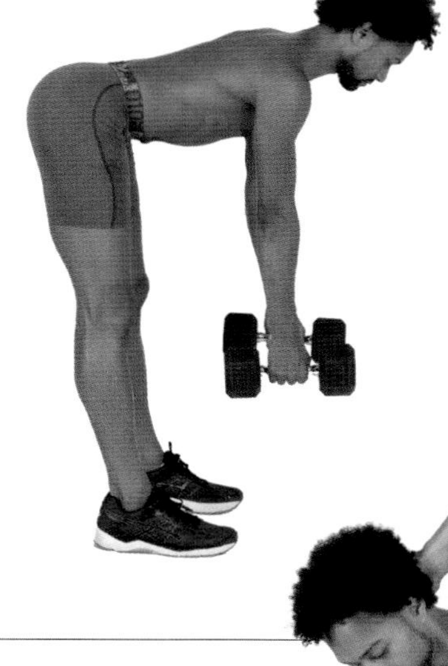

490 Single-Arm Dumbbell Deadlift

Start by standing with your core pulled in tightly, with a dumbbell by your right foot. Deeply bend the knees and hinge the hips back as you squat down. Grasp the dumbbell with your right hand, and perform as you would a Deadlift (#485).

491 Single-Arm Kettlebell Deadlift

Stand with your feet shoulder-width apart, with a kettlebell between your feet. Lean over to grasp the weight with one hand, and perform as you would a Deadlift.

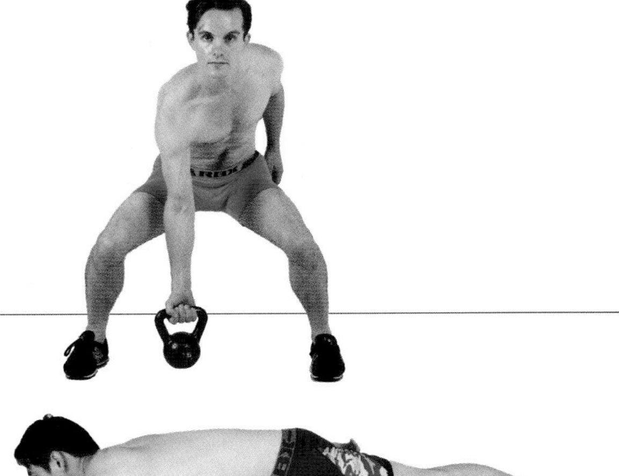

492 Single-Arm Stiff-Legged Kettlebell Deadlift

With the kettlebell in your left hand, bend forward, extending your left leg back behind you. Allow the kettlebell to pull your weight forward and down into the floor. Keep your abs engaged deeply. This is a great step for defining the legs!

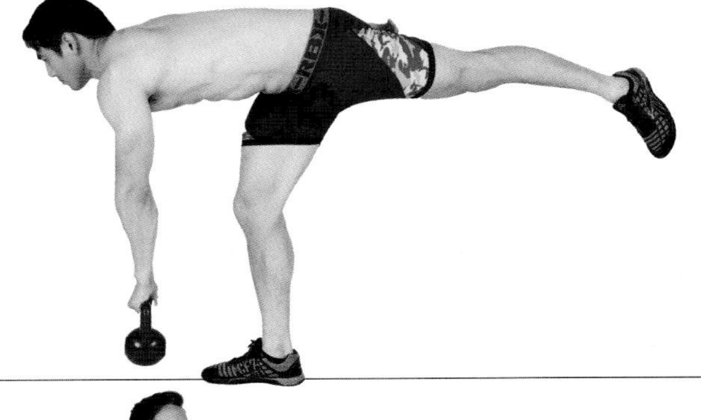

493 Good Mornings

Start by standing tall with the legs wide apart. Take your barbell and let it lie across the shoulders. Engage the hamstrings and glutes and pull the core up and in as you bend at the hips. Keep the back straight as you bend forward.

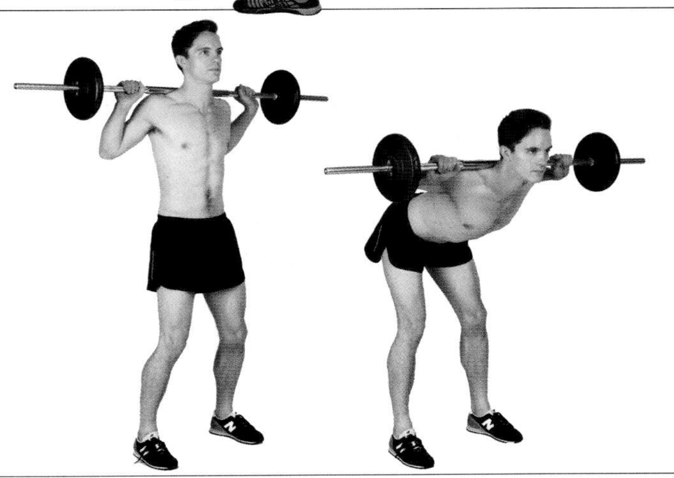

494 Good Mornings with Dumbbells

Start by standing tall with the legs wide apart. Take your dumbbells and bring them to either side of your upper shoulders. Engage the hamstrings and glutes and pull the core up and in as you bend at the hips. Keep the back straight as you bend forward.

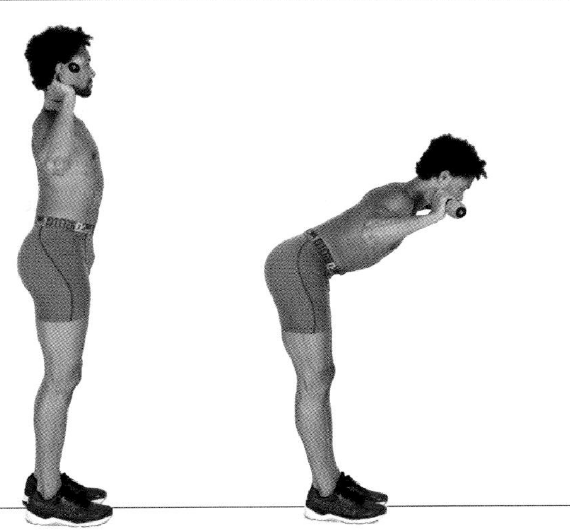

495 Standing Calf Raise

Well-developed calves help to track the ankle and knees underneath the hips, giving us a well-aligned gait and balance for standing, running, and walking. These calf raises also stabilize the ankle joints.

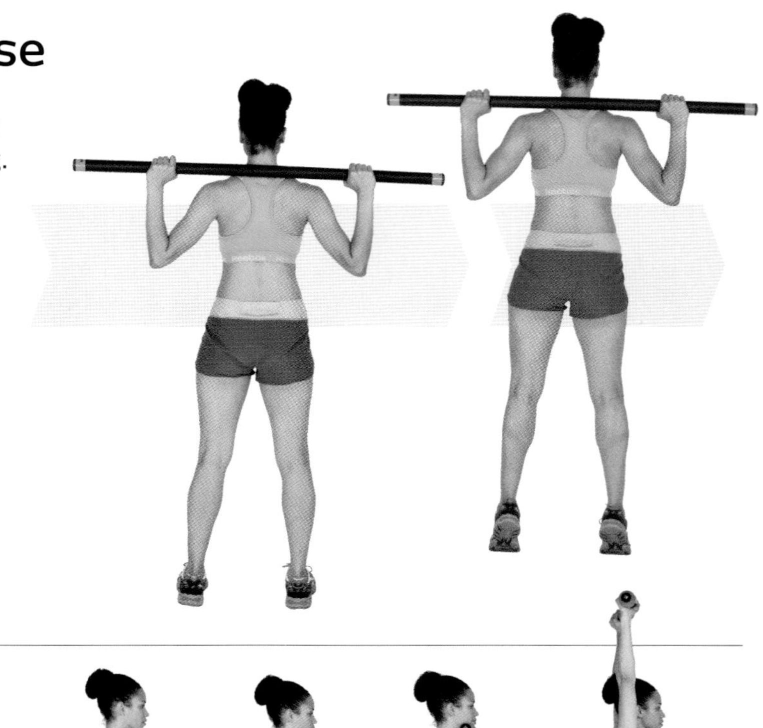

- Bring your feet open to shoulder-width. Hold a body bar across the shoulders for a weighted challenge.
- Shift the weight of your body onto the balls of your feet and lift the heels up off the ground.
- Hold the heels up away from the floor for a beat, and then lower down.

496 Calf Raise with Dumbbell Overhead Press

Stand with the feet shoulder-width apart and bring the weight of your body onto the balls of your feet. Holding a dumbbell in each hand, shift the body forward, raise the heels off the ground, and lift your dumbbells up along your sides and overhead.

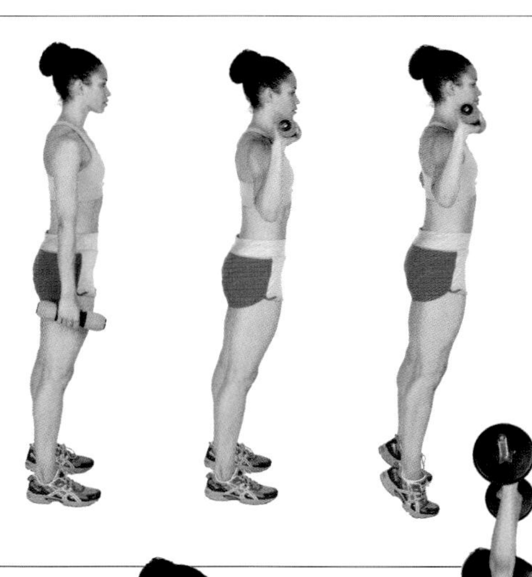

497 Calf Raise with Barbell Overhead Press

Stand with the feet shoulder-width apart and bring the weight of your body onto the balls of your feet. Holding a barbell at the shoulders, shift the body forward, raise the heels off the ground, and press the bar directly up overhead. Engage the core deeply for balance.

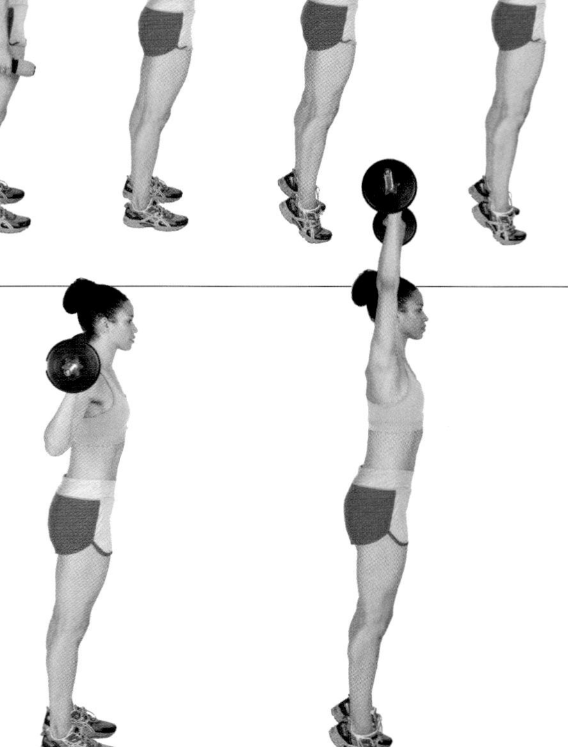

498 Toe Raise

Stand behind a weighted step box or elevated surface. With the spine straight and long, let your arms rest down at your sides. Place the left toes up against the side of the box in front of you, giving you a nice calf stretch. Alternate sides.

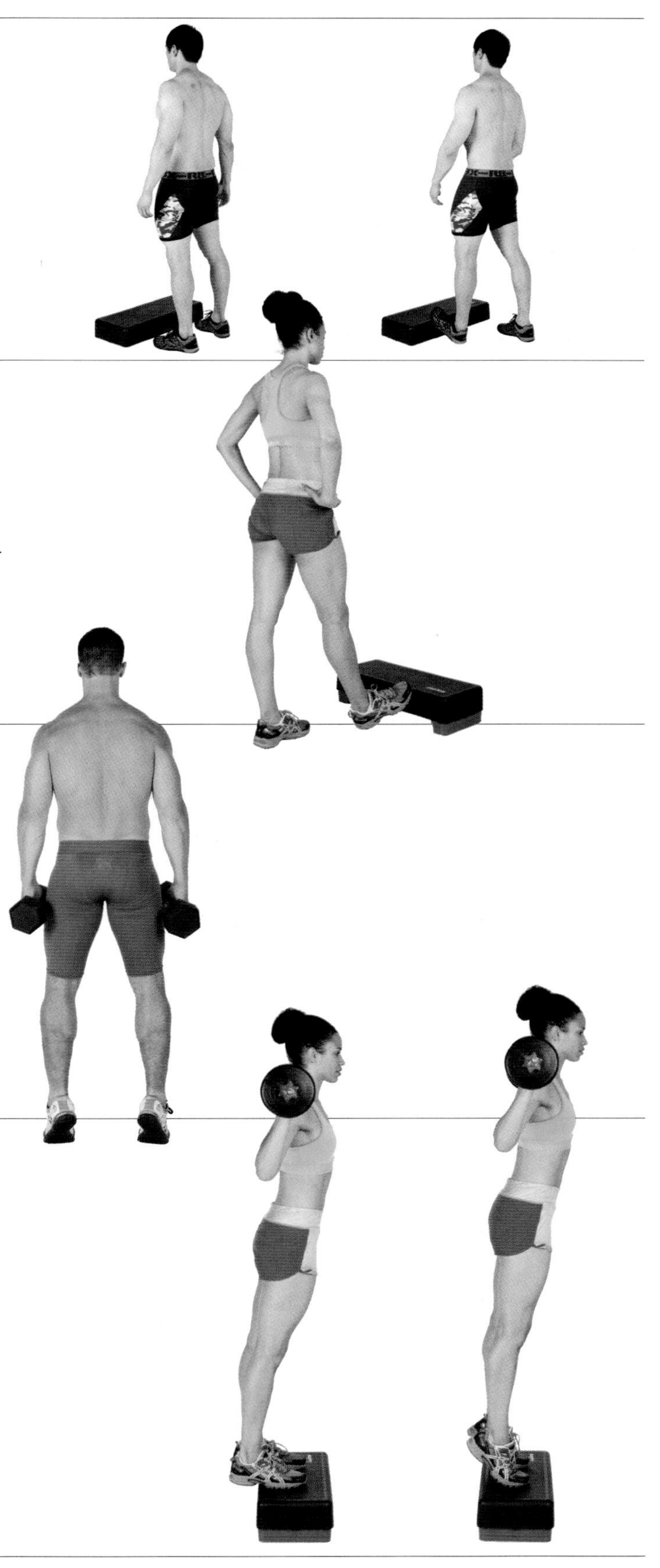

499 Toe-Up Heel Raise

Stand behind a weighted step box, or elevated surface in a Toe-Raise position (#498). Keeping your left foot planted, raise your right heel off the floor. You will feel the stretch shift from your calf to your hamstrings. Alternate sides.

500 Dumbbell Calf Raise

Stand with the feet shoulder-width apart and bring the weight of your body onto the balls of your feet. Holding a dumbbell in each hand, shift the body forward and raise the heels off the ground. Feel the work in the calves and ankles.

501 Heel Drop with Barbell

Stand with the feet shoulder-width apart on a step. Bring the weight of your body onto the balls of your feet, and drop the heels behind you off the step. Then raise your heels until you feel your calves contract strongly.

Index of Exercises

Bold type = main exercise (Numerals refer to page numbers not exercise numbers)

T

U–V

W

Credits

Photography

Naila Ruechel

Photography Assistant

Finn Moore

Models

Natasha Diamond-Walker
Abdiel Jacobson
Jessica Gambellur
Philip Chan
Anzie Dasabe
Lloyd Knight
Roya Carreras
Alex Geissbuhler
Daniel Wright

Additional Photography

Page 7 Uber Images / Shutterstock.com
Page 8 Rasulov / Shutterstock.com
Page 10 UfaBizphoto / Shutterstock.com
Page 11 Wavebreakmedia / Shutterstock.com
Pages 14/15 Wavebreakmedia / Shutterstock.com
Pages 116/117 Wavebreakmedia / Shutterstock.com

Illustration

All anatomical illustrations by Hector Diaz/3DLabz Animation Limited

Full-body anatomy and insets by Linda Bucklin/Shutterstock.com